Health Assessment in Clinical Practice

Health Assessment in Clinical Practice

KENNETH R. BURNS, R.N., M.S.

ASSISTANT PROFESSOR
SCHOOL OF NURSING
UNIVERSITY OF MINNESOTA

NURSE CLINICIAN/PRACTITIONER
ST. PAUL RAMSEY HOSPITAL
ST. PAUL, MINNESOTA

PATRICIA J. JOHNSON, R.N., M.S.

CLINICAL INSTRUCTOR
DEPARTMENT OF PEDIATRICS
SCHOOL OF MEDICINE
UNIVERSITY OF MINNESOTA

NEONATAL NURSE SPECIALIST
CHILDREN'S HOSPITAL
ST. PAUL, MINNESOTA

Prentice-Hall, Inc., Englewood Cliffs, New Jersey 07632

Library of Congress Cataloging in Publication Data

Burns, Kenneth R
 Health assessment in clinical practice.

 Bibliography: p.
 Includes index.
 1. Physical diagnosis.   2. Nursing.   I. Johnson,
Patricia J., joint author.   II. Title.
RT48.B87   616.07′5′024613   79–15907
ISBN   0-13-385054-4

© **1980 by Prentice-Hall, Inc., Englewood Cliffs, N.J. 07632**

Printed in the United States of America

10   9   8   7   6   5   4   3   2   1

Editorial/production supervision by Guy Lento
Interior design, cover design, and illustration supervision by Janet Schmid
Composition by York Graphic Services, Inc.
Page layout by Rita K. Schwartz
Illustrations by B. Andrew Mudryk and Bert Schneider
Acquisitions editor: Fred Henry
Manufacturing buyer: Cathie Lenard

Prentice-Hall International, Inc., *London*

Prentice-Hall of Australia Pty. Limited, *Sydney*

Prentice-Hall of Canada, Ltd., *Toronto*

Prentice-Hall of India Private Limited, *New Delhi*

Prentice-Hall of Japan, Inc., *Tokyo*

Prentice-Hall of Southeast Asia Pte. Ltd., *Singapore*

Whitehall Books Limited, *Wellington, New Zealand*

Contents

SECTION 4

358

Appendix Tables:
Clinical Assessment Guides
for Various Age Groups

Index

Preface

This text is intended to fulfill three basic purposes: First, to introduce to and familiarize the beginning level practitioner of nursing with the basic skills and tools of subjective and objective data collection; second, to assist practicing nurses with the integration of these skills into their practice, either through continuing education endeavors or in-service education with appropriate clinical supervision; and third, to provide a resource for the established nurse practitioner who already possesses expertise in assessment skills. Although this text is directed primarily at the student of nursing at various levels, the content, we hope, will be beneficial to a more diverse population of health care professionals.

The development of assessment skills, with appropriate clinical supervision, we believe, will increase the validity of data that direct the health care team's interventions. Nursing has recently demonstrated an intellectual readiness to expand the previously limited and nonsystematic data collection process. The use of physical assessment tools and skills will increase the nurse's effectiveness and efficiency as a contributing member of the health care team.

The content provides the information necessary for assuming a higher level of responsibility in the provision of health care, using a more complete data base. At no time should the content of the book serve as a replacement for skills and tools already used by the student or practitioner of nursing; rather, the book should be an addition to the method of data collection, using a systematic process.

The content presented is one model of a systematic process and is organized into four sections. Section 1 is a description of a systematic nursing process. The purpose of this section is to promote the student's understanding of the derivation and appropriate integration of subjective and objective data collection within the nursing process.

Section 2 begins with a set of behavioral objectives that the reader may expect to accomplish. This section describes a systematic methodology for collecting subjective data and discriminates between a nursing and a medical model of history taking.

Section 3 is organized according to body systems. Each chapter begins with a set of objectives and is then divided into three parts. Part 1 presents a brief review of the structure and function of that particular system, and Part 2 presents a systematic process of performing the physical assessment. Part 3 is a summary in the form of study guide questions that are based on the objectives at the beginning of the chapter. The assessment content is built around the developmental stages, from infancy through old age. The purpose is to provide understanding of each system, and acquisition and performance of the skills necessary for establishing a data base.

Section 4 is an appendix containing clinical assessment guides. The clinical assessment guides are tables that summarize normal and abnormal findings for the various developmental stages of life. These tables are organized according to the presentation of content in each chapter and can be used as guides in many clinical settings.

The text is neither intended to cover extensively all the necessary knowledge needed to make complete assessments, nor is it intended to provide detailed differentiation between all normal and abnormal findings. Emphasis on abnormal findings is provided primarily for the purpose of comparison and contrast.

In using this text as a guide for organizing data collection, we suggest that the reader also refer to other sources to enhance his or her depth of knowledge while proceeding as personal readiness dictates.

The authors acknowledge the help of their colleagues who reviewed the manuscript:

Bettie W. Hooks, R.N., M.A.
Associate Professor
School of Nursing
East Carolina University
Greenville, North Carolina

Sue E. Huether, R.N., M.S.
Assistant Professor
Family Nurse Clinician Program Director
University of Utah
Salt Lake City, Utah

Eleanor A. Schuster, R.N., D.N.Sc.
Director of Graduate Program, Department of Nursing
Wichita State University
Wichita, Kansas
Codirector and founder, Life Enrichment Opportunities, Inc. (a corporation for the independent practice of nursing)

KENNETH R. BURNS
PATRICIA J. JOHNSON

Health Assessment in Clinical Practice

SECTION 1

1

Data Collection and Its Relationship to the Nursing Process

THE NURSING PROCESS

Assessment, or the collection of data, is a process. A process generally involves a number of steps, methods, modes, or actions utilized or performed in a particular manner for a given purpose. A specific systematic process utilized by nurses is referred to as the nursing process. The nursing process generally consists of five basic components: (1) assessment, (2) interpretation, (3) diagnosis, (4) intervention planning and implementation, and (5) evaluation. Although there are many ways to label and describe each step, the process is basically the same. Utilization of this process enables identification of the client's need for intervention, the type of intervention needed, and the method for implementing intervention for the client or in consultation with the client and the evaluation of client outcomes. The five components of this process are discussed in detail in the following pages.

1. Assessment The assessment component of the process consists of obtaining subjective and objective data. Exploratory and direct questioning and listening are used to elicit subjective data. Subjective data are those data that only the client can relate, as they consist of the individual's perceptions and interpretations of reality experiences and sensations, including biological, psychological, sociological, cultural, and spiritual phenomena. These perceptions and interpretations are the motive for the desired health-care service sought, and they give temporal, spatial, and individualized importance to the data. This results in a holistic structure specific to each client, which the examiner uses as a guide throughout the process of assessment.

Objective data are collected utilizing the skills of inspection, palpation, percussion, and auscultation, as well as other instrumentation. Inspection refers to much more than cursory observation. It involves a detailed sensory intake performed in a logical, systematic manner. Frequently, an individual perceives only a fraction of what is actually presented. When inspecting a specific physical aspect of the client, such as the skin or a behavior, failure to assess all the necessary variables can impede the remaining steps in the nursing process, thus invalidating the data base.

Inspection is generally performed prior to the use of any objective data-collection skills to avoid disrupting the more valid undisturbed or resting state of the client. Comparative reliability of data obtained through inspection varies with the age of the client and the system of the body being assessed. Depending upon the setting in which the nurse is practicing, nursing observations would include (1) the client's interaction in social situations with family, friends, and other individuals; (2) behaviors when alone; (3) personalized space; (4) response to stimuli, functional performance, environmental effects on the client, and physical body characteristics that are observable, such as the skin, pulsations, and surface characteristics of the thoracic cage.

Palpation is "tactile perception" that yields data concerning the physical status of the client. Light pressure and firm pressure yield different types of data. Light palpation always precedes deep palpation. Light pressure applied to the body yields data concerning surface and superficial body characteristics; firm pressure yields data concerning characteristics of deeper structures. The motion of the hands in circular or horizontal movement in a longitudinal or horizontal plane affects the type of data collected. The type of pressure used immediately upon contact and throughout the data-collection process may also communicate different messages to the client, depending upon cultural background. For example, if the first contact made is with excessive pressure, it may communicate roughness and an attitude of carelessness. The use of such pressure may also cause pain.

Percussion is used for two purposes. One purpose is to differentiate the density and size of underlying structures. This is accomplished by striking a surface directly or indirectly, thus sending vibrations into the body to receive a meaningful auditory and tactile response. Percussion performed with various degrees of striking pressure affects the type of sound obtained. The greater the striking pressure, the more distorted the sound returned; extremely light striking pressure yields a flat muffled sound.

The second purpose of percussion is to stretch certain tendons of the body and obtain a deep tendon reflex, such as the knee jerk. This is generally accomplished with the aid of a percussion hammer. The pressure used in striking the tendon affects the type of reflex obtained. Bilateral inequality in the pressure used to strike the tendon will produce two distinct levels of reflex activity. If light pressure is used in the strike, a hypoactive reflex may result, whereas greater striking pressure on the opposite tendon may produce what appears to be a hyperactive reflex.

Auscultation is an instrumental method that uses a stethoscope to transmit sound waves not ordinarily heard by the ear to discriminate sound phenomena produced by movement within the body. The three major systems evaluated by auscultation, at least in part, are the pulmonary, cardiovascular and gastrointestinal systems. The stethoscope can yield valuable information only

if it meets certain criteria and if it is utilized appropriately. The following are factors that promote optimal functioning in sound transmission:

1. The tips of the earpieces must fit the external auditory meatus snugly, occluding it but not entering into the structure.
2. The earpieces should be able to be worn comfortably for at least 5 minutes. To achieve this, the examiner needs to experiment with several types and sizes of ear tips.
3. The binaurals or metal tubing leading up to the earpieces should possess a slight curvature. Placement of the stethoscope in the ears is done with the binaural curvature directed anteriorly toward the nose.
4. The earpiece tension spring constructed on the outside of the tubing, as opposed to one with a structural component inside the plastic tubing, promotes clearer sound transmission.
5. The tubing of the stethoscope should be composed of hard plastic or vinyl that is resilient enough to permit flexibility. The tubing thickness serves to filter out environmental noise.
6. The intraluminal diameter of the tubing should be smaller at the chest piece than at the binaurals.
7. Tubing length should be at a maximum of 25 to 30 cm. Tubing longer than this causes sound distortion.
8. The chest piece usually has two components: the diaphragm and the bell.
   a. The diaphragm is flat and broadly shaped. It transmits all sound, especially high-pitched sound.
   b. The bell transmits all sounds, but especially low-pitched sound.

Throughout the assessment process, other instruments are utilized by the examiner, including percussion hammer, tongue blades, cotton-tipped applicators, paper or metal measuring tapes, tuning forks, a time watch, pen light, otoscope, ophthalmoscope, and vaginal speculum. Oral and rectal thermometers are also necessary for measuring body temperature.

The assessment component of the nursing process is complete when the total client and the client's environment have been investigated and a data base is formulated.

2. Interpretation This component consists of cognitive subcomponents, the analysis and synthesis of the data collected. Based on the nurse's knowledge fund, an understanding of the data evolves. Interpretation of the data is prerequisite to the next component, diagnosis. However, during the interpretation of the data, it may be discovered that inadequate data are presented to formulate an understanding. This results in the necessity of returning to the assessment component for more data. Most frequently, data inadequacy is not recognized until the intervention and evaluation components are reached and completed. When organized and systematic in the process of data collection, this error can be avoided.

3. Nursing Diagnosis Once the data are interpreted, descriptions or labels of high-level specificity are placed on the data. These specific statements are derived not only from collected data, but also from the content of the conceptual nursing framework utilized. A diagnostic statement of inability to sleep contains little, if any, specificity and descriptive power concerning the client's state. The nursing diagnosis is a concise statement that reflects the facts pertinent to the situation, and is descriptive enough to enable any reader of the statement to know exactly the state of the client. A more precise diagnostic statement is "inability to sleep resulting from disruptions of sleep preparations and a strange environment." The restrictive capabilities of the examiner to diagnose would be limited only by the individual's ability to collect and comprehend data of varying complexity. The formulation of a nursing diagnosis is prerequisite to planning and implementing nursing intervention.

4. Intervention Planning and Implementation Intervention is the action needed to assist the client in working with or through a problem, concern, or goal. The intervention may be differentiated into nursing action and client action and is different from advice giving. Nursing actions are those methods or means employed by the nurse to assist the client to achieve some predetermined outcome. Patient actions are actions that the client implements in assisting himself or herself to achieve a predetermined outcome. Intervention on a professional level is differentiated from advice giving in that it is based on a logical sequence of actions, thought processes,

and knowledge of an area. Advice giving is based on little, if any, data, and generally there exists a breakdown in logical development of an expressed need. Frequently, advice giving benefits the advisor's need for self-fulfillment rather than the advisee's need for assistance. The needs of the advisee are not taken into account when self-experiences rather than the other's experience becomes involved.

5. Evaluation The evaluation component consists of subcomponents. Evaluation requires the step of assessment, analysis, and interpretation of the results. This phase of the nursing process then demonstrates the cyclical nature of the nursing process. The recollection of data, both subjective and objective, enables analysis to determine if the desired change or predetermined outcome has been accomplished.

Upon completion of the evaluation phase, if the desired outcome has been achieved, the client's next order of priority may be dealt with, or termination of services may occur. If the evaluation demonstrates that the predetermined outcomes were not met, the data base collected for the evaluation may then serve as the first step of the nursing process, and the interpretation step may be reentered.

In summary, then, it is evident that the nursing process becomes fluent and efficient only when its first component, assessment, is performed in a predetermined, logical, sequential pattern to yield a thorough collection of the necessary data.

CONCEPTS THAT INFLUENCE A SYSTEMATIC ASSESSMENT PROCESS

A systematic assessment process is influenced greatly by two major concepts: health and illness (problems). The approach in the collection of data depends upon the assessor's conceptual orientation. One approach shall be called the *health-oriented* approach and the other shall be termed the *illness-* or *problem-oriented* approach. Presently, little stress is placed on a health approach in working with clients, and little is known about variables to be manipulated and nursing intervention designs that maintain and/or promote the health state of the client. When developing a systematic assessment for a health state, the concept of health must be described along with the associated values, assumptions, and beliefs.

The influence is felt in the type of data elicited and subsequent activities carried out in the nursing process. Emphasis is placed on health, not illness. Problems or illness are assessed as they are related to the person's past health status, any growth that may have occurred from the illness, the coping strategies, and level function. The health-oriented approach is marked by inquiries into the present health state: what it is, what the client does to maintain it, and what internal and environmental resources are available for growth beyond the present health state. Therefore, the process of data collection and intervention reflects the concept utilized by the nurse.

When the approach is disease- or problem-oriented, data are collected regarding the present illness or disease states, how the client experiences the state, what meaning it holds, and what coping strategies are being used. With the use of this approach, the information obtained reflects the client's experience and disease process. This information reflects the preferred concepts of illness, disease, and restoration of health.

Frequently in a health assessment, nurses utilize a combination of a health and illness approach, especially when the client experiences a disruption in a health state. This approach may reflect a holistic view of man. The use of a health approach alone may reflect a holistic view when the client is well or healthy (experiencing no disruptions in the psychosocial and biological states) during the contact. Exposure to such individuals is more frequently encountered in clinics when clients enter for yearly annual health maintenance examinations.

Whichever approach is utilized in a health assessment, that approach must be organized into a framework to provide a systematized, logical methodology. A systematic approach for the collection of subjective data is covered in detail in Chapter 2, and the following outline summarizes one example of a systematic approach for objective data collection. Variations in this approach are needed, as it includes variables that are generally assessed only in children, as well as variables that are frequently assessed only in older child, adolescent, adult, and geriatric client populations.

A SYSTEMATIC APPROACH TO HEALTH ASSESSMENT

GENERAL

INSPECTION
1. General body structure
2. Posture

BASELINE OR COMPARATIVE SERIAL MEASUREMENTS
1. Blood pressure
2. Pulse rate
3. Respiratory rate
4. Temperature
5. Height
6. Weight
7. Occipital frontal head circumference

HEAD

INSPECTION
1. Anterior fontanel
2. Posterior fontanel
3. Sutures
4. Scalp

5. Hair pattern and texture
6. Head circumference

PALPATION
1. Anterior fontanel
2. Posterior fontanel
3. Sutures
4. Scalp
5. Hair

EYES

INSPECTION
1. Gross visual screening (Snellen)
2. Peripheral visual fields
3. Extraocular muscle coordination
4. Cover test
5. Lid location, symmetry, and integument characteristics
6. Conjunctiva
   a. Palpebral
   b. Bulbar
7. Color and vascularity of sclera
8. Color of cornea
9. Corneal light reflex

10. Pupil size and shape
11. Consensual pupil reflex

INSTRUMENTAL INSPECTION
1. Red reflex
2. Optic disc
3. Vascular structures
4. Macula

PALPATION
1. Eyeball turgor

EARS

INSPECTION
1. Alignment of auricle with palpebral fissure
2. Structure and color of auricle
3. Bilateral symmetry of structure

PALPATION
1. Consistency of the auricle

PERCUSSION
1. Mastoid prominence

INSTRUMENTAL INSPECTION
1. Structure and color of the external auditory canal
2. Structure, color, and landmarks of the tympanic membrane
3. Gross hearing screening
   a. Spoken word
   b. Whispered word
   c. Watch tick
   d. Weber test
   e. Rinne test
   f. Bing test

NOSE

INSPECTION
1. External structure of the nose
2. Characteristics of the integument

PALPATION
1. Structure of the nose
2. Nasal patency

INSTRUMENTAL INSPECTION
1. Structure and color of the internal nares
   a. Mucous membrane
   b. Kiesselbach's plexus
   c. Inferior turbinate
   d. Middle turbinate

MOUTH

INSPECTION
1. Lip color and structure
2. Integrity of seventh cranial nerve

3. Vestibule
   a. Character of mucous membrane
   b. Stenson's duct
   c. Gums
4. Mouth cavity proper
   a. Teeth
   b. Gums
   c. Tongue
   d. Sublingual ducts
   e. Hypoglossal nerve integrity
5. Posterior oral pharynx
   a. Soft palate; ninth and tenth cranial nerve integrity
   b. Uvula, color, structure, ninth and tenth cranial nerve integrity
   c. Pillars
   d. Tonsils

NECK

INSPECTION
1. Symmetry of neck angles
2. Height of venous filling
3. Venous pulsations
4. Carotid pulsations
5. Lymph-node regions

PALPATION
1. Carotid pulsation
2. Cervical lymph nodes
3. Thyroid gland
4. Direction of venous filling

AUSCULTATION
1. Carotid arteries
2. Venous structures
3. Thyroid gland

INSPECTION
1. Active range of motion
   a. Flexion
   b. Extension
   c. Lateral rotation
   d. Lateral bending

PALPATION
1. Passive range of motion
   a. Flexion
   b. Extension
   c. Lateral rotation
   d. Lateral bending

CHEST: ANTERIOR

INSPECTION
1. Characteristics of the skin
2. Structure of anterior chest wall
3. Symmetry of structure during respiratory cycle and at rest
4. Characteristics of respiration

CHEST: ANTERIOR (cont.)

PALPATION
1. Skin, subcutaneous and muscular structures, as well as the bony structure
2. Chest expansion
   a. Apical
   b. Mid-thoracic
   c. Lower thoracic
3. Tactile fremitus

PERCUSSION
1. Symmetrical sites on chest wall

AUSCULTATION
1. Symmetrical site on chest wall for:
   a. Breath sounds
   b. Adventitious sounds
   c. Voice sounds

CHEST: POSTERIOR

INSPECTION
1. Skin color and turgor
2. Structure of posterior chest wall
3. Symmetry of structure during respiratory cycle and at rest
4. Characteristics of respiration

PALPATION
1. Integument, subcutaneous muscular structures, as well as the bony structure
2. Chest expansion
   a. Mid-thoracic
   b. Lower-thoracic
3. Tactile fremitus

PERCUSSION
1. Lung fields
2. Diaphragm excursion
3. CV angle tenderness

AUSCULTATION
1. Symmetrical sites on chest wall for:
   a. Breath sounds
   b. Adventitious sounds
   c. Voice sounds

BREAST

INSPECTION
1. Individual sitting, arms at sides, then with arms over head, and finally with contraction of the pectoral muscles
   a. Size of breast
   b. Shape of breast
   c. Bilateral symmetry

d. Skin characteristics
e. Vascularity
f. Shape and surface characteristics of areola
g. Nipple shape and position (protruding, inverted)

PALPATION
1. Individual sitting, arms at sides; breast tissue, areola, and nipple
   a. Elasticity
   b. Nodularity
      Unilateral
      Bilateral
      Mobility
   c. Masses
      Unilateral
      Bilateral
      Mobility
2. Individual sitting, arms behind head
   a. Axillary lymph-node region
   b. Supraclavicular lymph-node region
   c. Infraclavicular lymph-node region
3. Individual recumbent, arms over head, towel under shoulder
   a. Elasticity
   b. Nodularity
   c. Unilateral
   d. Bilateral
   e. Mobility
   f. Areola
   g. Nipple

HEART

INSPECTION
1. Individual sitting
   a. Point of maximal intensity
2. Individual leaning forward
   a. Point of maximal intensity

PALPATION
1. Individual sitting
   a. Point of maximal intensity
   b. Thrills, heaves, thrust
2. Individual recumbent
   a. Point of maximal intensity
   b. Thrills, heaves, thrust

AUSCULTATION
1. Individual sitting, then recumbent, and, if necessary, in the left lateral position
   a. Rate
   b. Rhythm
   c. Auscultatory valve sites (first with diaphragm, then with bell)
      (1) Aortic: s_1, s_2, systole and diastole
      (2) Pulmonic: s_1, s_2, systole and diastole
      (3) Tricuspid: s_1, s_2, systole and diastole
      (4) Mitral: s_1, s_2, systole and diastole

ABDOMEN

INSPECTION
1. Contour
2. Skin characteristics
3. Trauma line
4. Pulsations
5. Peristaltic waves

AUSCULTATION
1. Bowel sounds
   a. Right upper quadrant
   b. Right lower quadrant
   c. Left lower quadrant
   d. Left upper quadrant
2. Vascular sounds
   a. Area of the liver
   b. Area of the spleen
   c. Area of the aorta
   d. Area of the kidney

PERCUSSION
1. Each quadrant
   a. Right upper
   b. Right lower
   c. Left lower
   d. Left upper
2. Liver margins (upper and lower)
3. Spleen

LIGHT PALPATION
1. Skin turgor
2. Subcutaneous tissue structure
3. Inguinal lymph nodes

DEEP PALPATION
1. Liver edge
2. Spleen
3. Kidney
4. Intestinal structures
5. Aorta
6. Femoral pulses

MUSCULOSKELETAL

INSPECTION: NECK
1. Symmetry of angles
2. Characteristics of the integument
3. Muscle movement (voluntary and involuntary)
4. Active range of motion

PALPATION: NECK
1. Muscle mass
2. Muscle strength
   a. Sternocleidomastoid muscle
3. Passive range of motion

INSPECTION: UPPER EXTREMITIES
1. Bilateral symmetry
   a. Muscle mass
   b. Extremity length
   c. Posture of extremities
2. Carrying angle of the arms
3. Joint contours
   a. Shoulder
   b. Elbow
   c. Wrist
   d. Metacarpophalangeal
   e. Inter and distal phalangeal joints
4. Numbers of digits
5. Shape and contour of dorsal and palmar hand surfaces
6. Palmar creases
7. Active range of motion

PALPATION: UPPER EXTREMITIES
1. Muscle mass
2. Muscle strength
3. Joint characteristics
   a. Shoulder
   b. Elbow
   c. Wrist
   d. Metacarpophalangeal
   e. Interphalangeal
   f. Distal phalangeal
4. Arterial pulsations
   a. Radial
   b. Brachial
   c. Axillary

INSPECTION: BACK
1. Curvature of spinal column
2. Characteristics of integument
3. Vertebral processes
4. Bilateral symmetry of muscle masses
5. Scapula

PALPATION: BACK
1. Spinal column
2. Muscle masses

INSPECTION: LOWER EXTREMITIES
1. Gait
   a. Stance phase
   b. Swing phase
2. Bilateral symmetry
   a. Muscle mass
   b. Extremity length
   c. Posture of extremity
3. Plane of sacral triangle and pelvic crest
4. Angulation of lower leg
5. Joint contours
   a. Hip
   b. Knee
   c. Ankle
   d. Metatarsophalangeal joint
   e. Interphalangeal joint
   f. Distal phalangeal joint
6. Number of digits
7. Shape and contour of dorsal and plantar foot surfaces
8. Active range of motion

PALPATION: LOWER EXTREMITIES
1. Muscle mass
2. Muscle strength
3. Joint characteristics

MUSCULOSKELETAL (cont.)

   a. Hip
   b. Knee
   c. Ankle
   d. Metatarsophalangeal
   e. Interphalangeal
   f. Distal phalangeal
4. Joint stability
   a. Hip
   b. Knee
   c. Ankle
5. Arterial pulsations
   a. Femoral
   b. Popliteal
   c. Posterior tibial
   d. Dorsalis pedis
6. Passive range of motion

MALE GENITALIA

INSPECTION

1. Hair pattern
2. Symmetry of inguinal area
3. Skin characteristics
4. Urethral discharge

PALPATION

1. Muscle strength of inguinal area
2. Penis
3. Urethral meatus
4. Scrotum
5. Scrotal contents
   a. Testis
   b. Tunica vaginalis
   c. Epididymis
   d. Spermatic cord
6. Inguinal ring

INSPECTION

1. Skin characteristics of anal region
2. Anal ring with increased intra-abdominal pressure

PALPATION

1. Anal sphincter tone
2. Rectal mucosa
3. Prostate gland

FEMALE GENITALIA

INSPECTION: EXTERNAL GENITALS

1. Hair pattern
2. Skin characteristics
3. Spread-open labia
   a. Prepuce
   b. Frenulum
   c. Clitoris
   d. Vagina orifice
   e. Hymen
   f. Urethral orifice
4. Perineum

PALPATION

1. Paraurethral glands (Skene's glands)
2. Greater vestibular glands (Bartholin's glands)
3. Tone of pelvic muscles

INSTRUMENTAL INSPECTION

1. Cervix
   a. Cervical os
   b. Squamocolumnar junction
2. Vaginal mucosa

PALPATION

1. Cervix
   a. Size, shape, and surface characteristics
   b. Consistency (firm, boggy)
   c. Mobility
2. Uterus
   a. Position
   b. Length
   c. Consistency
3. Adnexa
   a. Position
   b. Size and shape
4. Rectovaginal area
   a. Anus
   b. Rectum
   c. Rectal–vaginal septum
   d. Posterior cul-de-sac
   e. Uteral–sacral ligaments
   f. Lateral posterior portion of the pelvis

NEUROLOGICAL

1. Mental status
   a. Grooming and hygiene
   b. Level of consciousness
   c. Feelings
   d. Thought processes
   e. Mood
   f. Orientation
   g. Memory (immediate and remote)
   h. Knowledge fund
2. Cranial nerve
3. Motor function
   a. Station and gait
   b. Cerebellar integrity
   c. Neuromuscular strength
   d. Muscle tone
   e. Coordination
     (1) Gross motor
     (2) Fine motor
4. Reflexes
   a. Deep
   b. Superficial
5. Sensory function
   a. Superficial
   b. Deep

SECTION 2

2 Health History and Subjective Data Collection

OBJECTIVES

1. Identify four core patient factors that influence the development of a relationship and interpretation of the health history and physical findings.

2. Identify the respective data components of subjective data collection.

3. Summarize the differences between a comprehensive (complete) health history and an episodic or focused health history.

4. Discuss the implications of the use and position of the history taker for the delivery of health care.

5. Identify differences in content and approach when collecting subjective data from children and older adults or others.

6. Identify the implications of collecting subjective data across the life span when gathering a health history from the episodic client.

RELATIONSHIP FORMATION

The collection of subjective data, frequently referred to as historical information, requires that two or more people form a relationship conducive to an open line of communication. Subjective data refer to that which the client has perceived as reality about his life experiences. These experiences or knowledge are known only to this individual client. The nurse–client relationship is the vehicle through which health-care interviews, concerned with subjective data collection, evolve.

Relationships grow when concern for the client's total being is demonstrated by the health-care deliverer. Self-awareness and awareness of others are essential in the formation and continuation of a relationship that results in rapport. Rapport is defined as a harmonious relationship in which mutual interest and respect for each other occur.

Some specific influential factors that the nurse may bring into the formation of a relationship are preconceived ideas, values, assumptions, beliefs, biases, predetermined goals, the tendency toward premature conclusion formation, ability to communicate, and the ability to work collaboratively with clients. Many of the above factors are transmitted nonverbally through body language, and may influence positively or negatively the direction of the relationship. What is important in relation to these factors is the nurse's awareness of them and the ability to analyze each

of them, and work toward changing, as needed, the effect of each factor on the relationship.

For most clients, entry into a health-care relationship is within a foreign environment. The client is generally in a dependent position, needing the expertise of another to assist in the resolution of a problem, or to assist in the maintenance or promotion of his or her health status. The dependency role of the client is gradually subsiding as people are taking more initiative and active control in exerting their rights and responsibilities toward the restoration, maintenance, and promotion of their health status.

Some of the influencing factors brought by the client are categorically similar to those of the nurse. The nurse's adaptability to the language level and communication skills of the client determines the quality and quantity of information that can be obtained and integrated into the data base. The client's previous experiences with the health-care delivery system, coupled with the nurse's ability to understand the experiential data shared about these experiences, will assist both parties in the development of the relationship. For example, the confidence held by the client in past nursing diagnoses and interventions may encourage or discourage future relationship formation.

Frequently, it is difficult for individuals to say, "I need help," as these words may connote inadequacy, thus affecting feelings of well-being, or acceptability to self and others. It is therefore necessary for the nurse to assist the client in maintaining a sense of adequacy.

The relationship is also influenced by the client's formulated goals, expectations, and predetermined criteria or what constitute effective achievement of proposed interventions. It is through these criteria that the client may significantly control the outcome of the relationship.

Relationships are also influenced by the setting in which the involved individuals are meeting, that is, the privacy or exposure felt by the client and the interruptions that may occur. Relationships are established more quickly if privacy and an intrusion-free environment is established. Demonstration of accessibility and availability to the client provides a substantial impact on the relationship formation.

PURPOSES OF THE INTERVIEW

The purposes of the interview are (1) to gather historical data about the client's health status that are not available from other sources, (2) to clarify the meaning of the client's terminology, and (3) to formulate a data base. The data base is then the foundation around which physical assessments and nursing interventions evolve. If the client is unable to communicate the essential data, interviewing significant others, such as parents, spouse, relatives, or the accompanying person, is necessary to gain the needed preliminary information. Furthermore, the interview provides the nurse with the opportunities for introduction of self, description of role, and description of services available within the health-care delivery system. This, in turn, provides the client with expected outcomes from the interaction.

COMPONENTS OF THE SUBJECTIVE DATA-COLLECTION PROCESS: A MEDICAL MODEL

The first component of any data-collection process is that of biographical data, sometimes referred to as preinterview data. Frequently, biographical data are available prior to meeting the client through admitting personnel notes or admission interviews in clinics or hospitals, or through medical records. Currency and correctness of these data should be reviewed with the client. Basic biographical data include name, age, sex, race, occupation, marital status, religion, and

address. Table 2-1 presents types of biographical data elicited, the associated "norm" expectations, and the potential each area possesses for health-problem information.

The second component of the historical data-collection process is the health history. This component is divided into several subcomponents: (1) the chief complaint, (2) present problem or present illness, (3) past health history, (4) review of systems, (5) family history, and (6) personal history.

In the medical model of history taking, the chief complaint refers to the phenomenon that causes or stimulates the individual to seek assistance. The chief complaint is purely subjective and relates to the specific event and its duration in a brief, concise statement close to, or, in the actual words of the client, as opposed to the interviewer's interpretation or diagnostic labeling. Several examples of a chief complaint are as follows:

1. "Stomach ache for three hours."
2. "No bowel movement since last Sunday."
3. "Stepped on a nail two hours ago."
4. "Baby has been colicky for three days and nights."

The present problem follows the chief complaint as a new sentence, which again concisely elaborates on the chief complaint. The following examples demonstrate the chief complaint (C.C.) followed by a present problem (P.P.) statement.

1. C.C. "Stomach ache for three hours."
   P.P. The client enters with severe lower abdominal pain, which has progressed in severity during the last 3 hours.
2. C.C. "No bowel movement since last Sunday."
   P.P. The client visits the clinic with the complaint of constipation of 1-week duration.
3. C.C. "Stepped on a nail two hours ago."
   P.P. The client enters after having stepped on a nail 2 hours prior to the clinic contact.
4. C.C. "Baby has been colicky for three days and nights."
   P.P. Mrs. S. enters the clinic with 4-week-old baby who has had colic for 3 days duration.

TABLE 2-1
Biographical Data

BIOGRAPHICAL DATA TITLE	NORM EXPECTATIONS BASED ON THE GENERAL POPULATION	POTENTIAL HEALTH PROBLEMS ASSOCIATED WITH BIOGRAPHICAL DATA TITLE AND NORM EXPECTATIONS
Name	Provides personal identity	Degree of differentiation from others
Age	Developmental phases and associated task	Common health-care problems relative to age
		Completion of, or working through, developmental phases
	Communication ability	Inability to communicate relative to age
	Cooperation	Inability to work cooperatively with others relative to age
Sex	Sexual identity and concept of associated role	Genetically sex linked problems
		Formation of a concept of maleness/masculinity and femaleness/feminity, relative to age
Marital status	Roles and associated responsibilities	Stressors resulting from role, and associated responsibilities
	Relationships with others	Stressors from maintenance of, or inability to maintain, relationships with others
Race	Cultural norms	Cultural attitudes toward health
	Physical norms	Statistical predisposition toward hereditary problems
Occupation	Newborn to 5 years, play directed by others	Dissatisfaction with occupation: dependence, interdependence, independence, semidependence
	5 to 19 years, student	
	19 to 62/65 years, student or full-time employment	
	62 to 65 years and above, retirement	Unemployment
		Exposure to environmental health hazards
Religion	Set of beliefs and values	The holding of beliefs and values that affect the general population norms for acceptable interventions, treatments, and procedures
	Sense of spiritualness	
Address	Specified geographic location identified as a personalized boundary	Geographical isolation from health care
	Climate	Statistical incidence of problems associated with geographic areas
		Environmental maladjustment

Following the chief complaint and present problem is the present illness, or P.I. The present illness consists of the chronological development of the problem that the client is experiencing. The chronology is developed beginning with the point at which the symptoms began and progresses through events to the present. It includes a complete description of the symptoms, their changes, their types, their locations, and the severity of the discomfort experienced. Also included are the effects the symptoms have on the client, events creating aggravation, the setting in which symptoms occur, and alleviating factors utilized and their effectiveness for the client.

The reason for the patient's contact does not necessarily need to be discomfort or pain, but rather may be due to the presentation of signs that the client perceives as a deviation from the expected normal. Signs are objective changes in the body that can be observed and perceived by others (e.g., jaundice), whereas symptoms refer to the individual's perceptions of phenomena affecting the self, such as pain.

Chronological development is again utilized to gain an understanding of the events. The types of signs, their locations, variations in how they present themselves, their effect upon the individual, and any factors found to aggravate or alleviate the signs are included.

If the chief complaint involves a particular symptom or sign within a single system (e.g., pulmonary system, cardiac system), then the entire system is explored, as opposed to data concerned only with the sign or symptom. The data concerning the particular system, other than those related to the chief complaint, are summarized at the conclusion of the description of the present illness. An example of a recorded present illness follows:

Example
On August 3, the client awoke with the onset of mild periumbilical pain, which increased in intensity over 2 hours. The pain migrated to the right lower abdomen and was associated with nausea, followed by emesis of bile-stained material and fever of 101°F (38.5°C). Pain increased with walking, and decreased by lying still, slightly flexing at the waist, or with flexion of the right leg. The client denies changes in dietary intake prior to onset of distress, and denies change in bowel pattern, constipation, diarrhea, bloody stools, and hemorrhoids.

Subsequent to the present illness is the past history, or P.H. Obtaining data about the client's past can help the examiner to draw possible associations between the present chief complaint and what has occurred in the past, predispositions toward specific problems, degree of resistance to health problems, experiences with and type of health-care delivery systems and agencies, and exposure to geographical regions that are statistically associated with specific health problems.

To obtain data about the client's past history, the interviewer's questions must be explicit enough to ensure comprehension by the client, and yet stated in a manner that provides for open responses. Deliberate questions maintain the direction needed for a smooth and efficient flow of information. Global terms, such as the "usual medical or childhood diseases," yield no information for the interviewer, as what may be usual for one client may be extremely unusual for another.

The past history is frequently organized into categories and may be sequenced as follows: medical history, surgical history, childhood diseases, accident/injuries, allergies, medications, immunizations, military health history, and recent travel. Past medical history data may be elicited by asking, "Have you had any major medical problems?" or "Other than surgical pro-

cedures, have you had any major problems that required medical care?" When requesting historical information about past surgical experiences, it is frequently necessary to remind clients of the surgical procedures of tonsillectomy and appendectomy, as many times they are forgotten by the adult client. During the exploration of childhood diseases, the interviewer may ask, "What childhood diseases did you have?" or ask the client to respond to the childhood diseases he or she had as you list them, the age or approximate age at which they occurred, and any complications associated with each of them. For example, "Which of the following have you had?"

1. Rubeola (regular measles)
2. Rubella (German measles)
3. Mumps
4. Chicken pox
5. Scarlet fever
6. Whooping cough
7. Rheumatic fever

Injury or accident data are obtained by asking, "Have you had any injuries that required medical care?" and "Have you had any injuries for which you didn't receive medical care, but you thought that you should have?" or "Were you ever in an accident in which you sustained an injury?"

In the subcomponent of allergies, questions asked might be, "Do you know if you have any allergies?" or "Are you allergic to any of the following:"

1. Animals
2. Foods
3. Prescribed or over-the-counter medications
4. Plants
5. Pollens
6. Dust
7. Anything other than what I previously identified

If a positive answer is received to any of the inquiries, obtain an established pattern and description of the event. Allergies may follow a seasonal pattern, such as fall or spring. The signs and symptoms experienced may be burning and/or watering of the eyes, sneezing, and rhinitis.

Medications can be the next area of data collection. Inquiries are made into the current use, the frequency of any drugs used, and whether prescribed by a physician or not.

The type and date of immunizations are important to explore (i.e., diphtheria, pertussis, tetanus, smallpox, polio, and any others obtained). Military service health history is a brief inquiry that includes years in the service, branch of the service, location of the tour of duty, and the type of activity engaged in while on active duty. It is obvious that this component is not applicable when collecting subjective data from certain individuals, for example, a 14-year-old male client or an 84-year-old female client. Military service and recent travel data can give the examiner information related to exposure to statistically significant health problems in specified geographical locations, as well as an accounting of stressors experienced and the reaction to them.

The data presented in the past history may be narrated in several ways, but a consistent, systematic method of recording is maintained throughout the report. One method is to state the date or year of the occurrence. This is then followed by the problem, and finally the current status of that problem (i.e., resolved, recurrent, or ongoing). An example is: 1950 pneumonia, resolved. Another method is to state the age at which the event occurred. Again, as in the previously identified method, it is followed by the problem and the resolution or continuance of the problem. To illustrate: Age 20, pneumonia, resolved. The last method to be described is that of stating the problem first, which is then followed by date or age, and the present status of the problem. An example is: pneumonia, age 20, resolved. Tables 2-2 through 2-4 illustrate the narrative of the three types of past history recording methodology.

Following the past health history is the family history. In the review of these data, hereditary and familial predisposition factors are considered. When obtaining a family history, discrimination between biological relatives and relatives through marriage (e.g., step-parents and grandparents) must be made. The health status and relationships of step-relatives to the client are important factors that have impact on the client, but have no bearing on hereditary factors for the client. Maternal and paternal grandparents, siblings, spouse, children, and, at times, individuals

TABLE 2-2

Health History Data Systematically Presented by Area of Investigation, Date, Problem Statement, and Present Status of Identified Problem

AREA OF INVESTIGATION	NARRATED DATA
Medical	1950, pneumonia, hospitalized, resolved 1951, acute mastoiditis (L), hospitalized, resolved
Surgical	1952, tonsillectomy, without sequela 1960, appendectomy, without sequela
Childhood diseases	1947, rubeola 1947, rubella 1948, chicken pox 1964, mumps rheumatic fever denied
Accidents/injuries	1970, fractured left tibia (skiing), healed without sequela
Allergies	None
Medications	No prescribed medications ASA tabs $\bar{\text{ii}}$ for occasional headache One-a-day multivitamin
Immunizations	1974, diphtheria 1974, typhoid 1974, tetanus –0– smallpox 1974, pertussis 1974, polio
Military history	No military history
Recent travel	None

TABLE 2-3

Past Health History Data Systematically Presented by Area of Investigation, Problem Statement, Date, and Present Status of Identified Problem

AREA OF INVESTIGATION	NARRATIVE DATA
Medical	Pneumonia, 1950, hospitalized, resolved Acute mastoiditis (L), 1951, hospitalized, resolved
Surgical	Tonsillectomy, 1952, without sequela Appendectomy, 1960, without sequela
Childhood diseases	Rubeola, 1947 Rubella, 1947 Chicken pox, 1948 Mumps, 1964 Denies rheumatic fever
Injuries/accidents	Fractured left tibia, 1970, skiing, healed without sequela
Allergies	None known
Medications	No current prescriptions ASA tabs ṫ ṫ, occasional headaches One-a-day multivitamin
Immunizations	Diphtheria, 1974 Typhoid, 1974 Tetanus, 1974 Smallpox, –0– Pertussis, 1974 Polio, 1974
Military history	No military history
Recent travel	None

TABLE 2-4

Past Health History Data Systematically Presented by Area of Investigation, Age of Occurrence, Problem Statement, and Resolution

AREA OF INVESTIGATION	NARRATIVE DATA
Medical	Age 5, pneumonia, hospitalized, resolved Age 6, acute mastoiditis (L), hospitalized, resolved
Surgical	Age 7, tonsillectomy, without sequela Age 10, appendectomy, without sequela
Childhood diseases	Age 2, rubeola Age 2, rubella Age 3, chicken pox Age 14, mumps Denies rheumatic fever
Accidents/injuries	Age 20, fractured left tibia, skiing, healed without sequela
Allergies	None known
Medications	No current prescriptive medications ASA tabs ṫ ṫ, occasional headaches One-a-day multivitamin
Immunizations	Age 24, diphtheria Age 24, typhoid Age 24, tetanus Age –0–, smallpox Age 24, pertussis Age 24, polio
Military history	No military history
Recent travel	None

other than blood relatives (such as housing partners) are assessed. Generally, these data include age, sex, and health status of each. If family members are deceased, the age, date, and causative factors are recorded. A written narrative of a family history follows, and Figure 2-1(a) and (b) represents two methods of diagramming the family history.

Family Health History
Paternal grandparents:
GF* deceased, age 80, CVA
GM† living, age 85, adult onset diabetes mellitus
Maternal grandparents:
GF living, age 78, arteriosclerosis
GM living and well, age 76
Father, age 50, living and well

* GF, grandfather.
† GM, grandmother.

Mother, age 49, adult onset diabetes mellitus, insulin control
One sister, age 16, living and well
One maternal uncle, age 45, hypertensive

Another component of the health history is the systems review (S.R.) or the review of the systems (R.O.S.). The systems review is an organized, systematic approach to obtaining data about each of the body's major physiological systems (e.g., integument, cardiac, and pulmonary) and psychological state. The review of systems enables the examiner to (1) cross reference symptoms with systems other than those communicated by the client, (2) ascertain whether several problems exist but are being expressed as a single problem by the client, and (3) elicit pertinent data that may be related to the problem and not expressed by the client.

FIGURE 2-1

Pictographic representation of a family health history (a) including only paternal grandparents and (b) including both paternal and maternal grandparents.

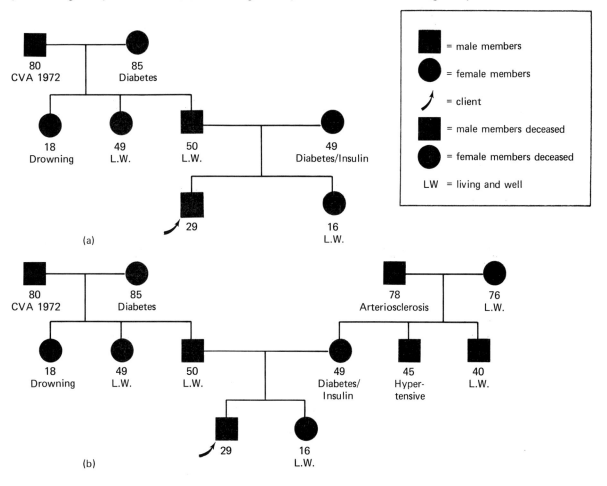

TABLE 2-5

Common Methods for Review of Systems

METHOD I	METHOD II	METHOD III
General	Body weight	Head
Skin	Skin/hair/nails	Eyes
Head	Head	Ears
Eyes	Eyes	Nose
Ears	Ears	Mouth and throat
Nose/sinus	Nose/nasopharynx/ paranasal sinuses	Cardiorespiratory
Oral cavity		Gastrointestinal
Neck	Mouth/throat	Genitourinary
Nodes	Neck	Venereal
Breast	Cardiorespiratory	Menstrual
Respiratory	Gastrointestinal	Neuromuscular
Cardiovascular	Genitourinary	Bone and joint
Gastrointestinal	Venereal	Endocrine
Genitourinary	Menstrual/obstetric	Adrenal Gonadal insufficiency Pituitary Pancreas
Extremities	Nervous system	
Back	Musculoskeletal system	
Central nervous system		
Hematopoietic		
Endocrine		

The narrative presentation of the R.O.S. can take several forms. Three commonly used formats are presented in Table 2-5. In the review of systems, questions are asked more directly, thus facilitating efficiency in the data-collection process. Any pertinent positive responses are clarified with the client in a manner similar to that in the development of the history about the present illness.

Presented next is an example of a recorded review of systems:

Skin/hair/nails: Denies rashes, pruritus scaling, or lesions.

Head: Denies headaches.

Ears: Denies pain, discharge, or loss of hearing. Low-pitched tinnitus noted upon retiring at night, does not interfere with ability to sleep.

Eyes: Corrective lenses for myopia. Denies pain, discharge, blurred, double vision, or night blindness.

Nose: Denies trauma, discharge, epistaxis, or sinus problems.

Mouth: All teeth present, good repair. Denies lesions or pain in mouth.

Throat: Denies pain or lesions. No history of strep infections.

Neck: Normal range of motion. Denies swelling of lymph nodes.

Respiratory: Denies pain, shortness of breath, orthopnea, dyspnea, nocturnal dyspnea, cough, sputum production, and hemoptysis.

Cardiovascular: Denies pain, unusual sensations, hypertension, edema, varicosities, claudication, or history of thrombophlebitis or phlebothrombosis.

Breast: Denies pain, nipple discharge, changes in skin characteristics and masses.

Gastrointestinal: Denies pain, nausea, vomiting, diarrhea, constipation, hemorrhoids, changes in stool color or pattern of evacuation.

Genitourinary: Denies pain, frequency, dysuria, nocturia, difficulty starting or stopping stream, discharge, and history of venereal disease.

Menarche age 14, cycle 28 days, 4 days of moderate flow. Two pregnancies, two live full-term births, no abortions, stillbirths, or neonatal deaths. (G_2P_{2002}) Birth-control pills used for contraception.

Joints/bones: Without limited range of motion, swelling, or pain in joints or bones.

Neuromuscular: Denies muscular pain, fatigue, tingling, or numbness. Denies insomnia or changes in sleep pattern.

Metabolic: Denies intolerance to cold, marked increases or decreases in weight, jaundice, unusual fatigue, sweating, polyuria, polydypsia, polyphagia, or history of glycosuria.

Social history, living patterns, or personal profile are several titles used to label a subcomponent of the medical history that describes how the client views personal daily living activities, such as personal habits, smoking, alcohol intake, stressors, adaptability to situations, occupational role, sexuality, exercise, modes of relaxation, nutritional intake and pattern, and social activities. The following is an example of a narrative social history.

Example

Mr. Patrick Lavel is single, lives with parents, attends Farnsworth Community College. Socially active with peer group, heterosexual relationships, and physically active in intramural college sports. The client smokes three-fourths pack of cigarettes per day, drinks a six pack of beer per week, and denies use of other addictive drugs.

The medical history, as described and illustrated, demonstrates that there is no one absolute method in which to record a health history.

COMPONENTS OF THE SUBJECTIVE DATA-COLLECTION PROCESS: A NURSING MODEL

A nursing history may follow the same format as that used in the medical model, or it can be different, depending upon the setting and the role that the nurse is fulfilling. The role may be one of health restoration, health maintenance, or health promotion.

Health restoration is defined as returning something that has been lost from the client's original health state. This loss may be malfunction or maladaptation of the functioning individual. Restoration, then, implies that the client is characterized as one who is seeking assistance to regain a former level of functioning or one seeking to regain certain types of behaviors that are adaptive.

Health maintenance is defined as sustaining the existing or continuing in the same state of health without decline or disruption. Maintenance activity, then, indicates a client's desire to continue on as he/she is presently able to do. Assistance from the health-care deliverer may be affirmation of present activities, support of the present functional pattern, and exploration of alternatives with the client that will maintain the present status. Promotion is defined as increasing or furthering the growth and development of health, or improving the present adequate health status. In promotional behavior, clients seek assistance in activities that will create and establish growth and increase their health status above its present level.

Within a nursing history, several components generally remain the same as in the medical model. They are the biographical data, past health history, and family health history. The other components of chief complaint, present problem, present illness, personal profile, and review of systems may differ.

If health maintenance is the client's purpose for contact, the chief complaint may be replaced by a concern or area of interest or importance. Goal statements may be used if health promotional activity is presented by the client as the purpose for the contact. Examples 1 and 2 demonstrate a concern; example 3 demonstrates health promotional activity with a goal statement.

Example 1

Mr. Bill Jones, a 24-year-old black male, enters with the concern of maintaining present weight.

Example 2

Mrs. Kathleen Melrose, a 70-year-old widowed, Caucasian female, enters with the intent of maintaining present level of independent functioning in her own home.

Example 3

Mrs. Kathy Barbo, a 30-year-old married Caucasian female, enters with the goal of planning a family with two children.

The present problem statement may or may not be used, depending upon the geographic location in which the nurse works. It is not included here as it is believed to add little information. If concerns or goal statements are used, a present problem would be inappropriate. The word problem, as defined, is a question related to the loss of function or maladaptation of the functioning individual for which a solution is required. It therefore may connote something other than maintenance or promotional activity on the part of the client and nurse.

The present illness is utilized if entry into the health-care system by the client is for restorative purposes. Maintenance or promotional entry into the health-care delivery system requires the use of an appropriate title thereby providing continuity of client activity. Appropriate titles for this component may be (1) the development of present concern, or (2) the development of present goal.

Regardless of the title used for the subcomponent, the same principles utilized for organization and presentation about the present illness are employed. The chronological development of events that promoted health-seeking behavior is associated with the particular or broadly defined area that is to be maintained or promoted. Chronology of development may be ascertained by

having the client describe his or her concept of health, and on a health continuum identify where he or she is at now in relationship to that definition, where he or she was 5 years ago, and what changes, if any, have been noted, and where he or she expects to be in 5 years (Table 2-6). It is also important to elicit data concerning influencing factors that inhibit or stimulate behaviors oriented toward the maintenance of his or her present status or growth-promotional activity.

To establish a subjective data baseline of physiological status, the basic review of systems may remain the same as in the medical model. This "model" is elaborated upon by including in each system information related to the total person, that is, ability to function, established patterns of functioning, loss of function, activities undertaken to maintain present status, and coping behaviors and their effectiveness.

In practice, a systems review, inclusive of all the aforementioned, would be devoid of individualized meaning for each client encountered. The type of needed data to be extrapolated by the nurse from the client varies with the purpose established for the contact. For example, it would be inappropriate to subject a client to a comprehensive review of systems when the purpose of entry into a health-care delivery system was for health restoration (e.g., chief complaint of severe abdominal pain).

A systems review, which is not all inclusive of every type of data one may need to know, but can be used as a beginning guide for the entering-level practitioner of nursing, is presented in Table 2-7. The type of questions stated are not meant to be followed in the strict sense of the word, since they were structured to decrease the bulkiness of the table and to be illustrative of the discrimination between a nursing and a medical format. The stated questions need to be adapted to the interviewer's personal style.

The nursing personal profile differs from the medical model in that a broader exploration is made with regard to growth and development, self-concept, major stressors, and coping mechanisms or behaviors related to the identified stressors and life goals. Frequently, in the medical personal profile, interpretation of the client's verbal and nonverbal communication and environment is made as part of the profile. In a nursing model, the interviewer's interpretation of data is placed in a summary statement after the collection of subjective and objective data has been completed. The personal profile therefore

TABLE 2-6
Health–Illness Continuum

Scale of 1 to 10, with 10 being "perfect" health	
At present	1 2 3 4 5 6 7 8 9 10
Five years prior	1 2 3 4 5 6 7 8 9 10
Five years from present	1 2 3 4 5 6 7 8 9 10
Patient's perception of meaning of 10 or "perfect" health	

consists only of the subjective data presented to the interviewer by the client. A personal profile of a client is as follows:

Mr. Patrick Scott has been married for three years, lives with his wife, and works an average of 8 hours per day for Dye Chemical Institute as a chemist. The client has an educational background of a B.S.

He considers his marital relationship satisfactory: both share household activities and both voice differences without lasting traumatic effects. When discrepancies arise, states "they put on the coffee pot and over coffee frankly discuss the issue until resolutions occur. Rarely are disruptions unresolved as both give and take." Mr. and Mrs. S. have chosen a nonparenthood state to facilitate their career goals and to allow for maximal individuality and sharing with each other.

Socially, the client and his wife are active with peer group, going out two nights per week to theatrical and sports events or parties. Individualized physical activity for him includes tennis and racquet games one evening per week with occasional weekend fishing.

Mr. Scott identifies as his strengths the ability to be flexible and make rapid adjustments in working or socializing with others. The greatest stressor experienced is in dealing with management's demands of accepting more tasks when other employees leave, as this affects his productivity as well as the quality of his product.

Mr. Scott smokes 20 cigarettes per day, alcohol intake of three to four drinks when socializing, uses a one-a-day multivitamin, and denies use of other over-the-counter, prescriptive, or addictive drugs.

Dietary pattern consists of three meals per day, breakfast, lunch, and dinner. Breakfast consists of cereal, milk, orange juice, and three cups of coffee. Lunch is composed of a meat sandwich, a fruit, potato chips, and three cups of coffee. Dinner consists of a vegetable (preferably green), bread, broiled meat, dessert (preferably ice cream), milk, and four cups of coffee. His fluid intake consists mainly of coffee and milk, with only occasional water intake. The client does not snack between meals.

TABLE 2-7
Systems Review

SYSTEM	DATA BASE	ABILITY TO FUNCTION, MAINTENANCE BEHAVIORS, COPING STRATEGIES
SKIN		Pattern of bathing skin Use of soaps Use of deodorants or antiperspirants Use of powders and lotions (body talcum, foot powder)
	Rashes Pruritis Scaling Lesions Turgor	How does rash, pruritis, scaling, or lesion or loss of turgor affect ability to follow through with hygiene patterns? How is this coped with (application of different ointments, cessation of bathing, increased bathing)? How effective have these coping strategies been? How do these changes affect ability to function socially, at work, and at home?
HAIR		Pattern of hair care Types of shampoos, hair sprays, and oils used
	Rashes, pruritis, scaling Lesions in scalp Brittleness Oiliness Loss of hair	How do these factors affect ability to follow through with established hygiene pattern? What coping behaviors are employed? How effective are they? How do these factors affect ability to function socially, at work, and at home? What coping strategies are utilized? How effective are they? What is the influence on self-concept?

TABLE 2-7 CONTINUED

SYSTEM	DATA BASE	ABILITY TO FUNCTION MAINTENANCE BEHAVIORS COPING STRATEGIES
NAILS		Pattern of nail care (trimming, cleaning)
	Brittle Soft Abnormally formed Cyanosis of nail beds	How have changes affected ability to function socially, at work and at home? Have changes affected ability to walk, work with hands, wear shoes? How is it coped with? Are coping strategies effective? Are there predisposing factors to biting or chewing on nails? What changes in your tolerance to stressors have there been?
HEAD	Headaches	Do headaches cause cessation of activity? Does the irritability decrease your ability to handle situations that otherwise call for little effort? Do the headaches alter perception? Are there factors that occur prior to the headaches? What is the pattern of coping with the predisposing factors or situations? How effective are the coping strategies?
EARS		What is the type and pattern of hygiene? Are invasive instruments used to clean the ears? Is there exposure to, or avoidance of, high-decibel noises? Is there periodic evaluation of hearing? Are nonprescriptive medications utilized in the ear?
	Pain	Does the pain alter perception? How does the pain affect ability to function socially, at work, and at home? What is the response to the pain? What methods of coping have been implemented? How effective are coping strategies?
	Discharge	How does the discharge affect ability to function socially, at home, and at work? Are cotton plugs used in the ear? How do you dispose of the drainage and materials used for cleaning the ear? What methods are used to cope with the discharge? How effective are these coping strategies?
	Tinnitus	How does tinnitus affect ability to function socially, at work, and at home? Does tinnitus affect ability to think, respond to others, or sleep? Are there predisposing factors? How effective are the coping strategies?
	Hearing, decrease or increase in hearing sense	How long has the decrease/loss been noted? Has the hearing decrease changed in any way since it began (hear better in noisy environments)? How has the decrease/loss affected ability to function socially, at work, and at home? How has the decrease/loss been coped with (hearing aid, reading lips, standing closer to others, requesting others to speak louder, or repeat words, increase sound intensity of radio, TV)? How effective have these coping strategies been? What have been the responses to unsuccessful attempts to cope? How does the hearing decrease/loss affect self-concept?

TABLE 2-7 CONTINUED

SYSTEM	DATA BASE	ABILITY TO FUNCTION, MAINTENANCE BEHAVIORS, COPING STRATEGIES
EYES		What is the general pattern of caring for the eyes? Pattern of eye and visual examinations Pattern of coping with "bloodshot" eyes
	Pain Discharge	How does pain/discharge affect ability to function socially, at work, and at home? In what way does pain/discharge cause cessation of activity? What hygienic measures are utilized in removing discharge from eyes? How are the materials used for cleansing and handling discharge disposed of? What are the coping strategies employed? How effective are they?
	Vision Corrective lenses needed Blurred vision Diplopia Night blindness Color vision	Do corrective lenses allow for fulfillment of functions carried on throughout the day? If able to read, does vision permit such activity? Do corrective lenses maintain or increase mobility? Do corrective lenses maintain or increase use of motorized transportation? How are visual changes coped with (rely more heavily on tactile sensations, books with larger print, use of braille, audio recorded books, maintain sameness of environment)? How is loss of depth perception adjusted for (walking, driving, stair climbing)? How has the lack of color vision affected your functioning socially, at work, and at home? How has it affected mobility patterns? What coping strategies are used? How effective are the coping strategies? How has the visual loss affected self-concept? What are the fears of complete loss of vision? How is this fear being dealt with?
NOSE		Pattern of hygiene (blowing nose) Any invasive agents used in the nose (fingers, tweezers)? Frequency of use of nose drops or nasal sprays
	Pain Trauma	Does the pain and trauma restrict any functions? What methods of coping have been used (cold packs, medications)? How effective were these coping strategies? What are the resulting effects of the trauma (deviated septum, loss of smell, decreased appetite)? What effect has this had on self-concept? How is the effect on self-concept coped with?
	Congestion	How does the congestion affect ability to function socially, at home, and at work? How does the decreased nasal patency affect ability to breathe? Has it decreased ability to smell? Is there awareness of predisposing factors to the congestion? How has the congestion been coped with (breathing through mouth, sit up to sleep, self-administered over-the-counter medications, control of environmental humidity)? Does congestion annoy others?
	Discharge	How does the discharge affect ability to function socially, at home, and at work? Has the discharge affected ability to breathe? Has it decreased ability to smell?

TABLE 2-7 CONTINUED

SYSTEM	DATA BASE	ABILITY TO FUNCTION MAINTENANCE BEHAVIOR COPING STRATEGIES
NOSE (cont.)		Is there awareness of predisposing factors? How is the discharge coped with (self-administered over-the-counter medications, nasal sprays, control of environmental humidity)? What hygienic measures are used with the nasal discharge and its disposal?
	Epistaxis	How do the episodes of epistaxis affect ability to function socially, at work, and at home? Is there awareness of predisposing factors? If predisposing factors are known, how are they coped with? What coping strategies are used (ice packs, pinching or clamping nose, retiring from setting, self-packing of nose)?
	Olfaction, Hypersensitivity Decrease or loss	Describe usual olfactory sense. Has the decreased ability to smell affected ability to function socially, at work, and at home? Has it affected the appetite? How is the change in olfaction coped with (force self to eat, cover up the loss, remove self from settings with strong odors)?
MOUTH		Pattern of oral hygiene Frequency of dental examinations
a. Teeth	All teeth present Extractions Repair Cavities	Does pain affect ability to function socially, at work, and at home? Does pain affect the ability to ingest hot or cold substances, or solids versus liquids? Does pain affect the ability to chew? What coping behaviors are used (ingestion of liquids versus solids, self-directed medications)? How effective are these coping strategies?
	Dentures/partials	Do dentures increase, maintain, or decrease ability to function socially, at work, and at home? Frequency of use of the denture? Is the ability to chew increased, decreased, or does it remain the same? What coping strategies are used when dentures create lesions? How effective are those coping strategies? How do the dentures affect self-concept?
b. Gums		Pattern and type of hygiene used in caring for the gums.
	Pain Lesions Bleeding Infections	Does the pain or lesions affect ability to function socially, at work, and at home? Does the pain or lesions affect the ability to ingest foods, or to chew? What coping strategies are used? Are they effective?
c. Tongue	Pain Lesions Movement	Does it affect the ability to function socially, at work, and at home? How does the pain or lesion affect chewing? How does pain or lesion affect the use of tongue in word formation? How does the pain or lesion affect the ability to ingest foods or wear dentures? Are there predisposing factors to tongue lesions?

TABLE 2-7 CONTINUED

ITEM	DATA BASE	ABILITY TO FUNCTION MAINTENANCE BEHAVIORS COPING STRATEGIES
MOUTH (cont.) d. Buccae	Pain Lesions, painful or painless	Do lesions or pain affect food ingestion or chewing? How does the pain or lesion affect ability to function socially, at work, and at home? Are there any predisposing factors to the pain or lesion? How are the predisposing factors coped with? Are there any factors that irritate the lesion (smoking, food)? Do you suck or chew on cheeks out of nervousness?
THROAT	Pain Lesions Dysarthria	How does the pain, lesion or dysarthria affect ability to function socially, at home, and at work? Are there any special hygiene practices used for the throat? How does the decreased ability or inability to phonate affect social, work, and home functions? How does other's inability to understand or communicate with you affect you? How are these situations coped with? How does it affect self-concept?
	Dysphagia	How does it affect ability to function socially, at work, at home? In what way does dysphagia affect swallowing? How does it affect nutritional intake? How are these inabilities coped with? Are the coping strategies effective?
	History of strep* infections	Frequency of strep infections? Seasonal relationships? Preventative measures used? Prophylactic medications used and frequency of use? How does a strep infection affect ability to function socially, at work, and at home? In what way do the strep infections affect nutritional intake? Do the strep infections result in fever? How is the fever coped with (cool baths, medications, alcohol sponges, cooler environment)? Does the fever result in dehydration? How is the dehydrated state coped with (force fluids)? What is your resistance level?
NECK	Pain	How does pain interfere with ability to function socially, at home, and at work? In what way does pain interfere with movement of the neck? How does it interfere with ability to safely transport self? What compensatory mechanisms are used when splinting neck movement?
	Pain	How do the swollen nodes interfere with ability to function socially, at work, and at home? How are the swollen nodes coped with? How effective are these coping strategies?
	Range of motion	How much limitation to the range of motion is there? How does the limited motion affect ability to function socially, at work, at home?

27

TABLE 2-7 CONTINUED

SYSTEM	DATA BASE	ABILITY TO FUNCTION MAINTENANCE BEHAVIORS COPING STRATEGIES
NECK (cont.)		How has limited motion affected ability to transport self, including motorized transportation? How are these limitations coped with? What measures are used to ensure visualization of the environment? How effective are these coping strategies? How has it affected self-concept? How are these effects coped with?
RESPIRATORY		What are, if any, the practices and patterns of pulmonary hygiene?
	Pain	Does pain affect ability to function socially, at home, or at work? How does pain affect breathing, sleeping, and mobility? What are the coping strategies used? How effective are these coping strategies?
	Shortness of breath Dyspnea Nocturnal dyspnea	How does shortness of breath affect ability to function socially, at work, and at home? How does it affect ability to achieve adequate rest? How does it affect mobility? What are the predisposing factors? What coping strategies are used? How effective are they? What types of feelings are created by shortness of breath?
	Cough	How does cough affect ability to function socially, at work, and at home? How does coughing affect sleep? Are there identifiable predisposing factors? How does pain or discomfort created by coughing affect functioning? What coping strategies are used (control of environmental humidity, increased fluids, avoidance of smoke-filled environments)? Frequency of use of nonprescriptive cough lozenges or suppressants. How effective are these strategies?
	Sputum production Hemoptysis	How does the production of sputum affect ability to function socially, at work, and at home? What is the hygiene related to sputum production and disposal of secretions? What kinds of fears result from large amounts of sputum or bloody sputum? How is the sputum production coped with (control of environmental humidity, increased fluid intake, use of tissues or handkerchief, isolation of self from others)? Frequency of use of nonprescriptive cough expectorants and suppressants or other over-the-counter medications. What is the resistance level?
CARDIOVASCULAR		Any practices to maintain cardiovascular functioning (diet, exercise)?
	Pain	How does pain affect ability to function socially, at work, and at home? Are there identifiable predisposing factors (cold, energy expenditure, excessive intake—fluid or food)?

TABLE 2-7 CONTINUED

SYSTEM	DATA BASE	ABILITY TO FUNCTION MAINTENANCE BEHAVIORS COPING STRATEGIES
CARDIOVASCULAR (cont.)		What type of fears does the pain create? What are the coping strategies used (staying inside in cold weather, wearing face mask, pacing amount of energy expenditure)? How effective are the coping strategies? How does it affect mobility? How does it affect self-concept?
	Unusual sensations	How do these sensations affect ability to function socially, at work, and at home? How and when do unusual sensations occur? Are there identifiable predisposing factors? What are the coping strategies used? How effective are they? How do they affect self-concept?
	Edema	How does the edema interfere with the ability to function socially, at work, and at home? Any predisposing factors or activities identifiable (sitting down with legs crossed, standing for long periods of time, restrictive clothing—girdle, garters)? How does it affect ability to walk? Is the edematous area prone to tissue breakdown? How is the edema coped with (decreased fluid intake, elevation of the area, decreased salt intake)? How does the edema affect self-concept?
	Varicosities	Do varicosities affect ability to function socially, at work, and at home? Does the pain interfere with ability to walk? What coping strategies are used (support hose, elevation of legs, leg makeup, exercise)? How effective are coping strategies? Do esophageal varices affect nutritional intake? What are the feelings related to esophageal varices? How do the varicosities affect self-concept?
	Hypertension	Blood pressure at last reading. What affect has hypertension had on ability to function socially, at work, and at home? How is it affected by environmental stimuli? Have there been changes in ability to cope with stressors? How do you cope with the hypertension (diet, decreased salt intake, medication)? Are the medications taken as prescribed? Have there been any changes in physical functioning since taking the medication? How are these changes coped with?
BREAST		Type and pattern of breast hygiene? Frequency of breast examinations? Frequency of self-breast examinations? How do you examine your own breast?
	Pain	How does pain affect ability to function socially, at work, and at home? Are there identifiable predisposing factors to the pain (occurs toward end of cycle, trauma, pregnancy, associated with lumps)? How are the changes and predisposing factors coped with (support, hot/cold compresses, denial)? How effective are these coping mechanisms?

TABLE 2-7 CONTINUED

BREAST (cont.)	Skin changes Lesions Dimpling Lumps	How have changes in the skin of the breast affected ability to function socially, at work, and at home? How have skin changes affected ability to breast feed? What kind of concerns have the changes produced?
	Nipple discharge	How is nipple discharge and materials used for cleansing disposed of? What coping strategies have been used (warm or cold packs, ointments, padding, discontinued breast feeding, seeking health consultation)? How effective have coping strategies been? What fears do the breast changes bring about? What effect do breast changes have on self-concept?
	Mastectomy	How recent? How radical was the surgery? Fears about recurrent CA? How long was your physical recovery, psychological recovery? What are the reactions of significant others (spoken or presumed)? How have you coped with loss (use of prosthesis)? Has the loss changed your family life, social life, work? How has it affected self-image?
GASTROINTESTINAL		Describe a routine daily nutritional intake, including breakfast, lunch, dinner, and snacks. Describe daily fluid intake, type and amount.
	Pain	How has the pain affected ability to function socially, at work, and at home? Are there predisposing factors to the abdominal pain? How do you cope with the predisposing factors? How does pain affect nutritional intake? How do you cope with the pain (eating crackers, splinting of abdomen, application of heat or cold, wear loose, nonconstrictive clothing, bland foods, antacids)?
	Nausea and vomiting	How does the nausea/vomiting affect ability to function socially, at work, and at home? During travel? How is the nausea and vomiting related to vertigo? Are there predisposing stimuli (foods, smells, taste)? How has nausea/vomiting affected hydration status? What coping strategies are used (eat crackers, drink milk, Coke, 7-Up, cessation of oral intake)? How effective are the coping strategies?
	Diarrhea	How has diarrhea affected ability to function socially, at work, and at home? Are there predisposing factors to the diarrhea (stress, water supply, fruit juices, infectious agents, coffee, travel)? How has it affected your nutritional and fluid intake? What skin changes have occurred (generalized turgor, fissures, excoriation, and inflammation of rectal area)? What coping strategies are used (decreased fluid intake, avoidance of predisposing factors, sitz baths and ointments for irritated skin)?

TABLE 2-7 CONTINUED

SYSTEM	DATA BASE	ABILITY TO FUNCTION MAINTENANCE BEHAVIORS, COPING STRATEGIES
GASTROINTESTINAL (cont.)		Frequency of use of nonprescriptive drugs? Prescribed drugs?
	Constipation	Frequency of constipation? How has constipation affected ability to function socially, at work, and at home? How does it affect you generally (feel slowed down, bogged down, abdominal distress)? What are the coping strategies for constipation (use of enemas, suppositories, fruit juices, increased fluid intake)? Frequency of use of nonprescriptive laxatives, mineral oil, cathartics? How effective are these methods? How does pain on evacuation affect you? Are there predisposing factors related to constipation (decreased fluid intake, cheese, bananas, long rides, decreased activity)?
	Hemorrhoids	How do the hemorrhoids affect ability to function socially, at work, at home? Do hemorrhoids cause pain or itching? How do the hemorrhoids affect mobility? How do the hemorrhoids affect ability to evacuate bowels? How do you cope with the hemorrhoids (hot baths, ice packs, ointments)? Frequency of use of nonprescriptive medications? How effective are the coping strategies?
	Bowel evacuation pattern	What is the present pattern of normal bowel habits? Any particular activities used to maintain pattern (laxatives, prune juice, cereals, hot water)? Are maintenance activities effective?
	Stool characteristics Color Consistency	Changes in color or consistency associated with predisposing factors (high milk intake, types of foods eaten, iron intake, medications taken, prescriptive or nonprescriptive)?
	Acid indigestion	What activities are used to remain free of indigestion? How does acid indigestion affect ability to function socially, at work, and at home? Are there identifiable predisposing factors (stressors, certain types of foods, lack of foods)? What coping strategies are used (eating, use of bland foods, use of antacids and frequency of use, change in sleeping positions)?
GENITOURINARY: MALE		Type and pattern of hygiene. If foreskin is present, is it easily retracted? What is normal voiding pattern?
	Perineal rashes and irritations	How does rash or irritation affect ability to function socially, at work, or at home? Are there any identifiable predisposing factors (warm weather, exercise, soaps, constrictive clothing—support, jockstrap, rubber pants, nylon briefs)? When does the rash or irritated area become excoriated? How is the rash or irritation coped with (increased frequency of hygienic measures, warm baths, ointments, powders, leave off rubber pants, switch to cotton briefs or boxer shorts)? How effective are these coping strategies?

TABLE 2-7 CONTINUED

		ABILITY TO FUNCTION MAINTENANCE BEHAVIORS COPING STRATEGIES
GENITOURINARY: MALE (cont.)	Difficulty starting or stopping stream Force of stream Dribbling	How has the difficulty starting or stopping the stream or dribbling affected the ability to function socially, at work, and at home? What type of discomfort in the bladder area is there? How has it affected routine voiding patterns? What coping strategies are used (sitz baths, increased muscle force to void)? How effective are these coping strategies? How has the force of the stream changed? What effect do these changes have on self-concept?
	Pain or burning on urination	How has the pain or burning affected voiding patterns? What is the frequency of urinary infections? What is the frequency of prostate infections? Has there been contact with a venereal infection? What type of discomfort in the bladder area is there? What is the color and smell of the urine? What is the color, amount, and smell of urethral discharge? How are these changes being coped with (sitz baths, avoidance of voiding)? How effective are these coping strategies?
	Incontinence	How has incontinence affected ability to function socially, at work, and at home? Has there been a pattern to the incontinence? Are there any predisposing factors (stress, activity, cold, exhaustion, dreaming, laughing, coughing)? How has it been coped with? How effective are the coping strategies?
	Lesions on or pain in penis and scrotum	How do the lesions or pain affect sexual activity or urination? What factors seem to be predisposing to the lesion or pain? How have these lesions or pain affected ability to function socially, at work, and at home? What coping strategies are used? How effective are the coping strategies? What fears do either the lesions or pain create?
	Reproduction Number of offspring	Is there satisfaction with the number of offspring? Is there desire for more offspring? How does the number of offspring affect ability to function socially, at work, and at home? How does the number of children affect ability to follow through with parental responsibilities? If no offspring, how do pressures to have children affect ability to function socially, at work, at home? What coping strategies are used in working with the pressures of nonparenthood from significant others (support groups, avoidance)? How effective are these coping strategies? How does the number of children, nonparenthood status, and subsequent pressures affect self-concept?
	Birth control	What type of birth control is used? What method is preferred? Satisfaction with the method of birth control used? How does this method affect sexual activity and sexual satisfaction? Has it been effective for you?

32

TABLE 2-7 CONTINUED

SYSTEM	DATA BASE	ABILITY TO FUNCTION, MAINTENANCE BEHAVIORS, COPING STRATEGIES
GENITOURINARY: MALE (cont.)		If no children are desired, and no birth control is used, how is the possibility of pregnancy coped with?
	Infertility	How long have you been trying to have offspring?
		How has the inability to have children affected the ability to function socially, at work, and at home?
		Has there been a fertility work-up for self and spouse?
		How have marital relationships changed?
		What coping strategies are used (adoption)?
		What effect does infertility have on self-concept?
	Venereal disease	What type of venereal disease is or was it?
		Did it interfere with ability to function socially, at work, and at home?
		Was it treated and how?
		Did it result in any complications (sterility, atrophy of testis, urethral strictures)?
		How was the sterility discovered?
		What effect does this have on self-concept?
GENITOURINARY: FEMALE		Type and pattern of hygiene?
		What is the routine voiding pattern?
	Perineal rashes and irritations	How do rashes or irritations affect ability to function socially, at work, and at home?
		Are there identifiable predisposing factors (warm weather, exercise, soaps, douching solutions, constrictive clothing—bikini panties, nylon panties, rubber pants)?
		How is the rash or irritation coped with (increased frequency of hygienic measures, warm baths, ointments, powders, leaving off rubber pants, switch from nylon to cotton undergarments)?
		How effective are these coping strategies?
	Difficulty starting or stopping stream	How has the difficulty affected ability to function socially, at work, and at home?
	Force of stream	What type of discomfort in the bladder area is there?
	Dribbling	How has it affected routine voiding patterns?
		What coping strategies are used (sitz baths, increased muscle force to void, or prevent voiding, padding in underwear, protective panties)?
		How effective are these strategies?
	Pain or burning on urination	How has pain or burning affected voiding pattern?
		How has pain or burning affected ability to function socially, at work, and at home?
		Frequency of urinary infections?
		Has there been contact with a venereal infection?
		What type of discomfort is in the bladder area?
		What is the color, amount, character, and smell of the urine?
		How is the pain or burning coped with (sitz baths, avoidance of urinating, douches)?
		How effective are the coping strategies?
	Incontinence	How has incontinence affected ability to function socially, at work, and at home?
		Has there been a pattern to the incontinence?
		Are there predisposing factors (stress, activity, cold, exhaustion, dreaming, laughing, coughing)?
		How has incontinence been coped with?
		How effective are the coping strategies?

TABLE 2-7 CONTINUED

SYSTEM	DATA	COPING STRATEGIES
GENITOURINARY: FEMALE (cont.)	Pain or lesions on genitalia	How do the lesions or pain affect sexual activity or urination?
		What factors seem to be predisposing to the lesion or pain?
		How have these lesions or pain affected ability to function socially, at work, and at home?
		What coping strategies are used?
		How effective are the coping strategies?
		What fears do either the lesion or the pain create?
	History of vaginal infections	How do the vaginal infections affect ability to function socially, at work, and at home?
		What is the frequency of vaginal infections?
		Are the types of infections known?
		What methods of coping are used (douches, sitz baths)?
		How effective are the coping strategies?
	Reproduction	How do premenstrual tension, dysmenorrhea, and menses affect ability to function socially, at work, and at home?
	Age of menarche	
	Age of menopause	
	Number of days in menstrual cycle	Frequency and use of nonprescriptive or prescriptive drugs for dysmenorrhea?
	Number of days in menses	How do hot flashes affect ability to function socially, at work, and at home?
	Type and amount of flow	
	Premenstrual tension	What color is postmenopausal or intermenstrual discharge?
	Dysmenorrhea	
	Hypermenorrhea/menorrhagia	What concerns does this discharge bring about?
		What are the concerns with the overdue period?
	Polymenorrhagia	What effect on your ability to function socially, at work, and at home does menorrhagia, polymenorrhea, or metrorrhagia have?
	Intermenstrual/metrorrhagia	
	History of pregnancies	How did pregnancies affect ability to function socially, at work, and at home?
	Number of pregnancies	
	Number of live births	What strategies were used to cope with these effects?
	Number of abortions (less than 20 weeks gestation)	What effect did the abortion have on your ability to function socially, at work, and at home?
	Number of still births	
	Number of neonatal deaths	How were these effects coped with?
	High-risk pregnancies	In what way was the pregnancy high risk?
		What coping strategies were used to deal with the high risk?
		How did the high-risk status affect ability to function socially, at work, and at home?
		Is there satisfaction with the number of offspring?
		Is there desire for more offspring?
		How does the number of offspring affect ability to function socially, at work, and at home?
		How does the number of children affect ability to follow through with parental responsibilities?
		If no offspring, how do pressures to have children affect ability to function socially, at work, at home?
		What coping strategies are used in working with the pressures of nonparenthood from significant others (support groups, avoidance)?
		How effective are these coping strategies?
		How do the number of children or nonparenthood status and subsequent pressures affect self-concept?
	Birth control	What type of birth control is used?
		What method is preferred?
		Satisfaction with the method of birth control used?
		How does this method affect sexual activity and sexual satisfaction?

TABLE 2-7 CONTINUED

ITEM	SIGNS/SYMPTOMS	ABILITY TO FUNCTION / MAINTENANCE BEHAVIORS / COPING STRATEGIES
GENITOURINARY: FEMALE (cont.)		Has it been effective? If no children are desired, and no birth control is used, how is the possibility of pregnancy coped with?
	Infertility	How long have you been trying to have offspring? How has the inability to have children affected the ability to function socially, at work, and at home? Has there been a fertility work up for self and spouse? Have marital relationships changed? What coping strategies are used (adoption)? What effect does infertility have on self-concept?
SEXUALITY	Sexual orientation	Sexual orientation: heterosexual, homosexual, or bisexual? Is there satisfaction with sexual orientation? How does the sexual orientation affect ability to function socially, at work, and at home? What types of stressors result from sexual orientation? What coping strategies are employed with these pressures (avoidance, support groups)? How does sexual orientation affect self-concept?
	Frequency of sexual activity	What are the types of sexual activity? Are the modes of expression satisfactory? In what way does hypo- or hyperactivity affect ability to function socially, at work, and at home? What are the stressors received due to this activity level? Are there predisposing factors related to frequency of sexual activity (job, illness)? What are the coping strategies? How effective are the coping strategies?
	Satisfaction with sexual activity	What is it that creates sexual satisfaction? What is the nature of the dissatisfaction? Has the dissatisfaction affected ability to function socially, at work, and at home? Are you able to have an orgasm? What have been the coping strategies? How effective are the coping strategies? How does the level of satisfaction affect self-concept?
MUSCULAR	Pain	How does muscular pain affect ability to function socially, at work, and at home? Where is the limitation of motion, and what is the degree of limitation? Are there identifiable predisposing factors? What coping strategies are used (warm/cold compresses or baths, splinting braces, elevation of area, increased amount of rest)? How effective are the coping strategies?
	Fatigue	How does fatigue affect ability to function socially, at work, and at home? Are there identifiable predisposing factors? Where is the fatigue experienced (generalized, localized)? How does it affect mobility and transportation? What are the coping strategies related to fatigue? What is the effectiveness of the coping strategies?
	Paralysis	What body parts are affected by the paralysis and to what degree?

TABLE 2-7 CONTINUED

SYSTEM	SIGNS	ABILITY TO FUNCTION MAINTAINING BEHAVIORS COPING STRATEGIES
MUSCULAR (cont.)		How does paralysis affect ability to function socially, at work, and at home? How has it affected ability to administer self-cares? How has it affected ability to be mobile (self and motorized)? How has it affected sexuality? How effective are the coping strategies? How is self-concept affected? What are the coping strategies (scheduled rehabilitation, use of mechanical aids—walk with cane, crutches, walker, braces, give up some of independence, isolation of self)?
BONES/JOINTS	Pain Swelling Stiffness Limited range of motion Sprain joints easily	How has pain, swelling, stiffness, or limited range of motion affected ability to function socially, at work, and at home? How has the pain, swelling, stiffness, or limited range of motion affected mobility? How does exercise affect the joints? What motions are limited? Are there predisposing factors to pain, swelling, stiffness? What coping strategies are used (rest, heat, cold, exercises, ointments, control of dietary intake, prescriptive or nonprescriptive medications)? Frequency of use of nonprescriptive or prescribed medications? Frequency of sprained joints? Are there identifiable predisposing factors (loss of depth perception, awkward gait, hurried motion)?
NEUROLOGICAL	Numbness Tingling Hypersensitivity (or hyposensitivity) Discrimination between heat, cold, and touch pressures	How does the occurrence of any of these signs or symptoms affect ability to function socially, at work, and at home? Are there any identifiable predisposing factors (crossing legs while sitting, hyperventilation, exposure to extreme cold, prolonged excessive pressure to an area)? If loss of sensation, what coping strategies are used (thermometer in tub water, someone else test warmth of substances)? How effective are coping strategies? How do these signs and symptoms affect self-concept?
	Tremors Seizures Dizziness Loss of consciousness Memory changes Sweating	How does the occurrence of any of these signs or symptoms affect ability to function socially, at work, and at home? Are there identifiable predisposing factors (heat, cold, quick changes in position, tremor when attempting to reach for something)? What coping strategies are used for awkward movements? Is the occurrence of seizures, dizziness, or loss of consciousness predictable? How are these factors coped with? What safety precautions are taken? What are the most difficult areas of recall or things to recall? How do these signs and symptoms affect self-concept?

TABLE 2-7 CONTINUED

SYSTEM	DATA BASE	ABILITY TO FUNCTION MAINTENANCE BEHAVIORS COPING STRATEGIES
ENDOCRINE	Intolerance to heat/cold Polyuria Polydypsia Polyphagia Thyroid Diabetes mellitus	In what manner does the occurrence of any of the symptoms affect ability to function socially, at work, and at home? Are there predisposing factors related to any of the symptoms? How are the predisposing factors coped with? Describe the intolerance to heat and cold. Describe the type and amount of nutritional intake, fluid intake for a typical day? How is this intake different from the previous pattern? What is the frequency and amount of the voiding? How has this changed from previous pattern? When was the thyroid condition diagnosed? What changes has this condition brought about? When was the condition of diabetes mellitus diagnosed? What changes has the condition brought about? What coping mechanisms are used? How effective are these coping strategies?

MENTAL HEALTH	Feelings of
	  Insecurity
	  Persecution
	  Nervousness
	  Depression
	  Insomnia
	  Mood changes
	  Suicidal thoughts
	Hallucinations: auditory or visual
	Tolerance to stressors
		How have these feelings, thoughts, changes in behavior, or sensory events affected ability to function socially, at work, and at home?
		How has insomnia affected the usual sleeping pattern?
		Are there predisposing factors to mood changes?
		What are the sensory events about?
		Have there been any behavior changes in relation to suicidal thoughts?
		How have feelings, thoughts, changes in behavior, or sensory events affected cognitive abilities?
		How are feelings, thoughts, changes in behavior, or sensory events coped with?

* Beta hemolytic streptococci.

Subjective Data Collection:
The Pediatric Client

The interview conducted to obtain subjective data regarding the pediatric client presents a special challenge for the nurse. Often the informant and the client are not the same, as the informant is the child's parent, guardian, or family member who either provides all the information, or at least provides additional information and clarification or verification of the child's responses. If the child is capable of responding to questions, he or she should be included in the interview and encouraged to communicate. However, the child's degree of participation will depend upon the parent's patience, the child's level of development, and the nurse's approach.

The nurse's approach becomes a very essential part of success in obtaining the necessary information and data from the parent or other informant. Proceeding successfully through the interview with an effective and nonthreatening approach is an acquired skill that requires much practice.

If the informant (other than the child) is the parent or primary caretaker (especially the mother), the nurse must remember that illness or environmental discord may be viewed by the parent as a social stigma of inadequate parenting. In such cases, the necessary information can be difficult to obtain if the approach is not an understanding one. Also, the anxiety level of the parent or caretaker must be assessed, especially if the child is presenting a health problem.

It is best to proceed by discussing with the parent or caretaker the details of the present situation (i.e., how the child is now and how the parents are handling the situation). Then the interviewer proceeds to the previous history, prenatal, pregnancy, mother's health, and family health, all of which to the anxious parent may seem unrelated to the child's history. Finally, explorations are made into what the parent's expectations are for the future, relative to anticipated health-care problems for this child.

The important factor in the interviewing process is the process itself and not the exact factual content. Although certain information is best obtained from the parent, the interviewer is interested in eliciting data from the child that add meaning to the identification of clues related to the needs, problems, or potential problems of the child. The information to be obtained is similar to that reviewed in the adult health history, with some additions and modifications as outlined next.

Chief Complaint

Distinguish and record the difference between factual observations of the informant from the impressions of physicians and other sources or from informant's interpretations of observations.

Present Illness

In the pediatric client population it is important to inquire about exposure to a contagious disease(s) within the last 3 weeks. If the present illness has been a chronic one, inquire about secondary disturbances of growth, personality changes, appetite changes, changes in sleeping pattern, weight loss, and hydration status.

Prenatal History

1. **Pregnancy** (brief if the child is over 2 years of age)
   a. Duration of pregnancy with this child, including expected due date versus birth date.
   b. Type and frequency of prenatal care.
   c. Maternal nutrition.
   d. Threatened miscarriage, infections, medications taken, bleeding, complications or problems.

2. **Birth**
   a. Labor: duration and intensity of labor.
   b. Where was child delivered and by whom.
   c. Medications during labor and delivery.
   d. Type of delivery and presentation.
   e. Child's birth weight and length.
   f. Problems during and immediately after delivery (needed oxygen or resuscitation).
   g. Anomalies or trauma observed at birth.
   h. How many days infant hospitalized? Mother hospitalized?

3. **Neonatal Period** (first 28 days of life)
   a. Jaundice in the newborn period: onset, degree of severity, treatment, and duration.
   b. Cyanosis or respiratory distress.
   c. Seizures.
   d. Bleeding problems.
   e. Feeding problems: vomiting, slow feeder, etc.
   f. Rashes or other skin eruptions.
   g. Infections.
   h. If child was a high-risk infant (required any special care) elaborate on problems, and the extent and duration of hospital care.

Developmental History

1. **Nutrition**
   a. If the client is an infant, is he or she being breast fed or bottle fed? What formula is used and how is it prepared? What is the infant's usual feeding schedule, how much is taken per feeding, and how much time does the infant require per feeding? Have solids been started; if so, what, when, and how much? Does the infant take a vitamin supplement, iron supplement, and/or fluoride supplement?
   b. Older child: Briefly review the child's nutritional intake during infancy for gross evidence of problems. When were solids started? When was child weaned from breast and/or bottle? When did child start eating table foods, finger foods, using a spoon, drinking from a cup? Then proceed with inquiry about child's present diet, including snacks, food preferences, and vitamin and iron supplements.

2. **Physical Growth**
   Inquire about problems or concerns relating to past growth. When did first tooth erupt and how many permanent teeth does child have if appropriate for age?

3. **Motor Development**
   As pertinent to child's present age, inquire when child first sat alone, stood alone, walked alone, spoke words (what words), and used phrases.

4. **Social Development**
   Inquire about weaning from bottle feedings, breast feedngs, and pacifier. Age and problems with toilet training, caring for self, adjustment in family and with playmates or schoolmates. Did child have any behavior problems such as temper tantrums, feeding difficulties, bed wetting, nail biting, unusual sleep habits, or pica? What is the child's present school grade and general achievement level (if appropriate for age)?

5. **Pubescence**
   Age of onset of puberty (i.e., breast development, menarche, pubic hair, and growth spurts).

Past Medical History

1. **General**
   Routine health care maintenance by whom, how frequent, and date of last visit.

2. **Immunizations**
   Describe any allergic reactions to immunizations.

3. **Illnesses**
   Along with inquiry about common childhood diseases and sequelae, inquire about infectious diseases and number of recurrences (i.e., pneumonia, ear infections, tonsillitis, and colds).

4. **Accidents**
   Inquire specifically about poisonings, head injuries, and fractures. Inquire about unusual illnesses of unknown origin relating to availability of poisons or drugs in the home.

Review of Systems

General: Weight loss, irritability, fever, slowness or retardation.

Skin: Eczema, urticaria, petechiae, purpura, easily bruised, change in texture or unusual dryness.

Head: Unusual shape, enlargement, injuries, headaches at home or at school.

Eyes: Strabismus, glasses.

Ears: Myringotomies, earaches and relationship to bottle feeding at night, discharge, responsiveness to sound.

Nose: Obstruction, discharge, mouth breathing, frequent colds.

Mouth: Condition and number of teeth, thrush, sores, sore throats (frequency and severity).

Respiratory: Chronic cough, asthma, bronchitis, croup, dyspnea, trachypnea, epiglottitis.

Cardiovascular: Cyanosis or blue spells, previously heard heart murmurs, clubbing of fingers, squatting during play, symptoms of rheumatic fever.

Gastrointestinal: Appetite, pain, vomiting, diarrhea, constipation, melena, usual bowel habits, use of cathartics, enemas, karo syrup, suppositories or other anticonstipation drugs, diet supplements or procedures. Jaundice.

Genitourinary: Frequency, problem with incontinence following toilet training or nocturia.

Neuromuscular: Fainting, seizures (with or without fever), staring spells, gait and coordination abnormalities, early right or left handedness, school performance, and behavior deviations.

Family History

Identify situations where present parents are not natural parents.

1. **Father**
   Age, health, occupation.

2. **Mother**
   Age, health, occupation.

3. **Siblings**
   Age, health, sex, biological relation to child.

4. **Familial diseases**
   Inquire about congenital defects, unusual diseases, causes of deaths during infancy or young childhood, and size of parents and siblings if child's size is unusual for age.

Personal Profile

Home environment
Obtain a brief description of the home, if urban or rural, size, conveniences, members of

household, pets (number and type), sanitation, water, milk and food supply. Where are poisons and medications stored? Is there any syrup of ipecac in the home?

Social History

Are parents living together? Is there known marital discord? Who cares for child primarily while parents are out or at work?

Subjective Data Collection: The Elderly Client

When interviewing the elderly, several considerations must be taken into account as numerous changes occur with the aging process. Each elderly client is at a different point in experiencing these changes, and therefore a single pattern of interaction should not preclude individualized interactions. Maturational changes do not produce a singular effect, but involve the total being of the person. A conscious awareness on the part of the interviewer is needed in elaborating on actions that may facilitate the collection of subjective data. Some of the interviewer's actions may serve as facilitators in more than one area in which the client is experiencing the effects of the aging process. Table 2-8 presents some broad categorizations of aging changes and the interviewer's actions that may facilitate the collection of data, as well as maintain the dignity of the individual.

TABLE 2-8
Aging Changes and Appropriate Interviewer Actions

CATEGORIZATION OF CHANGES RESULTING FROM AGING	INTERVIEWER ACTIONS BASED ON THE CHANGES OF THE AGING PROCESS
PHYSICAL CHANGES	
Decreased visual acuity	Sit close to the client Face client when speaking Occasional touching of the client's hand Ensure a good quantity of illumination
Decreased hearing acuity—conductive and sensorineural	Speak louder* Face the client Speak slowly Exaggerate use of the mouth and lips in the formation of words Sit closer to receptive hearing side, if one ear is affected to a lesser degree or not at all
Declining physical strength	Arrange environment to limit the need for increased energy expenditure (i.e., the process of becoming seated in a low chair and the thought processes related to getting out of it as well as the actual maneuver of getting up)
Increased time needed for reactions	Allow more time for nonverbal responses Observe closely for type and use of nonverbal behavior
Increased tolerance to internal stressors	Establish and reestablish the focus of discussion to ensure maximal description of concerns expressed
Decreased tolerance to environmental changes (i.e., heat and cold)	Ensure a warm environment Inform the client of any changes in the environment that will occur
PSYCHOLOGICAL CHANGES	
Decreased tolerance to changes in environment	Retain primary focus of the interview Change focus only after informing the client and an agreement has been reached

*Increasing voice intensity is ineffective in sensorineural loss.

TABLE 2-8 CONTINUED

CATEGORIZATION OF CHANGES RESULTING FROM AGING	INTERVIEWER ACTIONS BASED ON THE CHANGES OF THE AGING PROCESS
PSYCHOLOGICAL CHANGES (cont.)	
	Maintain consistency in pattern of eliciting data
Devaluation of self, resulting from changes in self-concept and body state.†	Listen to client's statement Be gentle and firm in moving on to the collection of related data Demonstrate empathic understanding
Loss of sense of identity	Call by full name and title Support dignity and worth
Suspiciousness related to decreased hearing acuity	Utilize same activities stated under hearing loss Ensure clarification of statements to client, as well as clarifying what the client means
COGNITIVE CHANGES	
Shortened attention span	May need to complete the interview over several sessions Maintain a consistent approach Direct special attention to cues of waning attention
Slowed mentation, increased time needed for reactions	Set focus of the interview Phrase questions concisely Ensure brevity of explanations Allow more time for responses Proceed with the interview at a slower rate in comparison with the young adult
Impaired memory recall of long past and immediate past	Consider the pertinence of each piece of data requested prior to asking for it Do not press for details Obtain details from other sources (i.e., family, past medical records, past nursing records)
Confusion	Set focus, and continue reiteration of the interview focus as necessary Be selective in the types of data elicited Obtain data and details from sources other than the client
SOCIAL/CULTURAL CHANGES	
**Loss of significant others	Allow time for verbalization of these losses, yet conduct gently and firmly an onward progression of the interview
Decrease in number and types of, or complete loss of, support systems	Allot a time period for verbalizations that normally occur with support system, and then move forward with the focus of the interview.
Changes in role expectations and attached significance as directed by self and others	Do not assign a role to the client Demonstrate respect for role Transmit dignity

† The interviewer must assess the priority of this area for the client; if it is a high priority, it must be dealt with before movement into other areas can occur.

** The interviewer must assess the priority of this area for the client; if it is a high priority, it must be dealt with before movement into other areas can occur.

PRACTICAL POINTS FOR THE HISTORY-TAKING PROCESS

Most clients cannot remember exact dates or exact details of past events. Asking more general nondirective questions first may give the interviewer clues whereby more specific questions for information can be posed.

1. Use a quiet, sympathetic but confident tone of voice.
2. Make your questions simple and brief.
3. Give the clients plenty of time to express themselves or explain before you clarify or continue. Use nonverbal and verbal gestures to indicate your listening and understanding.
4. Clarify inconsistencies between sources or interpretations in a nonthreatening or nonprosecuting manner.
5. Avoid asking clients for information that they are not likely to have; this may encourage mistrust or increase anxiety about the unknown.
6. Make it a point to ask appropriate questions (i.e., do not expect the client to remember details of the past that you would not be able to remember).
7. Avoid leading the client into misinterpretations, but do not expect them to anticipate the specific details that you are seeking. Use terminology that is appropriate to their social, cultural, and educational status.
8. Use the significant other, when present in the room, to clarify points that seem to be vague recollections: "Do you recall the incident?" or "Is that what you remember about it?" or "Do you have anything to add to his or her recollection?"
9. If a child is distracting the interview, provide some attention device and then later include the child as appropriate.

In communicating with a child, the interviewer should:

1. Speak quietly in a noncommanding voice.
2. Make questions simple but appropriate to the child's level of understanding.
3. Allow time for the child to respond.
4. Avoid negatives in your conversation (i.e., don't, not, doesn't).

In summary, time and experience in interviewing facilitate the growth of the interviewer's self-confidence. Frequently, the inexperienced interviewer finds himself or herself concentrating on learning the skills of interviewing, seeking the appropriate information, and not on the individual being interviewed, thus missing verbal and nonverbal cues. It is not only the verbal and nonverbal cues that are missed, but the person himself or herself. This may be perceived by the interviewer as the placement of high value on data and low value on the "I," resulting in feelings of dehumanization.

The interviewer formulates a personalized framework through which interviewing occurs. In essence, it is a composite of synthesized knowledge and the self. The interviewing process may include providing information to the client as appropriate. However, for some, the provision of information is not part of the interviewing framework and comes later, in order to ensure that premature conclusions are not formed.

BIBLIOGRAPHY

BERMOSK, LORETTA S., "Interviewing: A Key to Therapeutic Communication in Nursing Practice," *Nursing Clinics of North America,* June 1966, pp. 205–214.

———, and MARY J. MORDAN, *Interviewing in Nursing.* New York: Macmillan Publishing Co., Inc., 1964.

BERNSTEIN, LEWIS, ROSALYN S. BERNSTEIN, and RICHARD H. DANA, *Interviewing: A Guide for Health Professionals* (2nd ed.). New York: Appleton-Century-Crofts, 1974.

BROWN, MARIE S., "What You Should Know About Communicable Diseases and Their Immunizations, Part I," *Nursing 75,* September 1975, pp.70–72.

———, "What You Should Know About Communicable Diseases and Their Immunizations, Part II," *Nursing 75,* October 1975, pp. 56–60.

———, "What You Should Know About Communicable Diseases and Their Immunizations, Part III," *Nursing 75,* November 1975, pp. 55–60.

BURNSIDE, IRENE M., *Psychosocial Nursing Care of the Aged.* New York: McGraw-Hill Book Company, 1973.

———, *Nursing and the Aged.* New York: McGraw-Hill Book Company, 1976.

DEGOWIN, ELMER L., and RICHARD L. DEGOWIN, *Bedside Diagnostic Examination* (3rd ed.), pp. 11–32. Boston: Little, Brown and Company, 1968.

EDINBURG, GOLDA M., NORMAN E. ZENBERG, and WENDY KELMAN, *Clinical Interviewing and Counseling: Principles and Techniques.* New York: Appleton-Century-Crofts, 1975.

ENELOW, ALLEN J., and SCOTT N. SWISHER, *Interviewing and Patient Care.* New York: Oxford University Press, 1972.

FROELICH, ROBERT, and F. MARIAN BISHOP, *Medical Interviewing* (2nd ed.). St. Louis, Mo.: The C. V. Mosby Company, 1972.

HOCHSTEIN, ELLIOT, and ALBERT L. RUBIN, *Physical Diagnosis,* pp. 3–20. New York: McGraw-Hill Book Company, 1964.

JUDGE, RICHARD D., and GEORGE D. ZUIDEMA, eds., *Physical Diagnosis: A Physiologic Approach to the Clinical Examination* (2nd ed.), pp. 13–33. Boston: Little, Brown and Company, 1968.

LUCKROFT, DOROTHY, ed., *Black Awareness: Implications for Black Patient Care.* New York: The American Journal of Nursing Company, 1976.

"Patient Assessment: Taking a Patient's History," *American Journal of Nursing,* February 1974, pp. 293–324.

SECTION 3

3
The Integument

REVIEW OF STRUCTURE AND FUNCTION

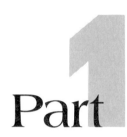

Part 1

STRUCTURE OF THE INTEGUMENT

The skin is the largest organ of the body. It is composed of two layers, the epidermis and the dermis. The subcutaneous tissue is frequently referred to as a layer of the skin, but anatomically it is not part of the integument's structure.

Epidermis

The epidermis (Figure 3-1) is the tough outer layer of the skin that is subdivided into the stratum corneum (horny layer) and stratum germinativum. The stratum corneum, composed of keratinized cells, is continuously being shed and replaced by newly generated cells from the lower cellular layers of the epidermis. These keratinized outer cells are flat, closely approximated, and serve as a protective barrier. The thickness of the epidermis varies with body location and the amount of pressure experienced by that region. For example, the palms of the hands and the soles of the feet experience greater pressure throughout the day as compared to other body regions, resulting in an increased thickness of the epidermis in these areas. The epidermis also adapts to excessive pressure by formation of callus, which is a circumscribed hypertrophic area of the epidermis, frequently found on the palms of the hands and the soles of the feet.

Contained within the epidermis are melanocytes, which produce the pigment melanin. Melanocytes of darkly pigmented races are no more numerous than in races of lighter pigmentation, but they are larger in size and are more densely approximated. The production of melanin is influenced by the melanocyte-stimulating hormone (MSH) and exposure to the sun.

Dermis

The dermis (Figure 3-1) layer of the skin, which lies beneath the epidermis, is often called the true skin. The dermis and epidermis are connected by elastic tissue, which gives the skin its resilience and increases its adaptability to body movements. Collagen, a fibrous protein, is the element of the dermis that toughens it. Contained within the dermis are blood vessels, lymph vessels, and nerve endings.

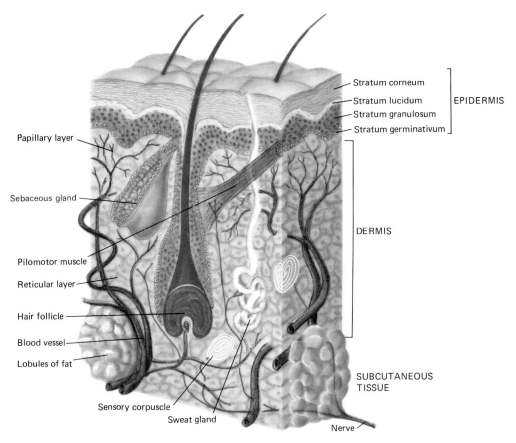

Papillary layer

Sebaceous gland

Pilomotor muscle

Reticular layer

Hair follicle

Blood vessel

Lobules of fat

Sensory corpuscle

Sweat gland

Stratum corneum
Stratum lucidum } EPIDERMIS
Stratum granulosum
Stratum germinativum

DERMIS

SUBCUTANEOUS
TISSUE

Nerve

FIGURE 3-1
The integument: the epidermis, dermis, subcutaneous tissue, and structures associated with each layer.

SKIN APPENDAGES

Hair

Embedded in the dermis are several append-ages of the skin. The hair root (Figure 3-1) forms in this layer at the third month of fetal develop-ment. The bulb of the hair is the germinal layer from which the tightly structured keratinized cells of the hair shaft are formed. Pigmentation of the hair shaft is determined by the functioning of the melanocytes, which are located in the bulb. Hair growth occurs in cycles. This cyclical growth is composed of an active and a resting phase that alternate in occurrence. All hairs do not enter the resting phase simultaneously and, therefore, while some are resting, others are growing. Vari-ations in the growth rate of hair occur with sea-sons of the year as well as body location. Fuzz is a type of hair that generally covers most areas of the body and is characterized by its fineness, light color, and short hair shaft. In comparison to fuzz,

terminal hairs are longer, coarser in texture, and darkly pigmented. Terminal hairs are located in the scalp and, in the biologically mature person, the face, pubic region, arms, legs, chest, and ab-domen.

Sebaceous Gland

Associated with the hair channel are the seba-ceous glands (Figure 3-1). These lobulated glands produce a fatty substance called *sebum,* which is secreted through the pathway of the hair follicle. Sebum secretions serve as an oiling substance for the skin. The sebaceous glands are distributed over the entire body, with the exception of the palms and soles. Lubrication of the integument of the hands and feet is accomplished through transference, which occurs when the hands or feet are rubbed on another body area that is lubri-cated. The greatest density of the sebaceous glands is in the scalp, face, periumbilical area, scrotal, and perianal areas.

Eccrine Gland

The eccrine or sweat gland (Figure 3-1) is innervated by cholinergic fibers. This gland responds to heat, secreting a dilute saline solution in an effort to maintain body temperature. Eccrine glands mature sufficiently after the first 2 months of life to function as a regulator of body temperature. Secretion of the eccrine gland is through the small pore openings. The forehead, palms of the hands, and soles of the feet have the greatest concentration of these glands, although the rest of the body is richly endowed with them also. Emotional stress also activates the eccrine glands. The amount of fluid secreted by glandular activity and lost from the body varies greatly in quantity.

Apocrine Gland

The apocrine gland, also associated with the hair follicle, produces a whitish fluid in small quantities. Apocrine fluid is odorless upon secretion, but, due to the action of body-residing bacteria, is responsible for body odors. The exact function of these glands is unknown and thus they are frequently referred to as vestigial glands. These glands respond to stress states following pubertal changes and decrease secretional activity in the aging process. The greatest concentration of apocrine glands is in the axillae, areola, periumbilical, perianal, and genital regions.

Nails

The nail is another appendage of the skin (Figure 3-2). It is composed of a nail plate, a colorless structure, that overlays the nail bed composed of epithelial cells. Covering the posterior nail plate is the posterior nail fold; the lateral borders are covered by the structures termed the lateral nail folds. The pinkish white color that shows through the nail plate is reflective of the highly vascularized nail bed. This nail bed does not contribute to nail formation or growth. The lunula, a semilunar whitish area generally found at the posterior border of the nail, especially the thumb nail, reflects the underlying nail matrix from which the nail originates. The nail plate possesses fine longitudinal ridges, which become accentuated in the elderly.

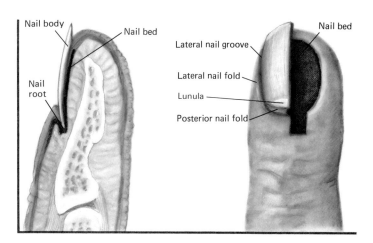

FIGURE 3-2
The nail, an appendage of the skin.

FUNCTIONS OF THE INTEGUMENT

The integument has multiple functions in the maintenance of the entire human system. Its importance cannot be underestimated. Many of the skin's functions can be categorized under the classification of protection. The following are some of these protective functions:

1. Protection from invasion.
2. Fluid regulation.
3. Thermal regulation.
4. Sensory reception: heat, cold, touch, pressure, pain (i.e., itching, burning, dullness, and sharpness).
5. Indicator of internal events: jaundice, cyanosis, exanthems, and edema.
6. Cosmetic and identity.
7. Expressive.

Protection from Invasion

An intact skin is the body's first line of defense. It serves to prevent penetration by foreign objects into the internal structures. During the activities of daily living, numerous blunt objects impinge against the hands, arms, and abdomen. Without the skin, direct penetration and damage to underlying structures, such as muscles, nerves, and organs, would occur.

The integument also acts as a host to bacterial colonization, most of which are not pathogenic. If the skin's continuity is broken, bacterial invasion can occur; when this occurs, the body's second line of the defense is activated and walls off the infectious agent, thus confining it to a specific area. As a result of this protective process, different types of lesions may be seen on the skin's surface. To further protect itself from pathogenic invasion, the skin maintains a slightly acid pH of 5 to 6, a level that is not conducive to bacterial growth.

Fluid Regulation

The intact skin is essentially an impermeable covering of the body, although a few substances are absorbed. Fat-soluble substances are absorbed through the skin at the follicular orifices. Absorption via follicular orifices demonstrates the necessity to rub in topical ointments so that they reach the follicular openings. Gases are another substance that can be absorbed directly through the skin, with carbon monoxide being one exception to this rule.

Fluid loss from the skin is called *insensible loss* and averages about 350 cc per day in the adult. The greatest loss of fluid through evaporation occurs when the skin is removed or destroyed, as in the case of a burn.

Thermal Regulation

The skin, through the blood vessels stimulated by the nervous system, regulates body temperature. In a cold environment vessels constrict, thus retaining the heat to maintain body temperature; in a hot environment, the blood vessels dilate, eliminating heat through convection, which results in a cooling of the body. In the infant, thermal regulation is limited, and maturation of this regulatory function occurs throughout childhood.

Sensation

The nerve endings embedded in the dermis yield sensations of heat, cold, touch, pressure, and pain.

Indicator of Internal Events

Internal events may be initially discovered or monitored by the progression or involution of what the integument presents to the observer. Jaundice, a yellowish-orange color of the skin, can indicate malfunctions of the liver or hemolysis of blood cells. Cyanosis, a bluish discoloration most easily observed in the oral mucous membrane and nail beds, can indicate problems associated with oxygen transport and delivery to the cells.

Exanthems, also known as rashes, may result from allergies to materials such as wool or drugs such as antibiotics. Exanthems also can indicate the presence of viral or bacterial infectious processes such as chickenpox, rubeola, rubella, or streptococcal infections.

Edema, or excess fluid in the intercellular spaces, is most frequently seen in the dependent segments of the body, such as the feet, ankles, lower legs, hands, face, or the sacral region. Frequently, edema is present when fluid-transport problems exist, or with shifts of electrolytes to the extracellular spaces, or with fluid overload.

Cosmetic and Identity

The skin serves as one basis upon which individuals can identify who they are. No one person looks exactly like another, with the exception of identical twins. Therefore, individuals can identify their person by what they see about themselves. Specific societies place high value on certain appearances and features that the skin presents to others. For ages, men and women have been striving toward a desired cosmetic appearance by perfecting their skin's appearance through the use of creams, lotions, and powders.

A burn to the skin, especially if it is a deep dermal burn that prevents regeneration of cells, or scarring from injuries such as lacerations, causes great emotional stress to the affected person and his or her significant others. This person suffers the loss of a body part, the skin, and frequently questions the personally held concept of physical identity. The psychological consequences of an abnormal appearance can be devastating to the person's total being. Many scarred individuals attempt to hide their abnormalities through dress or cosmetic substances, as scarring is thought to detract from their appearance on a personal and social basis. Scar hiding is culture dependent, as in some societies deliberate scarification is highly desirable.

Expressive

The integument, especially that of the face, serves to communicate to others, through expressions of the status of being, whether it be happy, sad, fearful, perplexed, or otherwise. The personal hygiene of the skin may also give an indication about the individual's attitude toward self. A clean, well-groomed person is thought to be satisfied with himself or herself and able to cope with life's daily stresses; a person who neglects his or her personal hygiene and appearance is thought to have devaluating ideas about his or her person and not to be able to cope with the stresses of daily living.

CHARACTERISTICS RELATIVE TO AGE AND SEX

During infancy, the skin is functionally immature, but contains all the structures of the normal adult's skin. The epidermis and dermis are thin and loosely bound together. The sebaceous glands are distributed over the entire body, except the palms of the hands and the soles of the feet. The apocrine glands are nonfunctional. The eccrine glands begin the activity of producing sweat in response to heat and emotional stimuli after the first few months of life. Thermal regulation through the infant's integument is limited.

Maturation of this regulatory function occurs throughout childhood.

By adolescence, the functions of the skin have matured. During puberty, the high levels of pituitary hormones secreted result in the secondary sexual characteristics of hair growth, fat distribution, and pigmentation. In the male, hair growth occurs primarily on the face, axillae, and pubic area, and frequently ensues on the arms, chest, back, and legs, although this is variable with individuals. Androgenic hormones produced in the male may result in loss of hair from the scalp.

In the female, hair growth occurs primarily on the axillae and pubic regions, although terminal hairs may be noted on the breast, arms, and legs. The density of hair in the female also varies with individuals as a result of genetic and hormonal influences.

Sebaceous gland activity varies according to climate. Individuals in tropical or hot climates tend to have higher levels of sebaceous-gland activity, creating oily skin; those in northern climates frequently have scaly skin as a result of lower levels of sebum production.

HEALTH ASSESSMENT OF THE INTEGUMENT

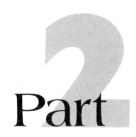

Part

Assessment of the integument is accomplished through inspection and palpation. Generally, inspection is the tool that yields the most significant data, whereas palpation yields supplemental data. Several systematic methods may be utilized to obtain the necessary data concerning the integument. First, the skin may be assessed as each area or region of the body is being assessed. In this method, the skin is assessed prior to any other structure in that particular region, as it is most external to the client and ensures that this important organ is not deleted from the assessment process. If the integument alone is assessed, a systematic method is again utilized. Two such methods used may be the cephalo–caudal or proximal–distal approach.

INSPECTION AND PALPATION OF THE SKIN

The skin is first assessed for color, which is then followed by assessment of the surface characteristics. In childhood through adulthood, the skin color varies with the client's genetic composition and exposure to the sun. The normal color of the integument is dependent upon the presence of melanocytes and the production of melanin. In the Caucasian newborn, the skin is normally pinkish in color, and the hands and feet may demonstrate physiological cyanosis. In the black newborn, the integumentary color is pink, with pigmented areas in deep crevices and creases such as the scrotal rugae, groin region, antecubi-

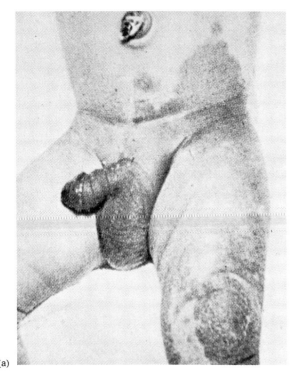
(a)

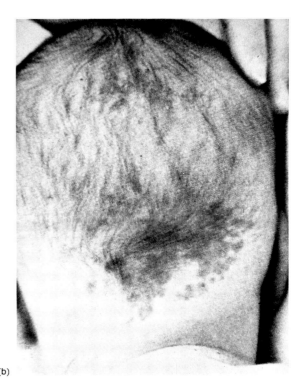
(b)

FIGURE 3-3
Capillary hemangioma: A flat, pink, red, or purple lesion. Part (a)
is a port-wine stain, and (b) is a "stork's-beak mark". (Photos courtesy of Mead Johnson.)

tal folds, neck folds, digital joint folds, and palmar creases.

Inspection of the integument during adolescence demonstrates a localized change in skin pigmentation of the areola and genitalia. The increased pigmentation of these areas remains throughout adulthood. In the elderly, the skin frequently may present a faded yellowish color as the number of melanocytes decreases with age. This decrease of melanocytes may also result in blotchy, uneven skin color in those areas exposed to the sun.

FIGURE 3-4
Strawberry mark, or nevus vasculosus.
(Photo courtesy of Mead Johnson.)

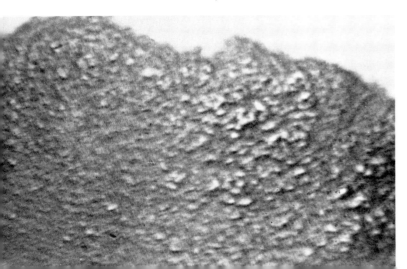

A variation of the integument's color can result from the presence of nevi. These congenital lesions may be present at birth, become visible shortly after birth, or occur later in life. Nevi are categorized according to the layers of the integument from which they arise. Epidermal nevi are categorized as nevus sebaceous, apocrine nevi, hair follicle nevi, and melanocyte-like nevi. Nevus or dermal origin are classified as vascular, lymphangioma, connective tissue, and melanocyte-like.

Hemangiomas are of dermal origin and fall under the category of vascular nevi. Capillary hemangiomas are also known as port-wine stains or nevus flammus (Figure 3-3). This vascular lesion, commonly present at birth, is flat and pink, red, or purplish in color. The most common site for capillary hemangiomas to occur is in the nuchal area. Fading or involution of this vascular lesion is infrequent. Strawberry marks or nevus vasculosus are immature hemangiomas (Figure 3-4). On inspection, they present as raised bright red lesions that do not blanch when pressure via palpation is applied. Nevus vasculosus may be present at birth or develop shortly after birth. This lesion consists of newly formed, dilated capillaries that occupy the dermal and subdermal layers of the integument. Immature hemangiomas may enlarge at a variable rate until about 8 months of age, after which they usually regress and disappear by approximately 7 years of age. Involution of the strawberry mark may be complete, although residual evidence of an atrophic area, such as brownish pigmentation or puckering, may be observed.

Mongolian spots (deep dermal melanocytes) are another variation of the normal skin's discoloration. Mongolian spots commonly occur in the neonate of darkly pigmented races. They are dark-blue or purple discolorations that are generally found in the lower lumbar region, buttock, and scrotal regions (Figure 3-5). Mongolian spots usually disappear spontaneously by 4 years of age.

Cafe au lait spots present yet another variation in the skin's color. This lesion appears as a light brown, nonraised patch on the skin. A single cafe au lait spot is generally of no significance, but when multiple spots are present, they are of concern as neurofibromas may develop.

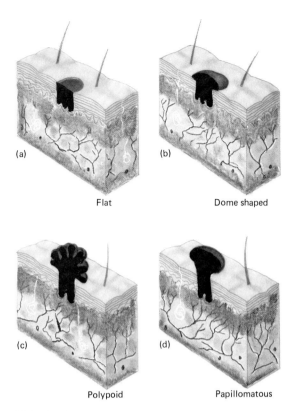

Flat   Dome shaped

Polypoid   Papillomatous

FIGURE 3-6
**Contours of moles: (a) flat; (b) dome-shaped;
(c) polypoid; (d) papillomatous.**

FIGURE 3-5
Mongolian spot.
(Photo courtesy of Mead Johnson.)

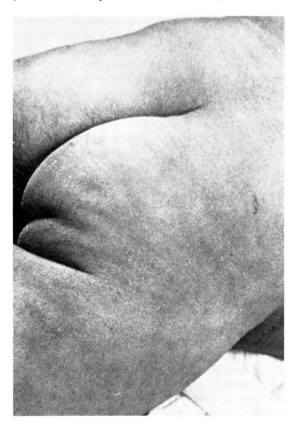

Lesions commonly known as moles are frequently termed nevus cell nevi and are formed from melanocyte-like cells. These lesions may appear flat or raised from the skin's surface. When inspected closely, the raised surface may be domed, polypoid, verrucoid, sessile, or papillomatous (Figure 3-6). Freckles or ephelids, another type of nevi, are commonly seen on the face or in other areas of the integument that are exposed to the sun. Lentigo or liver spots (Figure 3-7) can occur at any age. These lesions are small in diameter, flat, and light to dark brown in pigmentation.

Abnormally, the skin coloration may be jaundiced, cyanotic, erythematous, and hyper- or hypopigmented. Generally, in clients of light pigmentation, these color changes in the skin are readily observable, whereas in clients of dark pigmentation, these changes, with the exception of hypopigmentation, must be looked for more intently.

In the newborn, physiologic jaundice occurs with a high frequency. This phenomenon is due to the fact that there is no longer a need for the high number of red blood cells required during

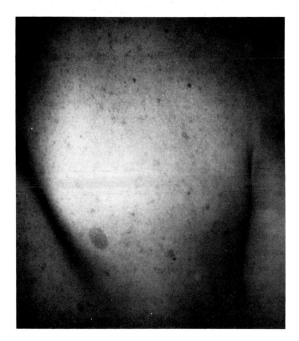

FIGURE 3-7
Lentigo. (Photo courtesy of the University of Minnesota, Health Sciences, Department of Dermatology.)

fetal development. The increased rate of red blood cell destruction produces bilirubin at a rate greater than the rate at which the liver enzyme glucuronyl transferase can convert insoluble bilirubin into conjugated or soluble bilirubin. When observed, normal physiologic jaundice develops slowly, becoming visually apparent in the full-term infant in approximately 36 to 48 hours following birth. It reaches maximal intensity in 3 to 6 days. This discoloration progresses from the head to the feet. Spontaneous remission of this physiological occurrence ranges between 7 to 10 days, although longer periods of time are not unusual.

Physiological jaundice appears as a yellowish-orange or yellowish-green discoloration of the skin in both Caucasian and black infants, since dark pigmentation is not fully developed. Jaundice may be visible in the skin, sclera, and mucous membrane of the mouth, especially the posterior side of the tongue, including the frenuli, posterior hard palate, and gum margins. The degree of bilirubinemia is predictable by the amount of skin area involved. If the entire skin is jaundiced, the higher the level of bilirubinemia. When observed, scleral discoloration is uniform throughout the sclera. A moderate level of bilirubinemia is associated with jaundice covering the head, chest, and trunk; a low level of bilirubinemia is associated with discoloration of the head or the head and neck.

The examiner can blanch the skin with pressure by using a glass microscopic slide. The pink color of the skin fades or blanches white. If jaundice is present, the yellow discoloration may remain.

Other causes of yellow discoloration of the skin in the infant are carotenemia, inflammation of the liver, biliary tract obstruction, hemolytic diseases, and excessive pregnanediol in breast milk. Carotenemia, a high level of systemic carotene, results in the deposit of carotene in the skin. Carotenemia results from ingestion of large amounts of yellow vegetables resulting in yellow-orange deposit in the skin of the forehead, nasolabial folds, palms of the hands, and soles of the feet.

Jaundice occurring in the first 24 hours of life may be associated with hemolytic processes and is indicative of pathology. Generally, this pigmentation of the skin occurs and progresses rapidly. Referrals must be made to the appropriate resources once this phenomenon is observed.

Jaundice in the Caucasian child and adult retains similar characteristics to those in the newborn. In blacks, jaundice appears more yellowish-brown or greenish-brown and is most visible in the sclera and oral mucous membrane, especially in the junctional area of the hard and soft palate. Abnormal pigmentation of the integument does occur, but intent inspection is needed to appreciate it. Several causes of jaundice in the adult are biliary tract obstruction and inflammation of the liver.

Cyanosis is observed as a bluish, bluish-gray, or purplish discoloration of the skin. Cyanosis is divided into peripheral and central. Peripheral cyanosis results from deoxygenated blood in the peripheral vessels and is observable in the nail beds. Central cyanosis results from an absolute level of reduced hemoglobin greater than 5 gms percent. This state can be a result of cardiac or pulmonary abnormalities or unusual hematologic problems, such as polycythemia and methemoglobinemia. During inspection, it is observed in the nail bed, lips, cheeks, ear lobe, oral mucosa, and the tip of the nose. Because peripheral and central cyanosis may be observed in the same areas, observation alone does not directly determine the type of cyanosis present. Circumoral cyanosis is normal in the crying newborn. As the infant grows, circumoral cyanosis is indicative of underlying pathology. In blacks, the easiest areas to assess for the presence or absence of cyanosis are the oral mucosa and the nail beds. When the observation of cyanosis is recorded, the location and any associated events are stated, as classifications of degrees or levels of cyanosis do not exist.

Erythema or redness of the skin is due to dilation of superficial blood vessels. Erythematous regions of the Caucasian integument are generally easily recognized, whereas in blacks these regions are more difficult to detect due to the dark pigmentation of the skin. Intense inspection and validated discrimination of the skin's color are required. In describing erythema, it is most helpful to record the actual color that is present, such as cherry red or dull red, and its exact location.

Other vascular-related skin discolorations are telangiectasis, venous and arterial spiders, angiomas, and purpura. Telangiectases are formed by dilation of small vessels. When observed in Caucasians, telangiectatic lesions appear bright red; in blacks they may be more of a reddish-brown color and linear or stellate in shape (Figure 3-8). Pressure applied to the dilated vessels may cause fading of the lesion's color. Telangiectatic lesions may occur on the face and nose of the elderly, on integument exposed to the sun over long periods of time, over scar tissue, irradiated areas, and mucous membrane, and during the presence of certain systemic disease processes or skin tumors. In the neonate, telangiectatic lesions are referred to as stork bites. Frequently, epistaxis originates from telangiectatic lesions on the mucous membrane of the nose, when they are located near Kiesselbach's plexus.

Small, slightly raised red lesions composed of blood vessels may be cherry angiomas or senile angiomas. Generally, these lesions are observed most frequently on the trunk of the body and extremities. Senile angiomas are not associated with pathology, but usually occur with the process of aging. In the elderly male, scrotal venous angiomas may be present. These lesions develop in the superficial veins of the scrotal integument and appear red or blue in color.

Venous stars are bluish-colored vascular lesions that radiate out from a central point, forming stellate or flaring patterns. The bluish discoloration fades when pressure is applied through palpation. A venous star is the result of either the aging process or the obstruction of a segment of the venous system. This lesion is commonly observed in female clients on the posterior neck, medial aspect of the thigh, and the leg.

Arterial spiders, vascular spiders, or spider angiomas (Figure 3-9) are deep red in color and resemble the shape of a spider. They are composed of radiations similar to spider legs, which extend from the body or central point. This vascular lesion fades when pressure is applied through palpation to the central body. It regains a deep red color, filling from the body to the radiations, after pressure is released. Arterial spiders may be observed on the face, neck, anterior chest, arms, and hands. The integument surrounding this lesion is erythematous.

Other altered colorations of the skin may be associated with disruption of the skin's surface characteristics. Frequently localized, although they may be generalized, are yellowish-white and silvery discolorations. Yellowish-white discolorations are most frequently associated with infectious processes. The lesions are generally well demarcated. Silvery discolorations are of epidermal scaling.

Alterations in the skin's pigmentation can be observed regardless of race, although it is generally more readily observable in darkly pigmented clients. In the newborn or adult, the genetic absence of melanocytes results in nonpigmented

FIGURE 3-8
Telangiectasis. (Photo courtesy of the University of Minnesota, Health Sciences, Department of Dermatology.)

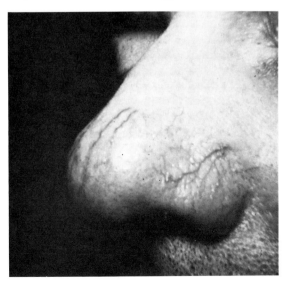

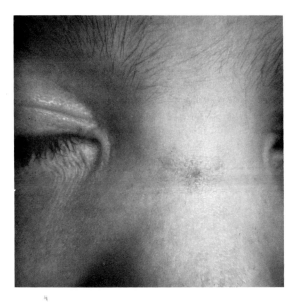

FIGURE 3-9
Arterial spider. (Photo courtesy of the University of Minnesota, Health Sciences, Department of Dermatology.)

skin. The absence of pigment throughout the integument is termed albinism. The skin of the Caucasian albino is whitish-pink; that of individuals who would otherwise possess darkly pigmented skin may appear white, cream, or tannish in color. Clients born with normally functioning melanocytes may experience a cessation of that function due to trauma to the dermis, chemical contact, physiological malfunction of the endocrine system, or inflammation. These factors may result in amelanosis, or complete loss of pigment in a circumscribed area. The surrounding skin is of normal pigment, bordered by erythema or hyperpigmentation.

Hyperpigmentation may be observed when the skin of a localized area is darker than the surrounding skin. Occasionally, during pregnancy or when oral contraceptives are used, hyperpigmentation may be seen over the forehead, bridge of the nose, and cheeks, forming an eye-mask-like pattern. This particular pigmented pattern is termed chloasma, melasma, or the mask of pregnancy. The deposit of melanin in the epidermis results in a brownish-black coloration, whereas melanin in the dermis results in a bluish-gray appearance. Hyperpigmentation is frequently associated with Addison's disease, hyperthyroidism, exposure to sunlight, and following inflammation and scar formation.

Exanthems are eruptions of the skin accompanied by the inflammation process. Inspection and palpation of the integument yields data that descriptively identify the lesion's color, size, metamorphosis, progression over the integument, and density. The color of the lesion is described as red, pink, white, or any combination of colors. The color of the integument surrounding the exanthem is inspected, as it may be erythematous, pale, or present no change. The size of the lesion's diameter is described in millimeters or centimeters unless it is minute, in which case it may be termed pinpoint. When multiple exanthems are observed, the average size of all lesions, with the range of the smallest to the largest lesion, is stated. Size approximation of lesions may be facilitated if the examiner measures the length of the index finger in centimeters and the width in millimeters. The index finger can then be held close to the lesion and used as a general measuring guide.

Two common exanthems in the neonate are erythema toxicum and diaper rash (which can occur throughout the entire non-toilet-trained period). Erythema neonatorum toxicum appears as an erythematous macular and/or papular exanthem, which most frequently occurs in the first 3 days of life. It may appear and disappear in less than a day, and is presently thought to be of no pathological significance. The most common body locations on which the exanthem appears are the cheeks, the chest, the back, and the buttocks.

Intertrigo, a mild type of diaper rash, presents as chafing of the skin and pinkish erythematous areas. Ammonia lesions are papulovesicular in nature, and may present as ulcerated, bleeding, and indurated areas. The surrounding skin of the ammonia lesion is pinkish in color. Monilial infections in the diaper-wearing child present as bright-red lesions that are scaly and papulovesicular in nature, with well-defined borders.

Exanthems vary in form, from macular, papular, and vesicular, to pustular. They may also proceed through various phases of change, such as macular to papular, or vesicular to pustular. Exanthems may appear as punctate or depressed lesions, as well as flat or raised. For a more complete description of changes in the integument associated with primary and secondary lesions, refer to Tables 3-2 and 3-3. The shape of a lesion is variable. The most commonly used descriptive terms for shape are presented in Table 3-1.

While examining the integument, determine if the eruption has a particular originating point on the body, such as the hair line of the face, the neck, the upper extremities, the trunk, or the lower extremities. It is also important to observe the distribution, the location and symmetry of areas involved, and where the greatest concentration of the eruptions exists. Deviations in the skin's normal color are noted, as well as any unusual discoloration that may not conform to the presenting pattern. One such discoloration is Postia's sign, in which dark red lines are present in the skin creases. When possible the examiner observes the exanthem and any unusual accompanying signs over a period of time in order to determine its duration, progression, and resolution.

The two major characteristics of the normal skin are smoothness and suppleness. Two other words frequently used to describe the suppleness of the skin are elasticity and resilience. During the assessment of the premature, the skin appears wrinkled and loose, frequently resulting in an appearance described as the "wrinkled old man." In the full-term infant, the skin appears smooth and taut, and may possess numerous skin folds, especially in the neck and groin, and, less frequently, in the popliteal and cubital regions. The presence of skin folds is dependent upon the birth weight of the infant. Various amounts of vernix caseosa may be present at birth, giving the skin an uneven, sometimes curdy appearance. Vernix caseosa, a white cheesy substance, is frequently most pronounced in the skin folds, and disappears owing to bathing and movements that rub it off. As the infant develops, the functions and structures of the skin mature. During adolescence, appendages within the skin mature, and the apocrine glands become active, while the sebaceous glands increase their production of sebum. Generally, the skin retains its smoothness and elasticity. As chronological age increases, environmental factors influence the skin's characteristics. Exposure to the rays of the sun causes definite aging patterns in the skin. The epidermis atrophies and becomes thin, thus predisposing the individual to invasion by foreign materials. The loss of elastic tissue gives rise to wrinkling of the skin, often noted first on the forehead and temporal to sides of the eye orbit. These wrinkles are frequently labeled "crow's feet."

The characteristic of smoothness can be interrupted by skin tags, decreased hydration, over-hydration of tissues, occlusion of pores and follicular openings, inflammation, and exanthems that may result from infectious processes. The density of the dermis can also be changed. This is frequently the result of vascular problems and scarring. Primary and secondary lesions change the normal skin characteristics and are frequently described in the terms presented in Tables 3-2 and 3-3. Primary lesions are those that appear first; secondary lesions are the result of a continuing disease process or changes in the primary lesions.

Projections from the skin's surface that are overgrowths of normal skin that form a stalk and head (or polyplike structure) are called *skin tags.* This tissue growth possesses normal skin coloration and most frequently develop on the eyelids, neck, axillae, trunk, and body creases. Other disruptions of the skin's smoothness may originate in the sebaceous and apocrine glands, through obstruction of their pores and secretion channels. During inspection of the follicular openings in the newborn, occlusions can result in the formation of milia. These lesions are most generally located on the face, especially the nose, chin, and cheeks, as small white papules. Milia spontaneously resolve by several weeks of age. Occasionally, this lesion is referred to as a miniature version of a wen.

A wen is a round or oval cyst that is filled with a whitish-yellow substance. Upon palpation, it is soft and mobile, and varies in size. The skin overlying the cyst appears domed and tense. Another lesion associated with the sebaceous gland is the comedo or acne. This lesion results from the occlusion of the follicular opening, and is more frequently observed during the preadolescent and adolescent phases of life, although it may be present throughout adulthood. Follicular orifices that appear dilated, filled with sebaceous secretions, and are black in color are termed open comedones or blackheads. Follicular orifices that are small in diameter or closed and are white or yellowish-white in color are termed closed comedones or whiteheads. It is the closed comedones that are frequently precursors to acne vulgaris, as the continual formation of sebaceous material in a closed channel can rupture it. Rupture of the closed channel exposes the epidermis and dermis to the bacterial-laden medium. The foreign material (sebum) and bacteria may create an inflammatory reaction, resulting in erythema and the formation of papules and pustules.

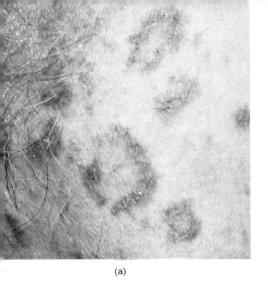

(a)

TABLE 3-1
Descriptions of Lesion Shapes

LESION SHAPE	DESCRIPTION OF SHAPE	ILLUSTRATION
ANNULAR	Circular, ring shaped	Figure 3-10(a)*
CORYMBIFORM	Clustered or grouped around a single, larger lesion	Figure 3-10(b)†
GEOGRAPHIC	Resembles the surface features of a region, area, country, or continent	Figure 3-10(c)*
GYRATE	In the form of a twisted spiral	Figure 3-10(d)*
IMBRICATED	Overlapping	Figure 3-10(e)†
IRIS	A circle within a circle	Figure 3-10(f)*
LINEAR	Resembles a line	Figure 3-10(g)*
OVAL	Oval or egg shaped	Figure 3-10(h)*
POLYCYCLIC	More than one ring or circle	Figure 3-10(i)*
SERPIGINOUS	Wavy margins, creeping, snakelike	Figure 3-10(j)*
TARGET	Circle within a circle, with the middle circle raised	Figure 3-10(k)*
UNIVERSAL	Involving the entire skin	Figure 3-10(l)*
VEGETATING	Fleshy or warty outgrowths	Figure 3-10(m)*
VERRUCOSE	Rough raised wartlike projections	Figure 3-10(n)*

*Photo courtesy of the University of Minnesota, Health Sciences, Department of Dermatology.
†From: "A Brief Course in Dermatology," Audio-visual program by the Institute for Dermatologic Communication and Education.

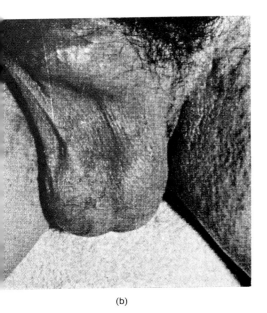

(b)

FIGURE 3-10

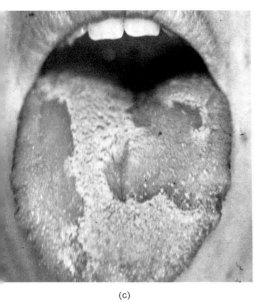

(c)

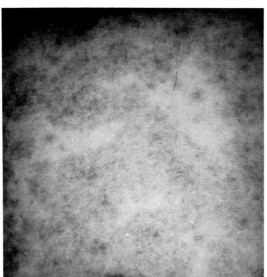

(d)

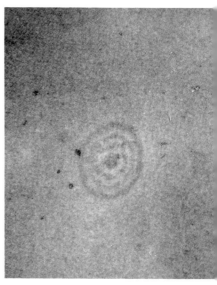

(e)

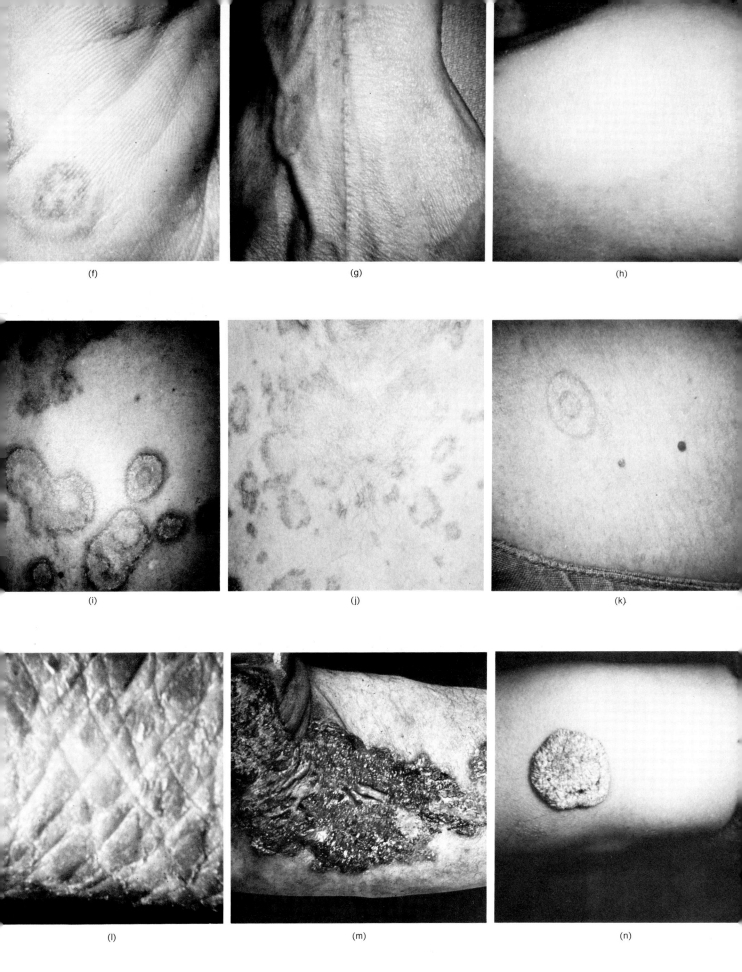

(f)

(g)

(h)

(i)

(j)

(k)

(l)

(m)

(n)

TABLE 3-2

PRIMARY LESION	DESCRIPTION OF INTEGUMENT DEVIATION FROM NORMAL	ASSOCIATED PHENOMENA	
MACULE	Discoloration of the skin variable (i.e., brown, faded, red, white) No elevation of the skin is present Texture characteristics are the same as the surrounding skin Variable in diameter	Cafe au lait spots Rubeola; rubella Petechiae; purpura First-degree burns Vitiligo; ephelids Moles; Mongolian spots Lentigo; erythema Neonatorum	Figure 3-11(a)*
PAPULE	Discoloration of the skin is variable Circumscribed elevation of the epidermis Firm in consistency Approximately 5 to 10 mm in diameter	Psoriasis Senile angiomas Eczematous Dermatitis; acne Elevated mole Erythema; neonatorum Diaper dermatitis	Figure 3-11(b)*
NODULE	Discoloration of the skin may or may not be present Circumscribed elevation of the skin Approximately 1 to 2 cm in diameter Firm in consistency	Lymphoma cutis Xanthomas Gouty tophi Erythema nodosum Deep hemongiomas	Figure 3-11(c)*
TUMOR	Discoloration of the skin may or may not be present Elevation of the skin may or may not be well demarcated Diameter is variable, but larger than a nodule Solid in consistency	Epithelioma Dermatofibroma Benign hyperplasia Neoplastic growths	Figure 3-11(d)*
CYST	Discoloration of the skin generally not present Elevation of the skin may or may not be present, dependent upon the depth of the lesion within the skin and its diameter Diameter is variable Consistency varies from firm resilient to fluctuant	Ganglion Epidermoid cyst	Figure 3-11(e)*
VESICLE	Discoloration of the skin results from epidermal transparency; presents color of underlying fluid Elevation of the skin is present Variable in diameter, generally small Consistency may be tense or fluctuant	Chicken pox Eczematous dermatitis Second-degree burn Varicella Variola Herpes simplex Herpes zoster (shingles)	Figure 3-11(f)*
BULLA	Discoloration of the skin results from epidermal transparency; presents color of the underlying fluid Elevation of the skin is present Variable in diameter, larger than a vesicle Consistency may be tense or fluctuant	Pemphigus vulgaris Contact dermatitis Second-degree burn Bullous impetigo	Figure 3-11(g)*
PUSTULE	Skin discoloration generally white or yellowish-white Elevation of the skin is present Variable in diameter, from minute to large Consistency may be tense, fluctuant, or boggy	Folliculitis Acne Furuncles Variola Diaper dermatitis Miliaria rubra	Figure 3-11(h)*
WHEAL	Skin discoloration generally red or pale Slight elevation of the skin is present Diameter is variable Consistency ranges between tense and fluctuant	Urticaria Insect bites	Figure 3-11(i)*

*Photo courtesy of the University of Minnesota, Health Sciences, Department of Dermatology.

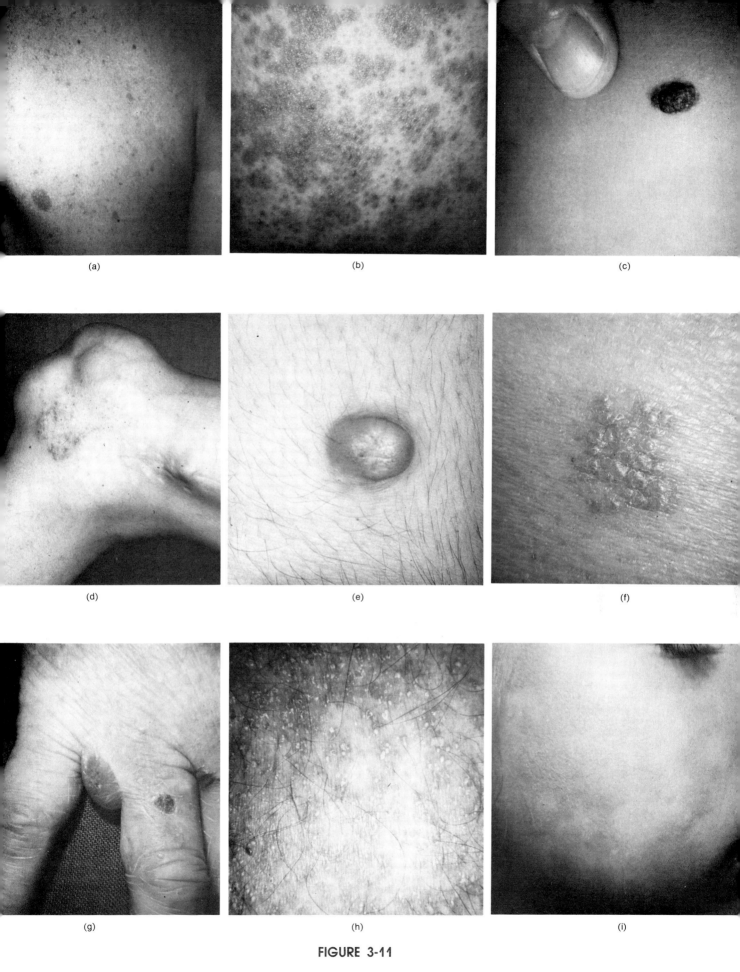

(a)

(b)

(c)

(d)

(e)

(f)

(g)

(h)

(i)

FIGURE 3-11

TABLE 3-3

SECONDARY LESION	DESCRIPTION OF INTEGUMENT DEVIATION FROM NORMAL	ASSOCIATED PHENOMENA	ILLUSTRATION
CRUST (scab)	Skin discoloration variable (i.e., brown, black, straw, or honey colored, yellow, red) May form a slight elevation above the skin's surface Diameter variable Hard and crusty in consistency; crust may be softened if lubricated	Rupture of vesicles, or bullae Impetigo Eczema	Figure 3-12(a)*
OOZING	Skin discoloration may be present from primary lesion Skin's surface may or may not be elevated depending upon type of primary lesion Diameter of oozing site is variable Wet characteristic; oozing or weeping may appear as droplets or moist appearing lesions	Contact dermatitis Infectious eczematoid dermatitis	Figure 3-12(b)*
PLAQUE	Skin discoloration variable (i.e., brown, reddish, silvery, yellow) Elevation of skin surface is present Diameter variable, generally considered to be large Firm in consistency, rough in appearance	Psoriasis Pityriasis rosea Discoid lupus erythematosis Seborrheic warts Xanthomas	Figure 3-12(c)*
SCALE	Skin discoloration is white, silvery, or ashen May or may not be elevated, dependent upon the type of primary lesion Diameter is variable Scales may be fine, sheetlike, coarse, or thick and loosely or tightly adherent to primary lesion	Pityriasis rosea Seborrheic dermatitis Dry skin Psoriasis Dandruff Exfoliative dermatitis	Figure 3-12(d)*
FISSURE	Epidermis appears red Integument disruption presents as a shallow incurvation of broken skin Small in diameter Appears as an open linear break in the skin; surrounding skin may appear thick, dry, and inelastic	Trauma Dehydration of skin Drooling	Figure 3-12(e)*
EROSION	Epidermis appears red Integument disruption presents as a wide and shallow incurvation of the skin Variable in diameter, larger than a fissure Appears as moist and glistening break in the skin	Rupture of vesicle and bullae Lacerations from rubbing Diaper dermatitis	Figure 3-12(f)*
ULCER	Tissue may appear red or bluish Incurvation is deep into the dermis, epidermis, subcutaneous tissue, or may penetrate muscular structures Diameter is variable Appears as an open area of the integument revealing lower structures	Trauma Third-degree burns Stasis ulcers Pressure Chancre	Figure 3-12(g)*
SCAR	Skin discoloration varies from red, pink, silver, to faded white May be elevated above the skin or appear concave to the horizontal plane Variable in diameter Appearance varies from a thinly elevated line to a thick protruding hypertrophy of tissue (keloid)	Trauma Burns Acne	Figure 3-12(h)*
ATROPHY	Skin may or may not be discolored Integument disruption is that of thinning of normal structures Variable in diameter Appears as thin, paperlike covering, shiny and translucent	Arterial insufficiency Striae	Figure 3-12(i)*

*Photo courtesy of the University of Minnesota, Health Sciences, Department of Dermatology.

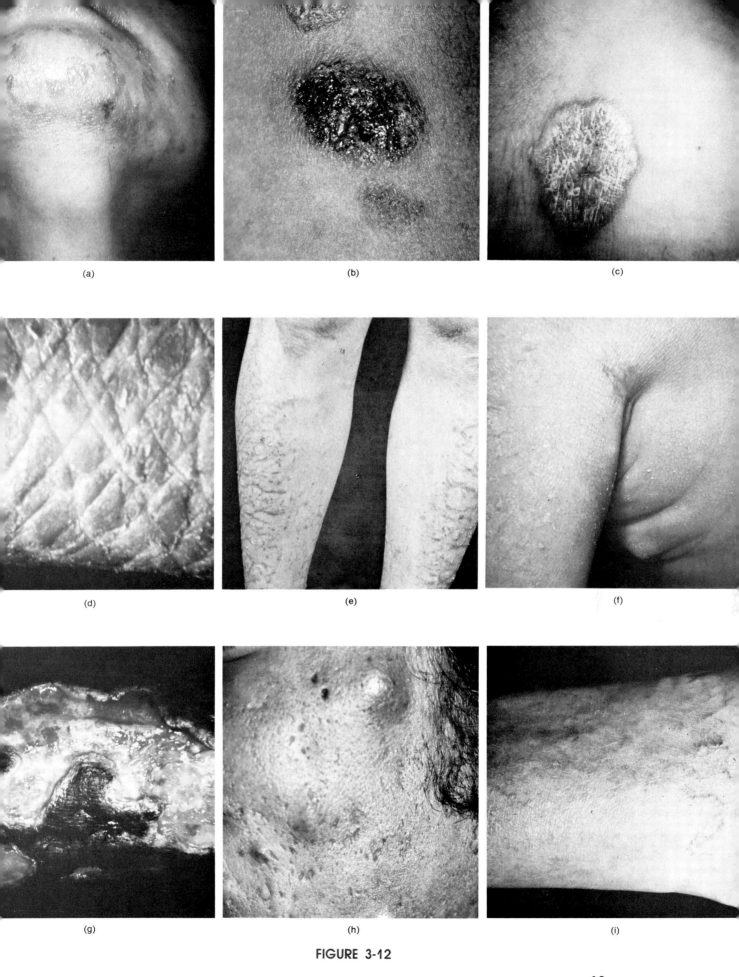

(a)

(b)

(c)

(d)

(e)

(f)

(g)

(h)

(i)

FIGURE 3-12

When present, obstruction of the eccrine glands yields papules or papulovesicular lesions. The surrounding skin of obstructed eccrine pores is edematous and erythematous owing to vasodilation. The most common process that affects the eccrine pore is miliaria rubra, heat rash, or prickly heat, and is most frequently observed involving the upper body areas.

Edema of tissue underlying the skin may cause the skin to appear puffy, taut, and distended when compared to surrounding skin. Excess fluid in the intercellular spaces is most frequently observed through the skin in the dependent segments of the body, such as the feet, ankles, lower legs, hands, or sacral regions and scrotum when a supine position has been assumed. The face and eyelids are also areas that may appear edematous, although edema in these locations generally signifies a pathological process in its late stages. In areas where hair is prominent, the hair may appear pitted in the skin, giving rise to the orange peel or pig-skin effect. This observable phenomenon is present only when there is a significant amount of edema. To determine the amount of edema, palpation is utilized. The index finger is placed over a bony prominence in the edematous area and pressure is applied, compressing the tissue against the bone. The depth of the depression is estimated in centimeters. Pitting can also be recorded in grades as 1+ (1 cm), 2+ (2 cm), 3+ (3 cm), and 4+ (4 cm). Generalized edema of the body is termed anasarca. This state exists when certain pathological processes are well established.

The integument itself may present edema to the examiner. Edema of the skin is in the form of blisters. In the neonate, the epidermis and dermis are thin structures and loosely connected to each other. Inflammation causes the two structures to separate from each other and form a blister. Because of the skin's immaturity, the transitional zone between the living and cornified cells is not an effective barrier to fluid loss in the presence of inflammation. This results in a greater evaporation of fluid.

In opposition to the edematous integument is the dehydrated integument, which appears rough, flaky, and less flexible. This status may lead to cracking and the formation of fissures. Flaky skin in blacks frequently appears ashen in color; in Caucasians, it is characterized by a dull white color. Loss of turgor is determined by pinching the skin. In dehydration, this activity results in the skin's remaining puckered and is described as tenting (Figure 3-13).

In the newborn, dehydration is related to percent of weight loss and is associated with the presenting signs observed during inspection. Moderate dehydration with weight loss of 10 percent is characterized by tenting; 15 percent is characterized by sunken orbitals, sunken fontanels, and dry mucous membranes. A newborn with moderate dehydration is in need of immediate referral to an appropriate resource. Mild dehydration with 5 percent weight loss is common.

FIGURE 3-13

Assessment of skin turgor: (a) gentle pinching of the skin; (b) tenting, a response associated with decreased skin turgor.

INSPECTION AND PALPATION OF SKIN APPENDAGES

The hair is assessed through inspection and palpation for amount, color distribution, and texture. In the neonate, the amount of hair is variable at birth. Lanugo, a fine, downy hair, is most evident on the back and shoulders of the premature infant, although it is present over the entire body. Lanugo is present on the skin of the full-term infant, but is not as prominent as in the premature infant. Scalp hair may also be present. Frequently, the newborn exhibits patchy loss of hair, especially in the occipital and/or temporal regions of the scalp. Regrowth of the hair in these regions, as well as growth over the other areas of the scalp, is frequently slow as the neonate's hair

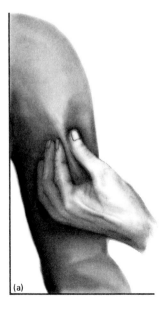
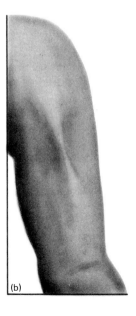

(a) (b)

is in a resting phase. Ectodermal abnormalities can yield the congenital absence of hair.

During adolescence in the male, some hairline recession occurs in the frontal and temporal regions. In the adult male, male pattern baldness may occur rapidly or gradually. Genetic and hormonal factors influence this hair loss, which is characteristically in a W shape (Figure 3-14). In the female, notable hair loss generally occurs in the aged and is characterized by a thinning throughout the scalp.

Abrupt patchy loss of terminal or coarse hair is referred to as alopecia areata (Figure 3-15). These lesions appear white, oval, or round, and are completely devoid of hair, except lanugo or fine "fuzz" hair. The lesion and surrounding skin are otherwise normal in appearance and characteristic. If numerous lesions are present, they may be in various stages of hair loss and hair regrowth. Patches of hair loss that exhibit broken or stubble hairs may be due to pulling at the hair or continual scratching of the scalp. This state is termed trichotillomania. Other forms of hair loss that may be observed are alopecia totalis, loss of all scalp hair, and alopecia universalis, loss of all body hair. Hair loss preceded by inflammatory conditions is referred to as scarring alopecia. Other factors that can influence thinning of the hair are endocrine disorders, pregnancy, febrile states, and medical regimes that alter the chemical homeostasis of the body.

Hirsutism, an abnormal amount of hair, can be localized or diffusely spread across the body. In females, coarse dark hairs prominent on the face, especially the upper lip and chin, may be a familial tendency. The male generally presents a wide range in amount and concentration of hair.

Hair color varies dependent upon one's genetic background. In congenital states where pigment is absent, such as in albinism, the hair of individuals of Caucasian background is white or yellow, whereas the hair of individuals of darkly pigmented parents may be reddish in color. Graying of the hair frequently begins in the temporal regions and progresses at a variable rate. Generally, graying begins in the third decade of life or later. Graying prior to this time is referred to as premature or senile graying.

Hair texture ranges from fine to coarse. Interruptions of a client's normal hair texture can be caused by bleaches, dying of the hair, and frequent use of harsh shampoos. The use of such chemical substances may result in brittle hair

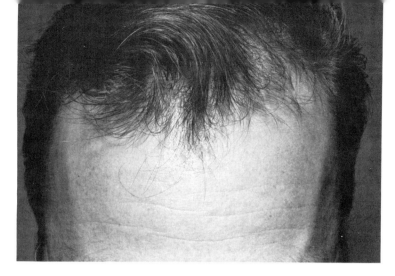

FIGURE 3-14
Male pattern baldness.

shafts. The aging process may also be a factor that contributes to the hair becoming brittle.

The nails of the digits, whether in the neonate, child, adolescent, or adult, are normally thin, firm, convex in shape, and present the underlying color of the nail bed, as the nail plate itself is clear. The normal nail also possesses an approximate angle of 160 degrees between the nail plate and the proximal portion of the digit (Figure 3-16). In the newborn, the nail may appear cyanotic for the first several hours of life, after which it should appear pink, unless the infant is stressed or crying. In the premature neonate, the nail length rarely reaches the end of the digits (fingers or toes) while the post mature neonate frequently has nails that extend beyond the end of the digits and may be discolored by a yellowish hue.

The lunula is generally present in the nails, especially in the thumb nail. The free edge of the nail appears grayish-white. The posterior and lateral nail folds should appear smooth to the examiner.

FIGURE 3-15
Alopecia areata. (Photo courtesy of University of Minnesota, Health Sciences, Department of Dermatology.)

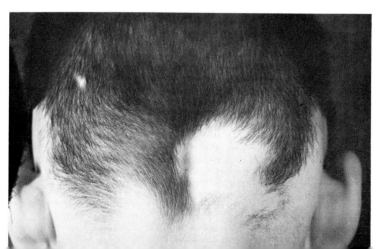

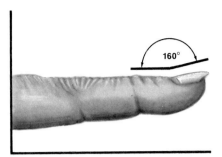

FIGURE 3-16
Approximate angle of the nail.

Deviations from normal can be manifested in the nail plate thickness, shape, and color, as well as the nail bed and posterior and lateral nail folds. The nail plate can atrophy, become thin, and assume a concave shape as opposed to the normal convexity. This change in shape may result in the lateral edges of the nail turning upward. Such a deviation from normal is termed a spoon nail. Hypertrophy of the nail results in an increased thickness of the nail. Hypertrophy may or may not be associated with an elongation of the nail and a curving over the end of the digit. In such cases it is known as a claw nail. Clubbing of the nails is a deviation in the angle between the nail plate and proximal portion of the digit (Figure 3-17). Clubbing is characterized by an increase in the angle (180 degrees). This angle change is created by an elevation of the proximal portion of the nail and a broadening and round-ing of the terminal phalanx. Clubbing of the nails is frequently associated with cardiopulmonary pathology.

The nail-plate color can also change. The nail plate may separate from the nail bed, producing a greater free edge. This increases the amount of grayish-white coloration of the free edge nail margin. This phenomenon is frequently associated with the type of manual labor a client performs. It is also seen with systemic disease, but is not a diagnostic sign of its presence. Beau's lines, a transverse white discoloration of the nail plate may be seen following trauma that impairs keratin synthesis. White spots in the nail plate leukonychia, frequently called love spots or fortune spots, may appear as centrally depressed lesions that are striated or streaked in shape. Other color changes of the nail plate may be caused by metal substances. Gold may produce a brownish-black appearance; silver produces a slate-blue color. Heavy smokers may present a yellowish-brown discoloration of the nail plate.

In blacks, the nail bed may possess a longitudinal column of pigment. In Caucasians, the presence of such pigment should alert the examiner to the need for referral, as this type of pigmentation may be a precursor to the formation of a malignant melanoma.

The lateral margins of the nail may grow into the underlying tissue. This ingrown nail, which has penetrated the skin, sets off an inflammatory reaction of the lateral nail fold. The lateral and posterior nail folds may form triangular tags of skin, known as hang nails. This tag of skin predisposes the integument to an inflammatory process, since the intact epidermis has been disrupted.

In summary, deviations in the integument's color and surface characteristics are assessed and described by the following:

1. Presence or absence of color change. If color change has occurred, it is then described.

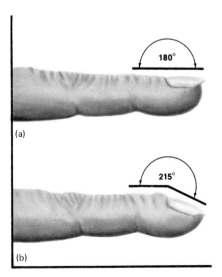

FIGURE 3-17
Clubbing of the nail:
(a) early clubbing at 180° angle;
(b) severe clubbing with an
angle greater than 180°.

2. Type of lesion: refer to descriptive terms for primary and secondary lesions.
3. Location or body area.
4. Distribution of change: localized, generalized, or universal.

5. Symmetry of areas involved: unilateral, bilateral, or symmetrical.

The healthy integument is described by its color and surface characteristics of smoothness and suppleness.

STUDY GUIDE QUESTIONS

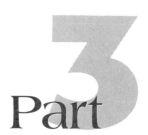

Part

In the following client situations, identify and describe the subjective and objective data to be collected, the specific tools and procedures to be utilized in the collection of those data, and the rationale for the nursing assessment.

1. Baby boy Neville is a 2-day-old infant that you are examining. You are ready to proceed with your assessment of his skin.
2. Anna Horwitz, a 72-year-old widow, is hospitalized. During your initial interview with her, she complains about her swollen legs.
3. Howard Mills is a 59-year-old male who comes to you, the industrial nurse, during his morning coffee break complaining of an itching rash on the inner aspects of his forearms.
4. Mrs. Rondus comes into the clinic with her 5½-month-old infant, Jason, complaining of patchy loss of his hair.
5. Nathan Wilson, an 18-month-old, is admitted to the hospital in your ward because of vomiting and diarrhea of 6 day's duration. You are to assess his hydration status.

SAMPLE FORMAT TO BE USED IN RESPONDING TO THE STUDY GUIDE QUESTIONS

SUBJECTIVE DATA TO BE COLLECTED	OBJECTIVE DATA TO BE COLLECTED	SPECIFIC TOOLS AND PROCEDURES TO BE UTILIZED	RATIONALE FOR NURSING ASSESSMENT

BIBLIOGRAPHY

ALLISON, J. RICHARD, and TOIVO RIST, "Skin Infections May Be Outward Signs of Inner Disorders," *Geriatrics*, February 1975, pp. 85–95.

BROWN, MARIE S., and MARY M. ALEXANDER, "Physical Examination, Part Three: Examining the Skin," *Nursing 73*, September 1973, pp. 39–43.

CARLSEN, RAY A., "Aging Skin: Understanding the Inevitable," *Geriatrics*, February 1975, pp. 51 54.

EVANS, WILLIAM F., *Anatomy and Physiology* (2nd ed.), pp. 37–45. Englewood Cliffs, N.J.: Prentice-Hall, Inc., 1976.

EVERETT, MARK A., and ROBERT L. OLSON, "Understanding Pigmentary Abnormalities," *Geriatrics*, February 1975, pp. 99–103.

FRITSCH, WILLIAM C., "Managing Age Related Vascular Skin Lesions," *Geriatrics*, March 1975, pp. 45–48.

HARMON, VERA M., and SHIRLEY M. STEELE, *Nursing Care of the Skin: A Developmental Approach.* New York: Appleton-Century-Crofts, 1975.

HOLLINGSHEAD, W. HENRY, *Textbook of Anatomy* (2nd ed.), pp. 139–143. New York: Harper & Row, Inc., 1967.

KATZ, HENRY, and KEITH G. REDDING, "Therapeutic Challenge of Premalignant and Malignant Skin Lesions," *Geriatrics*, March 1975, pp. 53–59.

KNOX, JOHN M., "Common-Sense Care for Aging Skin," *Geriatrics*, February 1975, pp. 59–60.

LANTIS, LARRY R., and SHARON D. H. LANTIS, "Allergic Dermatosis in the Older Patient," *Geriatrics*, February 1975, pp. 75–84.

LUCKROFT, DOROTHY, ed., *Black Awareness: Implications for Black Patient Care*, pp. 16–35. New York: The American Journal of Nursing Company, 1976.

MARROW, LEWIS B., "Hirsutism," *Primary Care*, pp. 127–136. Philadelphia: W. B. Saunders Company, March 1977.

OGAWA, CATHERINE M., "Degenerative Skin Disorders: Toll of Age and Sun," *Geriatrics*, February 1975, pp. 65–69.

PILLSBURY, DONALD M., WALTER B SHELLEY, and ALBERT M. KLEGMAN, *Cutaneous Medicine.* Philadelphia: W. B. Saunders Company, 1961.

POLEDNAK, ANTHONY P., "Connective Tissue Responses in Negroes in Relation to Disease," *American Journal of Physiological Anthropology*, July 1974, pp. 49–58.

RICE, ALICE K., "Common Skin Infections In School Children," *American Journal of Nursing*, November 1973, pp. 1905–1909.

ROACH, LORA B., "Assessing Skin Changes: The Subtle and the Obvious," *Nursing 74*, March 1974, pp. 64–68.

———, "Assessment of Color Changes in Dark Skin," *Nursing 77*, January 1977, pp. 48–51.

TINDALL, JOHN P., "Relieving Localized and Generalized Pruritus," *Geriatrics*, March 1975, pp. 85–92.

WEBSTER, STEPHEN B., "Vesiculobulbous Eruptions Can Cause Serious Problems," *Geriatrics*, February 1975, pp. 109–113.

WEXLER, LOUIS, "Gamma Benzene Hexachloride in Treatment of Pediculosis and Scabies," *American Journal of Nursing*, March 1969, pp. 565–566.

4

The Head

OBJECTIVES

1. Identify the cranial bones of the head.
2. List the major sutures of the head.
3. Identify the major fontanels and their intersecting sutures.
4. Identify the function of the fontanels.
5. Systematically examine the skull.
6. Describe the structural signs of:
   a. shape of the head.
   b. shape of the head.
   c. Cephalohematoma and caput succedaneum.
   d. Characteristics of abnormal sutures.
   e. Characteristics of abnormal fontanels.
   f. fontanels.
   g. sounds obtained on striking the head, see percussion.
   h. Abuse — the violent shaking and concussion.
   i. examination of the skull.

Part 1

REVIEW OF STRUCTURE AND FUNCTION

STRUCTURE OF THE HEAD

The head is composed of the cranium and the face. The cranial and facial bones are flat bones organized to provide a protective vault and support for the brain and other soft tissue structures within. The eight cranial bones include the frontal bone, right and left parietal bones, right and left temporal bones, the ethmoid, the sphenoid, and the occipital bones. These bones are joined by immovable joints called sutures (Figure 4-1). The major cranial sutures are listed in Table 4-1 with the adjacent bones.

The junctions of the major sutures form fontanels, which are membranous intervals prior to complete ossification. Ossification of the major sutures and their junctions is delayed until after birth and infancy to allow for vaginal delivery of the head and for brain growth later. The two most conspicuous fontanels are the anterior fontanel, occurring at the junction of the coronal and sagittal sutures, and the posterior fontanel at the junction of the coronal and lambdoidal sutures.

The four less conspicuous fontanels are the left and right anterolateral fontanels created by the junction of the frontal, parietal, temporal, and sphenoid bones, and the left and right posterolateral fontanels formed at the junction of the lambdoid, occipitomastoid, and parietomastoid sutures. The lateral fontanels close (ossify) shortly after birth. The posterior fontanel closes in the first year and the anterior fontanel in the second year of life, after which brain growth is less rapid. Premature or postmature ossification of the sutures or fontanels may lead to a spectrum of cranial abnormalities from cosmetic deformity to retarded brain growth.

FUNCTION OF THE HEAD

The 14 bones of the face are aligned to give support and protect the eyes, nose, and tongue. The facial bones also provide a structural orifice for the reception and mastication of food. Of the 14 facial bones, only the mandible is movable. The more conspicuous facial bones are illustrated in Figure 4-2.

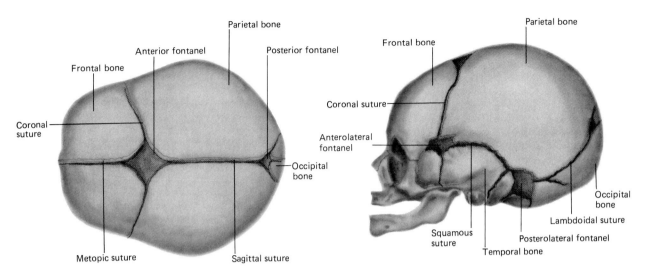

FIGURE 4-1
The major cranial sutures and fontanels that are readily assessed.

TABLE 4-1

Major Cranial Sutures and Adjacent Cranial Bones

SUTURE	BONES FUSED
Sagittal	Right parietal to left parietal down midline
Coronal	Anterior side of the right and left parietals to the posterior side of the frontal
Lambdoid	Posterior side of parietals to anterior side of occipital
Right and left squamosal	Superior side of temporals to lateral aspect of the parietals
Sphenofrontal	Sphenoid to the frontal
Sphenoparietal	Sphenoid to the parietals
Sphenosquamosal	Sphenoid to the temporals
Left and right occipitomastoids	Occipital to the mastoid processes

Structural air spaces called air sinuses are found within the facial bones. These serve to prevent overweighting of the head while adequate bony protection for the soft tissue structures within is ensured. The air sinuses of the face include frontal, sphenoidal, petrosal, transverse, and maxillary (Figure 4-3).

The air sinuses and air cells (spongy composition within many of the cranial and facial bones) begin to form early during gestation by means of a hollowing process called **pneumatization.** These sinuses and cells vary markedly in size. They are lined by a mucous membrane that is a continuation of the nasal cavity mucous membrane, making them prone to infections and an inflammatory condition called sinusitis.

The head is maintained erect and its movement controlled by the various muscles of the neck and shoulders. An even more complex group of muscles are the facial muscles of expression and mastication.

The surface of the cranium, the scalp, is composed of hairy skin, the subcutaneous layer containing fat lobules and numerous blood vessels, and the epicranius containing the occipitofrontal muscle, the galea aponeurotica muscles, the subaponeurotic layer composed of loose connective tissue, and the pericranium (outer periosteum). The skin of the scalp is said to be the thickest of the body.

The epicranius or muscles of the scalp control the wrinkling of the forehead and raising of the eyebrows; the subaponeurotic layer permits easy movement of the scalp.

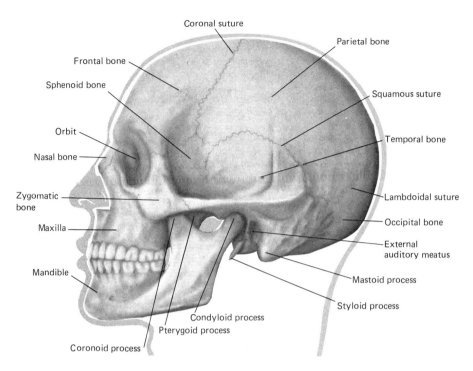

FIGURE 4-2

Facial and skull bones readily visible
from a lateral view.

FIGURE 4-3

The air sinuses of the skull.

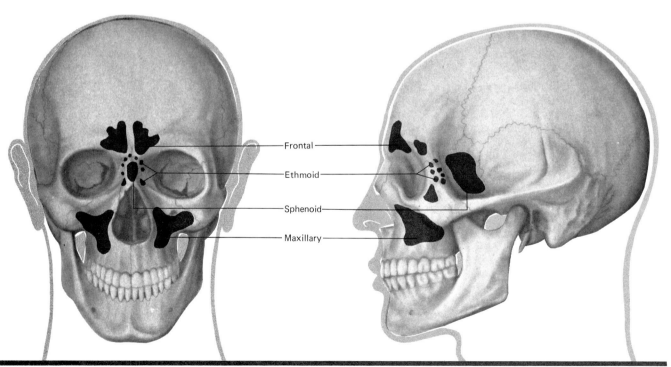

HEALTH ASSESSMENT OF THE HEAD

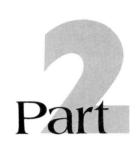

Assessment of the head and face generally precedes assessment of the senses (eyes, ears) in the cephalocaudal approach. These may be deferred to last in the child to prevent antagonizing the pediatric client. The assessment of the head incorporates primarily the skills of inspection and palpation, but also includes measurement and transillumination.

MEASUREMENT

If the occipitofrontal circumference (OFC) has not previously been obtained during the assessment, it is an essential measurement, especially in the child. The OFC is obtained by using a tape measure (metal or paper, not cloth), which encircles the head above the ears bilaterally over the occipital prominence posteriorly and above the brows anteriorly. After obtaining this measurement, it should be plotted on an appropriate growth curve (Figure 4-4).

A single measurement of the OFC in a child is of little value, but serial measurements demonstrate head growth and may indicate signs of inadequate head growth (microcephaly) or excessive head growth (macrocephaly). As with other body measurements, familial traits, growth spurts, and, in the neonate, gestational age and intrauterine growth should be accounted for.

The other important measurements to obtain in the child are the sizes of the anterior and posterior fontanels. The anterior fontanel ranges from 1 to 6 cm in each dimension at birth and the posterior fontanel is usually 0.5 to 1 cm in each dimension. This measure is usually deferred until palpation of the fontanels.

INSPECTION OF THE HEAD

Inspect the head at all angles for symmetry. Flattening of the occiput is occasionally seen in young children and infants who are supine sleep-ers. It is of no pathologic significance and can be reversible if identified in infancy. Other markedly abnormal shapes may be due to premature closure of the suture lines, as described in Table 4-2.

For the first week of life, molding of the head is commonly seen in newborns delivered vaginally in vertex presentation (Figure 4-5). Other observable variations or deviations of asymmetry in the head and face include bossing of the forehead or prominent foreheads. Bossing may be an early indication of rickets or syphilis in the infant, and prominent foreheads are associated with rickets, with Hurler's syndrome, and are a common positional problem in the premature infant.

In the normal adult, the head is usually described as round or normocephalic. Bilaterally, the mastoid processes, located in the postauricular region and the parietal regions of the skull, are prominences that distort the round appearance of the head. Bossing may also occur in the adult. The mandible may demonstrate hyperplasia, both in bone width and length, yielding a protruding lower jaw. This sign plus others may be an indication of acromegaly.

The head and face should then be inspected for masses or raised areas. These may indicate trauma, such as cranial or facial swelling with or without ecchymosis, petechiae, or lacerations. In the newborn, inspect the cranium for cephalohematoma or caput succedaneum (Figure 4-6). The cephalohematoma is due to extravasion of blood beneath the periosteum. It does not cross the midline, but rather localizes over one cranial bone or another (usually the parietal), and may appear reddish or bluish in color. It usually resolves spontaneously by 12 weeks and may be associated with fracture of the underlying bone. The caput resolves in about 1 week and is much more superficial, being only edema. Both conditions are associated with vertex vaginal presentations and seldom have long-term significance.

After inspection of the head, concentrate on inspection of the face. Note asymmetry of the facial expression and response. Facial expressions

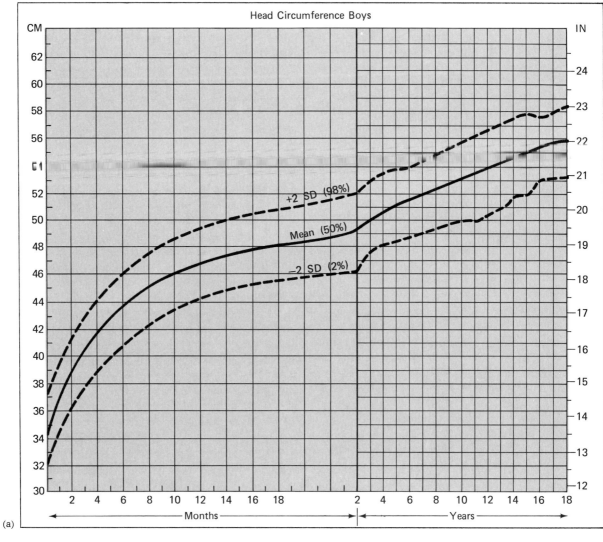

FIGURE 4-4

Growth chart of head circumference of (a) males; (b) females.
(From: National Center for Health Statistics;
published by Ross Laboratories: Columbus, Ohio, 1976.)

TABLE 4-2

Deviations in Cranial Contour

NAME	SHAPE	SUTURE SUTURE
Oxycephaly	Tower head	Coronal or lambdoid or both
Scaphocephaly (boat head)	Keel-like ridge along the top	Sagittal
Trigonocephaly (three-cornered head)	Triangle shape	Frontal
Plagiocephaly (oblique head)	Flattened anterior part of one side and posterior part of another	Positional, not due to suture closure

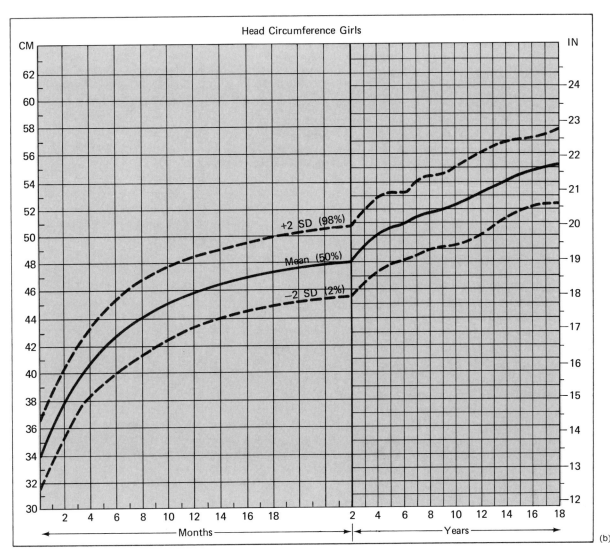

Head Circumference Girls

+2 SD (98%)

Mean (50%)

−2 SD (2%)

Months — Years

(b)

FIGURE 4-4 CONTINUED

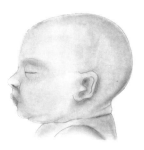

FIGURE 4-5

Molding of the newborn's head following vaginal delivery in the following vertex presentations:

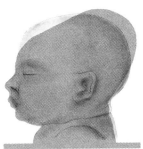
(a) Occiput anterior

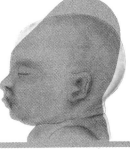
(b) Occiput posterior

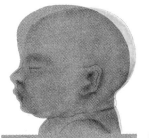
(c) Brow

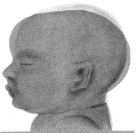
(d) Face

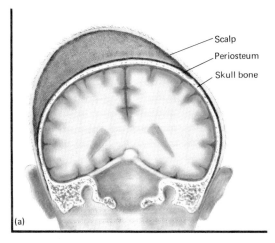

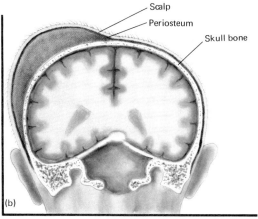

FIGURE 4-6
Deviations in head contour in the newborn due to vertex presentation: (a) caput succedaneum and (b) cephalohematoma.

frequently reflect the status of one's health. Expressions of the facial muscles may indicate alertness or dullness. In a wasting appearance, the face appears sunken away from the nose, giving it a sharply defined and prominent characteristic. The eyes may appear sunken (enophthalmos) or protruding (exophthalmos), closely set, or widely set, or the slanting plane of the eyes may be deviated from one's inherited characteristics or markedly pronounced. The cheeks and temple areas can also appear concave to the horizontal plane. Pathological processes involving the facial nerves can affect the facial muscles of expression, such as ptosis of the eyelids, sagging of the lower eyelid, and drooping at the corner of the mouth. Facial lines such as those of the forehead and the nasolabial fold may disappear. Changes in the texture of the skin, as when it becomes coarse and thickened, may pull the lips back, baring the teeth. The face may also

become rounded or "moonlike" or expressionless, as a masked face. Dimples and clefts should be identified as well as skin color and characteristics.

Next, move to inspection of the scalp and hair of the head. Usually, this requires palpation as well as inspection. While separating the hair to visualize the scalp in several areas, note a dry or flaky characteristic of the scalp that is associated with cradle cap in the newborn, or dandruff or seborrhea in the older child and adult. Inspect the scalp closely for signs of lesions, lacerations, or discoloration. Then inspect the hairline and distribution of hair. Uneven distribution of hair is found commonly in the occipital region in children who favor sleeping on their backs or in adult males due to balding, usually in the frontal region. Other causes of balding include therapeutic irradiation, some chemotherapy, and certain hormonal and metabolic disorders. Normally, hair grows in a direction toward the face and neck except when cowlicks are present. Hair growing toward the crown is often associated with chromosomal disorders and should be noted.

PALPATION OF THE HEAD

Palpation of the head should be organized and include scalp, hair, and surface structures. Begin in the front and palpate down the midline, using a gentle rotating motion with palmar surface of the fingers. Note the presence or absence of the fontanels. Usually, in the newborn, both anterior and posterior fontanels are palpable as soft spaces and may be communicating by a spread sagittal suture. Suture spaces or marked ridges should not be palpable after 5 to 6 months; however, coronal, sagittal, and lambdoid sutures can be identified normally as breaks in the skull throughout adulthood. Ridging of the sutures in the adult is abnormal and frequently occurs in acromegaly. Any other ridges or breaks are abnormal and probably represent fractures. Only two fontanels are generally palpable; the anterior until 18 to 19 months, and the posterior until 9 months; a third fontanel may be present along the sagittal suture. Although this may be normal, it has been associated with chromosomal syndromes. Palpate the size of each fontanel and note pulsations and the characteristic tension while the child is calm in an upright position. Bulging or sunken fontanels are significant, as are marked pulsations. Marked pulsations or a bulging fontanel may be associated with increased intracranial pressure. A sunken fontanel is an indication of dehydration of a moderate to severe degree.

After palpating down the midline, palpate each side of the head for ridges, scalp lesions, masses, or other unusual findings. In the occipital region, feel for the occipital lymph nodes, which are normally absent in the newborn. Other nodes on the head are intermittently detected and should be movable. Nonmovable or enlarging nodes are abnormal.

INSTRUMENTATION

Little instrumentation is indicated for assessment of the head; however, both auscultation and transillumination are recommended.

Following palpation of the head, proceed to auscultation over the fontanel, temporal, and orbital regions for bruits, which are associated with cerebrovascular anomalies (Figure 4-7). Then, in the young infant and child, proceed to transillumination of the head using a flashlight with rubber cuff over the light end. This procedure should be done on all newborns before discharge from the hospital, and then used as a tool to rule out specific pathology such as hydrocephalus, intracranial lesion, decreased brain tissue, or subdural effusion. It must be performed in a room absent of light. The nurse should wait about 3 minutes after turning out the room light to allow eye adjustment to the dark. Begin the test by firmly placing the unlit rubber-cuffed flashlight against the frontal region (Figure 4-8). Turn the light on and proceed by moving the light down the midline and then around each side. Note any marked light rings around the light or asymmetry of the light ring. The frontal region may illuminate a ring of 2 cm or less, and the posterior occipital region light ring is normally 1 centimeter or less. The remaining portions of the head transilluminate less than the frontal region. Premature infants often transilluminate in the frontal region and over the anterior fontanel. This should be followed, but not considered abnormal, for several months unless associated with other questionable signs of abnormality. An unusual transillumination should be validated by a more experienced examiner and then referred.

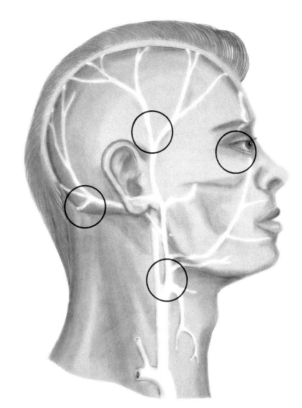

FIGURE 4-7
Auscultatory sites of the cranium.

FIGURE 4-8
Transillumination of the head.

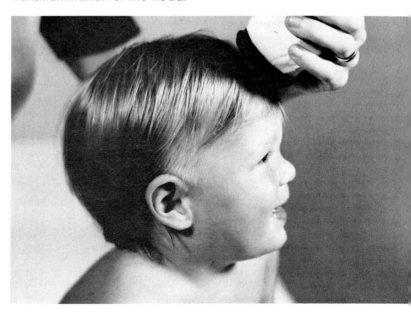

PERCUSSION

Finally, percussion of the head and face is done. It is seldom used and usually only to rule out sinusitis or intracranial pressure. Normally, percussion of the sinuses yields a resonant, painless response. A nonresonant or painful response indicates collection of fluid and inflammation of the sinuses. Macewen's sign is in response to percussion of the skull. It is a resonant "crackpot" sound, which may indicate intracranial pressure, but is normal before the fontanels close. The "crackpot" sound also occurs with fractures of the skull.

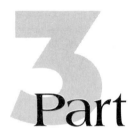

Part 3

STUDY GUIDE QUESTIONS

In the following client situations, identify and describe the subjective and objective data to be collected, the specific tools and procedures to be utilized in the collection of those data, and the rationale for the nursing assessment.

1. Johnny Thompson is a 2-week-old infant brought to well-baby clinic by his mother for his routine follow-up. You are ready to proceed with assessment of his head.
2. Baby girl Samson is a 4-hour-old infant you are called to see because of a fluctuant mass on the crown of her head.
3. You are charge nurse on the 3 to 11 shift when Mr. Klein is admitted for elective knee surgery. Prior to your admission assessment, the orderly comments to you that the 43-year-old Mr. Klein has a very blank expression and an unusually large head.

SAMPLE FORMAT TO BE USED IN RESPONDING TO THE STUDY GUIDE QUESTIONS

SUBJECTIVE DATA TO BE COLLECTED	OBJECTIVE DATA TO BE COLLECTED	SPECIFIC TOOLS AND PROCEDURES TO BE UTILIZED	RATIONALE FOR NURSING ASSESSMENT

BIBLIOGRAPHY

ALEXANDER, MARY M., and MARIE S. BROWN, *Pediatric Physical Diagnosis for Nurses,* pp. 33–45. New York: McGraw-Hill Book Co., 1974.

————, "Part 6: The Head, Face and Neck," *Nursing '74,* January 1977, pp. 47–50.

EWARDS, LINDEN F., and GEORGE R. L. GAUGHRAN, *Concise Anatomy* (3rd ed.), pp. 262–287. New York: McGraw-Hill Book Co., 1971.

EVANS, WILLIAM F., *Anatomy and Physiology* (2nd ed.), pp. 54–62. Englewood Cliffs, N.J.: Prentice-Hall, Inc., 1976.

The Head, Number Two of a Series on Variation and Minor Departure in Newborn Infants, Evansville, Ind.: Mead Johnson, 1971.

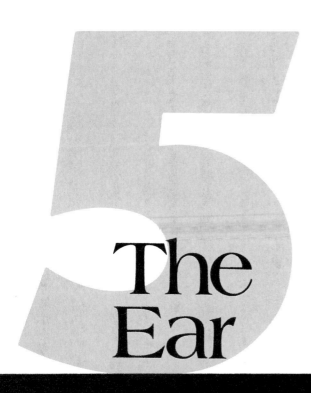

The Ear

REVIEW OF STRUCTURE AND FUNCTION

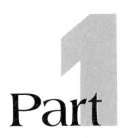

Part 1

The external ear is called the **auricle** or **pinna.** It consists of two parts, the prominent external ear structure and the external auditory canal. Structural composition of the auricle is skin and supportive cartilage, except for the lobule, which is composed of skin and intervening connective tissue. The prominent incurvations of the auricle are functionally significant for sound-wave entrapment. The folds are characteristically symmetrical in each person, but variations in patterns exist between individuals. Occasionally, Darwin's tubercle, a thickening along the upper ridge of the helix, may be present. The protrusion created by this structure may be directed (1) anteriorly, (2) laterally, (3) posteriorly, or (4) superiorly. Darwin's tubercles are a variation of the normal. Figure 5-1 illustrates the most prominent auricular features. The identified areas are used as landmarks to facilitate accurate and descriptive locations of any findings that may be observed.

The size of the auricle varies from individual to individual, as does the degree of abduction from the head. Distal displacement of the auricle may be increased significantly if enlargement of the parotid gland exists. This displacement can be either unilateral or bilateral. The lobule of the ear may be connected to the facial skin, or it may be a separate hanging structure, with the latter occurring most frequently.

The external auditory ear canal is approximately 2.5 cm in length and leads to the tympanic membrane (ear drum). It has an S-shaped pathway in the adult. The first section of the auditory canal is directed forward and upward; the second section is directed slightly posteriorly. Completion of the S-shaped canal is accomplished in the final section with a forward and downward direction. The distal third of the outer ear canal is lined with hair follicles and sebaceous glands. Cerumen, a yellowish waxy substance that serves as a lubricant and as a protective substance to the canal lining, is secreted by the sebaceous glands. Cerumen may be wet or sticky, or dry or hard. The moisture characteristic of cerumen is controlled genetically. Dry wax is prevalent in the Mongoloid race of Asia and in American Indians; wet or sticky wax is prevalent in American Caucasians and blacks.

In the newborn, the ear canal is very short, less curved, and is formed by the tympanic ring, a portion of the temporal bone to which the ear drum is attached at the periphery. As the infant

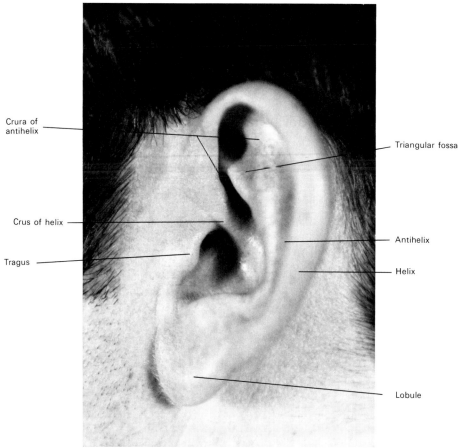

Crura of antihelix

Triangular fossa

Crus of helix

Antihelix

Tragus

Helix

Lobule

FIGURE 5-1
Auricular landmarks.

progresses through growth and development, the external auditory canal lengthens and eventually takes on adult characteristics.

The function of the auricle is to collect sound waves and transmit them through the external auditory canal to the tympanic membrane, which in turn transmits sound to the middle ear. The middle ear, often referred to as the tympanic cavity or tympanum, is a small sinus within the temporal bone. It contains the malleus, incus, and stapes, all of which are bones and all of which are involved in sound transmission from the tympanic cavity to the oval window, the opening to the inner ear. The malleus is attached to the tympanic membrane. When sound is conducted through the auditory canal, the tympanic membrane vibrates and in turn mobilizes the malleus. The malleus articulates with the incus, and the incus articulates with the stapes, which in turn rests on the vestibular window. It is in this manner that sound waves are conducted to the internal ear. Any decrease in the amount of mo-

bility of the tympanic membrane or the three bones inhibits conduction of sound waves. The middle ear is a chamber that serves to decrease the magnitude of vibrations, thereby protecting the internal ear from overstimulation due to intense sound waves of low frequency. Another protective structure is the eustachian tube or auditory tube, which extends from the pharynx to the middle ear. Generally, it is closed until swallowing or yawning occurs, at which time it opens. This structure allows for equalization of pressure in the middle ear,thereby preventing rupture of the tympanic membrane. The eustachian tube in the child is functionally less protective than in the adult owing to its shorter length, small diameter,and anatomical position.

The internal ear contains the cochlea, a structure of hearing, the vestibule and semicircular canals, which are concerned with equilibrium, and the auditory nerve. Figure 5-2 illustrates the structural divisions of the external, middle, and inner ear.

82

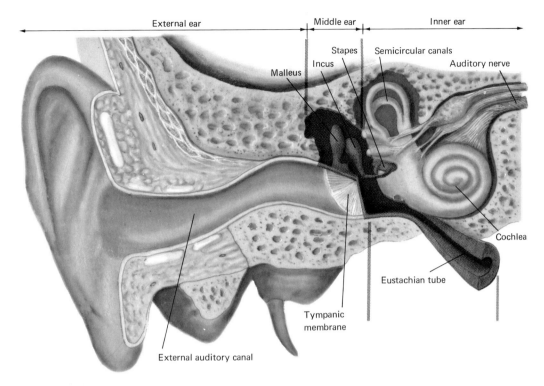

External ear | Middle ear | Inner ear

Stapes
Semicircular canals
Malleus
Incus
Auditory nerve

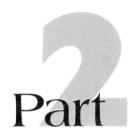

Cochlea

Eustachian tube

Tympanic membrane

External auditory canal

FIGURE 5-2
Structural divisions of the ear.

HEALTH ASSESSMENT OF THE EAR

Part 2

INSPECTION

Assessment of the ear begins with inspection of the auricle for color, size, and position. The ear is generally the color of the facial skin. If the auricle is bluish in color, this may indicate some degree of cyanosis, possibly associated with problems of the heart and lungs. Pallor or excessive redness may be due to underlying vasomotor instability, either vasodilation or vasoconstriction. Redness can also be due to a febrile condition that results in capillary dilation. Extreme pallor may indicate that the blood within the vascular system of the ear has been coagulated, as with frostbite.

Unusual size and shape of the ear may be a familial trait or an abnormality. It is important when such deviations are noted to obtain further historical data prior to making an interpretation of the physical findings. The most superior portion of the helix should cross a line approximated from the lateral angle of the eye to the occipital protuberance (Figure 5-3). The position of the ear should be almost vertical with, and not greater than, a 10 degree lateral posterior angle. Deviations in position or alignment of the auricle may be suggestive of abnormalities, such as chromosomal aberrations and renal disorders. It is most important to observe the position and alignment of the auricles in neonates, infants, and young children.

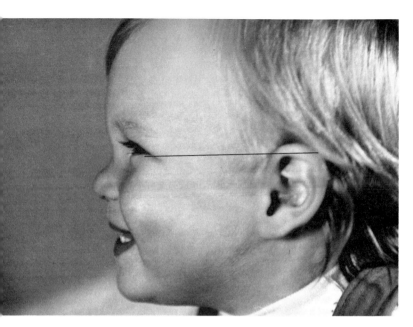

FIGURE 5-3

Alignment of the auricle with the lateral angle of the eye and occipital protuberance.

The auricle must also be inspected for lesions. Lesions of internal origin are tophi, which are small, whitish uric acid crystals seen along the peripheral margins of the auricle, moles, and cysts. A decubitus ulcer of the external auricle can result if pressure is placed on the auricle for a period of 2 hours without relief.

PALPATION

After inspecting the external ear, palpate the pinna to determine the consistency of its structure. It should be mobile and firm, not rigid, and without nodules. If folded forward, the pinna should readily recoil to its normal position. This quality of elastic firmness is due to the cartilage and is therefore absent in the immature newborn. A rigid ear structure can often be palpated after a person has experienced frostbite. Tugging gently on the ear lobule can elicit pain if an inflammatory process is occurring. This manipulation is generally performed in infants and young children to elicit an interpretable response.

FIGURE 5-4

Auricle manipulation in the adult: (a) manipulation of the auricle in preparation for an otoscopic exam; (b) positional changes of the external auditory structures with manipulation of the auricle in an upward direction.

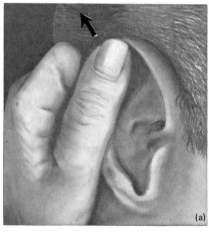
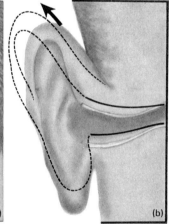

FIGURE 5-5

Auricle manipulation in the child: (a) manipulation of the auricle in preparation for the otoscopic exam; (b) positional changes of the external auditory structures with manipulation of the auricle in a downward direction.

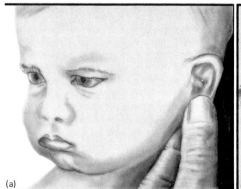
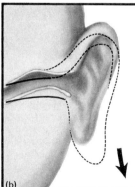

OTOSCOPIC INSPECTION

Complete inspection of the ear includes otoscopic examination. Competence of the examiner in this instrumental procedure is essential in maintaining client safety. For the adult, pull the auricle upward and back (Figure 5-4) as this straightens the S-shaped external auditory canal, facilitating visualization of the tympanic membrane. For the child, pull the auricle directly downward (Figure 5-5). In the newborn and young child it is essential to prevent movement during otoscopic examination. To accomplish this safety measure, the examiner may place the child in a prone position on an examining table, bed, or an adult lap (Figure 5-6). The cooperative parent can be helpful in restraining the child's movement. In the newborn, the tympanic membrane is difficult to visu-alize owing to the size and shape of the canal; however, patency of the canal must be determined.

The adult external ear canal is approximately 2.5 cm in length and is small in diameter. The otoscopic speculum used should be the largest that will fit the ear canal. A speculum too large causes considerable pain as it compresses the thin layer of tissue directly onto the bone. Pain is also generated if the speculum is directed in an acute downward or upward angle. Otoscopic observation occurs after the speculum is in place, as the procedure of insertion requires the full attention of the examiner. To accomplish insertion, hold the otoscope in one hand with your third and fourth fingers extending beyond the handle of the otoscope, so that it comes in contact with the person's head. This protects the drum or canal

(a)

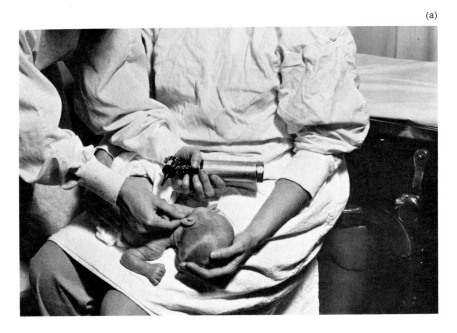

(b)

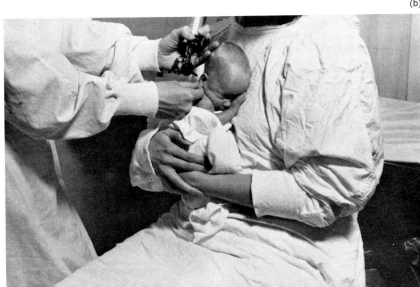

FIGURE 5-6

Safety positioning of a child in preparation for the otoscopic exam: (a) prone on the lap of an adult; (b) held upright against an adult's chest or shoulder.

from injury in case of quick movements of the head. The medial aspect of the other hand tilts the head to facilitate the inspection process and serves to control and prevent subsequent head movements. With children, the ulnar surface of the hand manipulating the otoscope is placed on the child's head. This method of protecting and stabilizing the client can also be used with an adult (Figure 5-7).

FIGURE 5-7
Positioning the examiner's hand during the otoscopic exam: (a) adult; (b) child.

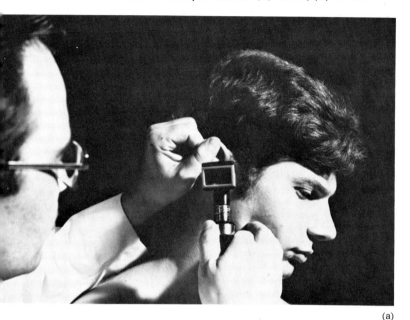

(a)

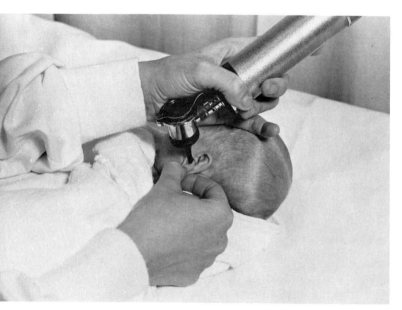

(b)

Upon examination of the external canal, note that the distal third of the canal contains hair follicles and sebaceous and cerumen glands. The amount of hair within the canal varies from person to person as does the amount of cerumen (ear wax). Dry cerumen is characteristically granular, scaly, and grayish-tan in color; wet cerumen is sticky and presents various shades of brown. Cerumen can occlude visualization of the tympanic membrane, and may be a factor in causing hearing loss and injury to the ear canal tissue. Earwax plugs may be symptomatic with sudden loss of hearing, full feeling in the ear, and tinnitus or dizziness. After wax has lodged in the canal for a variable period of time, it loses water content through evaporation and becomes firmer and darker in color until it is hard and black. Obstructive wax deposits require expertise for removal before further otoscopic assessment can be carried out. Inflammation, or scaling of the external canal, should be reported.

When an ear canal is unobstructed, the tympanic membrane is seen at the end of the external canal, and appears as a smooth, glistening, pearlish-gray screen. The inferior edge of the membrane is more posterior to the examiner, whereas the superior edge is more anterior (Figure 5-8). The annulus or tympanic ring is a peripheral fibrous structure located within the tympanic sulcus. It appears whiter and denser than the rest of the drum head. Perforations of the drum frequently occur at the periphery of the annulus, although not exclusively.

The malleus originates in the superior hemisphere of the drum and extends approximately to the center. It is visualized through the transparent membrane as a dense whitish streak. At the end of the malleus is the point of its attachment to the tympanic membrane. This point of attachment, from which the drum receives its conical shape and from which the light reflex results, is called the **umbo.** The light reflex is seen in the anterior inferior quadrant of the drum as a cone, with its point directed toward the umbo and its broad base at the periphery of the drum. This reflex is more diffuse in the young child owing to the shortness and decreased angles of the external canal as compared with the adult. Figure 5-9 illustrates the tympanic membrane and the associated landmarks.

For the purpose of describing findings, the tympanic membrane is divided into quadrants. The anterior superior quadrant indicates findings that are superior and anterior in position or to the nasal side of the drum; posterior superior indicates the superior region toward the occiput. The inferior quadrants are also referred to in a similar manner, anterior inferior and posterior inferior.

Table 5-1 compares several abnormal otoscopic findings with the normal. This table is not illustrative of all findings that could be associated with the identified abnormalities. When the data are utilized as a comparison to the normal, it provides the beginning practitioner with a basis for discrimination between normal and abnormal findings.

In children, drum vibrability is always evaluated with the use of a pneumatic otoscope when physical findings are equivocal. This special otoscope attachment allows the examiner to direct a light stream of air toward the drum. The directed air current should then cause the tympanic membrane to vibrate. Lack of vibrability can indicate a dysfunctional state of the eardrum.

Discharge is an external sign originating from the ear and indicating the presence of an abnormal condition. Frank blood or clear fluid may indicate a basal skull fracture following a traumatic incident. Serosanguineous or purulent drainage is consistent with a perforation of the tympanic membrane secondary to middle-ear infection.

ASSESSMENT OF HEARING

Gross hearing can be evaluated by several methods. Normally, a person can hear a word whispered 15 ft away and a spoken word from 20 ft away. When evaluating hearing through the use of whispered and spoken words, the sound should be directed toward one ear at a time while the other is kept covered. The examiner should take care to prevent lip reading. The client is requested to repeat the word or phrase immediately after it is spoken. Another screening method used necessitates the use of a ticking watch. The ticking-watch test is a high-frequency test. High-frequency sounds are best transmitted by the sensorineural path, whereas vocal sounds are lower pitched and transmitted via bone conduction. Neither the voice nor the watch-ticking test should be used alone, as separately they do not screen the high and low frequencies of hearing. The Weber and Rinne tuning fork tests may also be used to screen gross hearing.

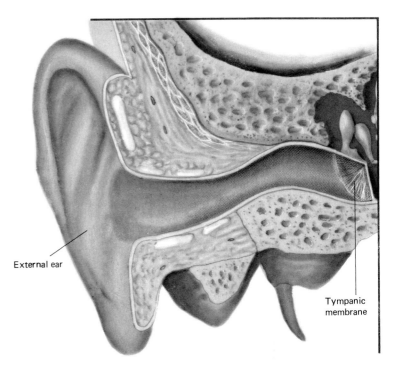

External ear

Tympanic membrane

FIGURE 5-8
The anatomic position of the tympanic membrane.

FIGURE 5-9
The tympanic membrane, its landmarks and quadrant divisions.

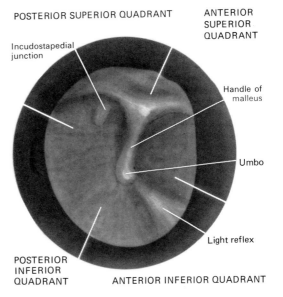

POSTERIOR SUPERIOR QUADRANT

ANTERIOR SUPERIOR QUADRANT

Incudostapedial junction

Handle of malleus

Umbo

Light reflex

POSTERIOR INFERIOR QUADRANT

ANTERIOR INFERIOR QUADRANT

87

TABLE 5-1
Otoscopic Findings in Normal and Abnormal States

	COLOR	MOVEMENT	DIMENSION	LIGHT REFLEX	UMBO	ANNULUS	MALLEUS	VASCULARITY
NORMAL	Pearlish gray, transparent	Vibratory	Slightly conical	Bright to dim	Appears regressed	Defined, whitish gray	Defined, whitish gray	Variable in number, regular, smooth
INFLAMMATION, MILD	Pink Opacification Beginning	Moderately impaired vibrability	Beginning loss of conical shape or normal	Dimmed	Appears regressed	Less well defined or normal	Defined	Hyperemic
INFLAMMATION, MODERATE	Deep pink opacified	Vibrability absent	Beginning loss of conical shape	Absent	Not visible	Poorly defined	Poorly defined to absent	Not visible
INFLAMMATION, SEVERE	Red opacified	Vibrability absent	Convex bulging	Absent	Not visible	Not visible	Absent	Not visible
SERUM IN MIDDLE EAR	Yellow-amber	Grossly impaired to absent	Bulging	Absent	Poorly visualized to absent	Variable dependent upon fluid level	Variable dependent upon fluid level	Variable dependent upon fluid level
BLOOD IN MIDDLE EAR (Hemotympanium)	Blue	Absent	Bulging	Absent	Not visible	May not be visible	Variable dependent upon blood level	Variable dependent upon fluid level
PUS	Dead white	Absent	Bulging	Absent	Not visible	May not be visible	Variable dependent upon pus level	Variable dependent upon pus level
PERFORATION	If minor, pearlish gray; within interrupted area may be black	Minor; normal; mildly impaired	Minor; normal if small	Minor; present or interrupted if perforation in interior anterior quadrant	Minor; visible behind membrane	Minor; visible or visualization interrupted if at periphery	Minor; present or interrupted	Minor; normal vascularity present
OBSTRUCTED EUSTACHIAN TUBE	Pearlish gray to slightly pink	Impaired	Retracted	Bent, broken, or absent	Appears smaller	Visible	Appears shorter, remains defined	Normal to injected
TYMPANO-SCLEROSIS	Pearlish gray with overriding dense white plaques	Normal or impaired if plaques are multiple	Conical	Present, may be broken if plaques in inferior anterior quadrant	Visible, unless plaques multiple and diffuse	Visible, unless plaques multiple and diffuse	Visible, unless plaques multiple and diffuse	Visible, unless plaques multiple and diffuse

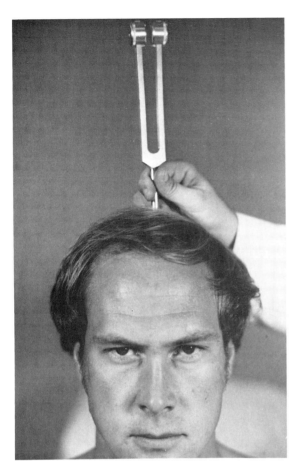

FIGURE 5-10
The Weber test. The tuning fork is placed midline on the vertex of the skull.

The Weber test, which tests bone conduction of sound, is performed by holding the stem of the tuning fork and striking the prongs against the palm of the hand with moderate pressure or snapping the prongs between the thumb and index finger. The client is requested to identify if sound is heard and indicate in which ear the sound is perceived the best. The vibrating tuning fork is then placed in a midline position on the skull at the forehead or vertex (Figure 5-10). The sound is normally of equal loudness bilaterally. In conductive loss, the sound is most readily perceived in the ear with the loss, whereas in sensorineural loss, the sound conducted via bone is heard best in the intact or good ear.

With the occurrence of sound lateralization, further problem refinement can be achieved with the use of the Rinne test. It is important to remember that the Rinne test is not exclusively a follow-up test to the Weber, but rather is performed in conjunction with it. The Rinne test (Figure 5-11(a) and (b)) is a comparative measure for air and bone sound conduction. Again, tuning fork prongs are stimulated with moderate pressure. The stem of the vibrating fork is placed on the mastoid process. The client is instructed to indicate when the sound (not the vibrations) is no longer heard. The tuning fork is then removed

FIGURE 5-11
The Rinne test, a comparative measure of air and bone sound conduction: (a) placement of the tuning fork on the mastoid process to test bone conduction; (b) placement of the tuning fork in front of the ear to test air conduction.

(a)

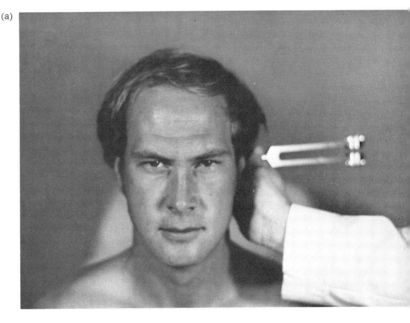

(b)

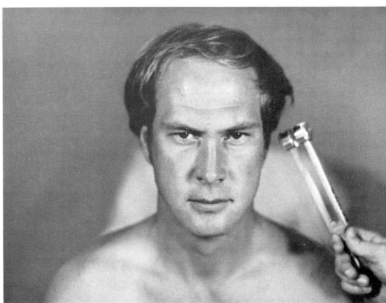

from the mastoid area, and the lateral surface of the prongs is placed near the anterior surface of the ear, taking care not to touch it as this would result in early cessation of sound emitted from the tuning fork. The client is requested to state when the sound is no longer heard. Normally, air-conducted sound is heard approximately twice as long as bone-conducted sound. Determination of sound ratio requires timing of the duration for which sounds are heard. Frequently, the results are recorded as a positive Rinne test, indicating normal results, or a negative Rinne test, indicating abnormal results. Further descriptive time data can be recorded and are calculated in the following manner:

$$
\begin{array}{ll}
\text{Air conduction} & 40 \text{ seconds} \\
\text{Bone conduction} & \underline{10 \text{ seconds}} \\
& 30 \text{ seconds}
\end{array}
$$

The results are then recorded as +30 second Rinne test. When bone conduction is of longer duration than air conduction, the results are recorded in the negative, such as −10 second Rinne test. A negative Rinne test may indicate a conductive hearing loss.

The Schwabach tuning fork test is performed by alternately placing a vibrating tuning fork on the mastoid process of the client and examiner. Normally, the cessation of sound occurs at approximately the same time for both individuals. Sound duration for the client that is shorter than the examiner's may indicate nerve-impaired hearing; a longer duration of sound may indicate conductive loss, although the latter is under controversy.

Another test employed is the Bing test. Similar to the Weber, the tuning fork is placed midline on the vertex of the skull. The ear being assessed is occluded and normally hears the sound conducted. Such results indicate that a normal conductive mechanism exists, and hearing loss may be related to nerve deafness.

Hearing in the newborn is difficult to evaluate in the first 24 hours. However, by a few days of age, the newborn should respond to loud noises such as clapping the hands together. The common neonatal responses include the Moro reflex, eye movements or blinking, and cessation of movement. Between 6 and 8 months of age, the child will turn the head in the direction of the sound, and by 9 months of age, may identify the sound originating object by staring at it. As the child grows older, his responses become consistent with his stage of growth and development. Indications of hearing deficits at any age should be referred to an individual with expertise and more sophisticated methods of testing.

Part 3

STUDY GUIDE QUESTIONS

In the following client situations, identify and describe the subjective and objective data to be collected, the specific tools and procedures to be utilized in the collection of those data, and the rationale for the nursing assessment.

1. While making a family home health visit with Mr. and Mrs. Brian Carls, who have two children, ages 4 years and 1 week, you observe that the 4-year-old is irritable and sporadically tugs at his right ear.
2. Mr. Peter Able is a 67-year-old married male who enters the Seniors' Health Care Clinic and states he has noted a decrease in his hearing.
3. During your cursory exam of 1-hour-old baby girl Steel, you questioned the level of ear placement and degree of pinnae abduction. The infant is now 8 hours old and stable, so you are ready to proceed with a more in-depth assessment.

SAMPLE FORMAT TO BE USED IN RESPONDING TO THE STUDY GUIDE QUESTIONS

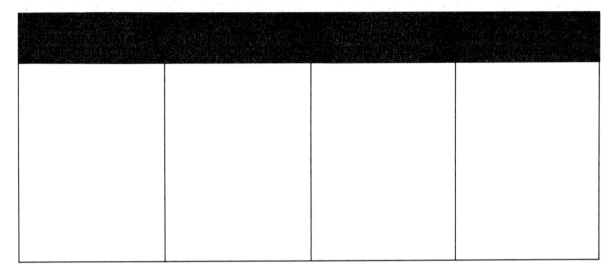

BIBLIOGRAPHY

BATES, BARBARA, *A Guide to Physical Examination,* pp. 62–63. Philadelphia: J. B. Lippincott Company, 1974.

BROWN, MARIE S., and MARY M. ALEXANDER, "Physical Examination, Part 7: Examining the Ear," *Nursing 74,* February 1974, pp. 48–51.

———, "Physical Examination, Part 8: Hearing Acuity," *Nursing 73,* April 1973, pp. 61–65.

BUSIS, SIDNEY N., HYMAN M. PAISNER, and ROBERT J. WOLFSON, "Pointers for Detecting Hearing Loss," *Patient Care,* August 15, 1977, pp. 174–202.

CHINN, PEGGY, L., and CYNTHIA J. LEITCH, *Handbook for Nursing Assessment of the Child.* Salt Lake City, Utah: University of Utah Printing Service, 1973.

CHUSED, JOSEPH G., ed., *Correlative Neuroanatomy and Functional Neurology.* Los Altos, Calif.: Lange Medical Publications, 1970.

ELLIOT, DEAN, and others, "Sorting out the Vagaries of Otitis," *Patient Care,* January 1976, pp. 60–85.

HELLER, MORRIS F., *Functional Otology.* New York: Springer Publishing Company, Inc. 1955.

HOLLINSHEAD, W. HENRY, *Textbook of Anatomy* (2nd ed.), pp. 886–901. New York: Harper & Row, Inc., 1967.

KOBRACK, HEINRICH G., *The Middle Ear.* Chicago: University of Chicago Press, 1959.

MALKIN, E. A., "The Middle Ear Cleft and Its Acute Infections," *Nursing Times,* September 19, 1974, pp. 1466–1468.

MYERS, DAVID, and others, "Otologic Diagnostic and the Treatment of Deafness," reprint from *Clinical Symposia,* 22, no. 2, 1970.

NEWBY, HAYES A., *Audiology* (2nd ed.). New York: Appleton-Century-Crofts, 1964.

MECHNER, FRANCIS, "Patient Assessment: Examination of the Ear," *American Journal of Nursing,* March 1975, pp. 1–24.

PETRAKIS, NICHOLAS L., "Dry Cerumen—A Prevalent Genetic Trait Among American Indians," *Nature,* June 14, 1969, pp. 1080–1081.

———, and others, "Evidence for a Genetic Cline in Earwax Types in the Middle East and Southeast Asia," *American Journal of Physiological Anthropology,* July 1971, pp. 141–144.

PRIOR, JOHN A., and JACK S. SILBERSTEIN, *Physical Diagnosis* (4th ed.). St. Louis, Mo.: The C. V. Mosby Company, 1973.

ROSE, DARRELL E., ed., *Audiology Assessment.* Englewood Cliffs, N.J.: Prentice-Hall, Inc., 1971.

6

The Eye

REVIEW OF STRUCTURE AND FUNCTION

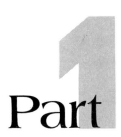

The eyeball is housed in the protective bony structure of the skull called the orbit. Positional areas on the orbit are referred to as superior, inferior, medial or nasal, and lateral or temporal. The orbital structure contains several fissures and a channel through which the optic nerve passes from the eye to the brain. Anteriorly and laterally on the superior margin, the orbit contains a smooth depression that houses the lacrimal glands. Figure 6-1 illustrates the bony structures protecting and housing the eye.

EYELIDS

The eyelids or palpebrae are loose folds of skin that maintain their shape through muscle and ligament structures, one of which is the tarsal plate. The margin of the lid contains hair follicles or eyelashes and sebaceous glands. On the posterior surface of the lid is the palpebral conjunctiva, a clear transparent membrane that is continuous with the skin. It is due to this transparency that the underlying pinkish coloration of the tissue is presented. Meibomian glands can be observed as yellowish striations extending from the tarsal plate; lymph vessels may be seen as grayish white dots. Meibomian glands produce and secrete a fatty material with a surface tension that prevents tears from flowing onto the facial surface. Lymph drainage is generally directed downward and backward to the parotid nodes, while, medially, this drainage is in the direction of the submandibular lymph nodes. The upper eyelid overlaps the limbus 1 to 3 mm; the lower lid margin is just below the inferior margin of the limbus. The distance between the upper and lower eyelids in an open position is called the palpebral fissure.

LACRIMAL GLANDS

The lacrimal glands extend from the superior anterior lateral margin of the orbit into the superior conjunctival fornix. These glands secrete tears. Tears are approximately 88 percent water with a pH of 7.35 and contain lysozyme, a bacteriostatic enzyme. Blinking of the upper eyelids serves to evenly distribute tears over the eyeball,

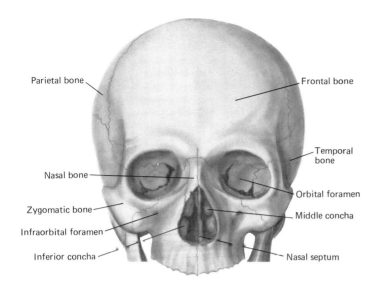

FIGURE 6-1

Bony structures protecting and housing the eye.

thereby maintaining a moist and cleansed surface. In the medial angle of each eye is the lacrimal papilla, which contains the punctum of the lacrimal canaliculus. This structure serves to drain the tears to the nasolacrimal duct and finally into the nasal cavity. The aging process creates involution of the lacrimal glands, resulting in decreased fluid secretion, dryness, and burning. Figure 6-2 illustrates the anatomical location of the lacrimal glands and associated structures.

EXTRAOCULAR MUSCLES

The eyeball is controlled by the muscles of the orbit. There are six major voluntary muscles. The innervation and directional control of these voluntary ocular muscles are described in Table 6-1, and the direction of eye movement is illustrated in Figure 6-3. The muscles of both eyes are coordinated for simultaneous movement in the same direction. This is referred to as conjugate movement.

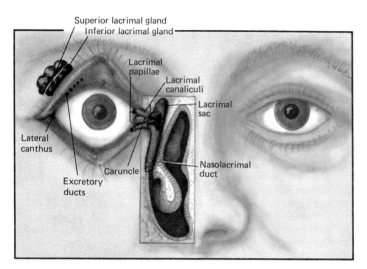

Superior lacrimal gland
Inferior lacrimal gland
Lacrimal papillae
Lacrimal canaliculi
Lacrimal sac
Lateral canthus
Caruncle
Nasolacrimal duct
Excretory ducts

FIGURE 6-2
Anatomical location of the lacrimal structures.

TABLE 6-1
Extraocular Muscles: Source of Innervation and Associated Direction of Gaze

Muscle	Source of Innervation	Direction of Gaze
Superior oblique	Trochlear nerve (IV cranial nerve)	Downward and lateral; medial rotation of eyeball
Inferior oblique	Inferior branch of oculomotor (III cranial nerve)	Upward and lateral; lateral rotation of eyeball
Superior rectus	Superior branch of oculomotor (III cranial nerve)	Upward movement
Inferior rectus	Inferior branch of oculomotor (III cranial nerve)	Downward movement
Medial rectus	Abducens (VI cranial nerve)	Lateral movement
Lateral rectus	Abducens (VI cranial nerve)	Lateral movement

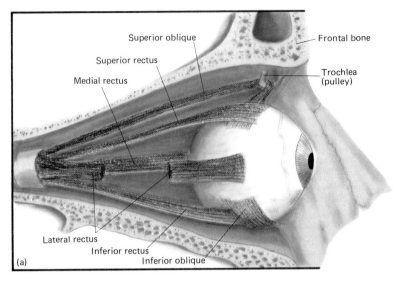

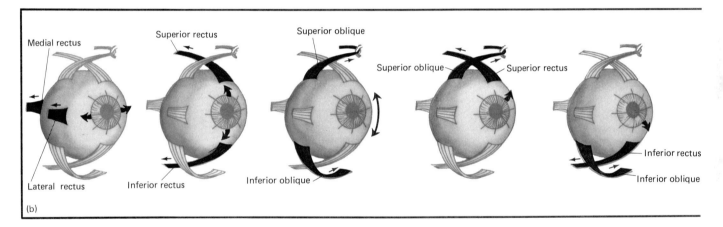

FIGURE 6-3

**Ocular muscles and eye movements:
(a) extrinsic muscles of the eye;
(b) ocular movement associated
with muscles.**

EYEBALL

The eyeball consists of three layers. The outer layer of fibrous tunic consists of the sclera and cornea. The medial vascular tunic consists of the choroid, ciliary body, and iris; finally, the tunical interna composes the sensory portion of the retina (Figure 6-4).

The sclera, which is composed of connective tissue, appears as a whitish opaque area with visible blood vessels near the peripheral margin. The sclera is continuous with the transparent cornea. The corneal structure is avascular and receives nutrients through the process of diffusion. Lack of vessels throughout the cornea permits transmission of visual images without interruption of the incoming light rays.

The iris, a part of the choroid, lies behind the cornea. Its central portion is the pupil, which develops its permanent color from the age of 6 months to 1 year of life. At the periphery of the iris is the ciliary body, a structure composed of muscle fibers that relax and contract and thereby control the amount of light allowed to enter the internal portion of the eye. Immediately behind the cornea is the anterior chamber, which is filled with aqueous humor. The production and drainage of aqueous humor must remain constant in order to maintain the normal intraocular pressure, which is in the range of 15 to 25 mm of Hg. Aqueous humor is probably produced by the epithelium of the ciliary body and drains from the anterior chamber into the canal of Schlemm (Figure 6-5).

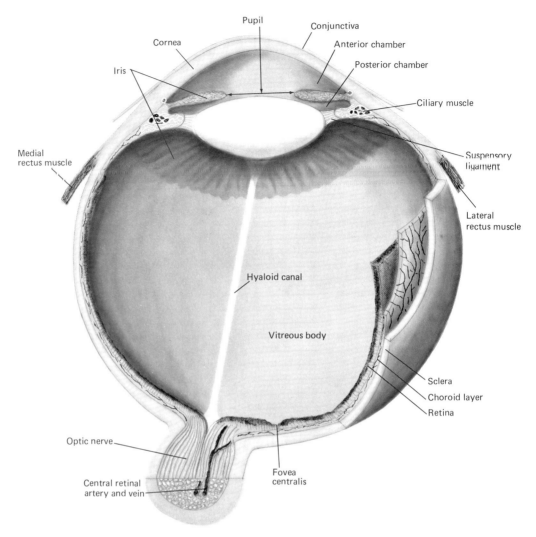

FIGURE 6-4
Structural components of the eyeball.

Labels (Figure 6-4):
Pupil
Cornea
Conjunctiva
Anterior chamber
Posterior chamber
Iris
Ciliary muscle
Medial rectus muscle
Suspensory ligament
Lateral rectus muscle
Hyaloid canal
Vitreous body
Sclera
Choroid layer
Retina
Optic nerve
Fovea centralis
Central retinal artery and vein

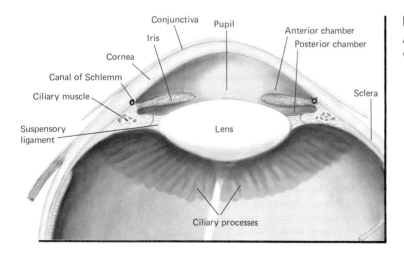

Labels (Figure 6-5):
Conjunctiva
Pupil
Iris
Anterior chamber
Posterior chamber
Cornea
Canal of Schlemm
Ciliary muscle
Sclera
Suspensory ligament
Lens
Ciliary processes

FIGURE 6-5
Anatomical location of the canal of Schlemm.

The lens lies posterior to the iris and is a biconvex disc of transparent fibers. Transparency of the lens allows passage of light, while the convexity controls the point of light focus on the retina. The lens accommodates to near and distant images through the contraction or relaxation of the ciliary muscle, which increases or decreases the convexity of the lens.

Posterior to the lens is the vitreous chamber or vitreous body. The gelatinous inner mass filling this chamber is formed very early in development and is not replenished. It is capable of transmitting light because it is clear and avascular. It also supports and maintains the appropriate placement of the retina. Any damage to the eye that permits the loss of vitreous humor can lead to blindness, as retinal support is lost and retinal detachment can occur.

The retinal surface or inner nervous layer of the eye transforms light waves into neuronal impulses and then relays these impulses to the brain for interpretation. Located within the retina are chemical substances termed **rods,** which are for vision in darkened or dimly lighted environments, and **cones,** which are for brightness and color vision. The greatest concentration of cones is located in the macula, an area that is predominately free of vessels and lies to the temporal side of the retina. Within the macula exists an area approximately 0.5 mm in diameter called the *fovea,* the most sensitive part of the eye as well as the central focusing point of the eye's optic system.

On the posterior surface of the retina is the optic disc or optic nerve, which is encompassed by a sheath. This encapsulation is continuous with the dura and arachnoid membranes. The optic disc transmits sensory data to the brain.

HEALTH ASSESSMENT OF THE EYE

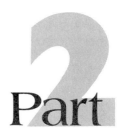

Part 2

Objective data collection of the eye begins with visual testing, and proceeds to the external structures and, finally, the internal structures. The internal assessment or funduscopic exam is presented for the purpose of developing awareness of the procedure rather than the actual performance of this instrumentation.

VISUAL TESTING

Visual perception is most frequently tested using the Snellen letter eye chart (Figure 6-6). A standardized Snellen chart is placed at eye level and at a distance of 20 ft from the chart a line is marked on the floor. The client, either standing with heels on the line or sitting in a chair with the chair's back on the line, is requested to read a specified chart line with one eye, the other eye being covered and with glasses or contacts in place if worn. The examiner must instruct the client to keep both eyes open while reading the specified letter being pointed to. Generally, the examiner first points to the 40-ft line on the chart and, with appropriate interpretation, uses the subsequent lines. If the 40-ft line is inaccurately interpreted, begin at the 200-ft line and progress downward. If the client misses several letters in one line, do not continue on. Visual perception is recorded in numerical figures, with the numerator indicating distance from the chart and the denominator representing the distance a person with "normal" vision could see and interpret the symbols. For example, if the score is recorded L 20/40, the client is 20 ft from the chart and reads with the left eye at 20 ft what the "normal" eye visualizes at 40 ft. Children are tested with the Snellen letter chart beginning at age 7 or 8. Children

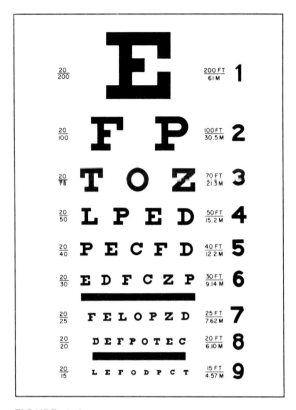

FIGURE 6-6

The Snellen letter eye chart used for testing visual acuity.

for this test. The examiner must first confirm the child's ability to identify the pictures correctly by name. Then the child is placed 15 ft from the examiner. The child places the eye occluder over one eye first and later over the other as the examiner holds up each picture to be identified. To pass, the child must identify three of five pictures correctly in each eye. This test material and instructions can be obtained from the Denver Developmental Testing Bureau.

The third test, the fixation test, is used to screen vision in children 6 months to $2\frac{5}{12}$ years and for those children up to 3 years who cannot be tested with the picture cards. The materials used are a flashlight (penlight) and a colorful spinning toy. First the light is used to test the child's ability to track or follow it. Cover one eye and hold the light $1\frac{1}{2}$ ft from the child. Move the light from midline, right then left, and observe the child's eye movement. The spinning toy replaces the light if the child loses interest in the light. The test is repeated with the opposite eye

FIGURE 6-7

The Snellen symbol eye chart used to test vision in children under the age of seven and illiterate individuals.

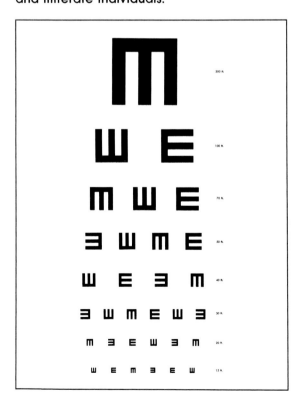

younger than this are tested using the Snellen symbol chart (Figure 6-7) or symbol cards. The symbol chart or cards are needed for modified distant vision screening in adults and children (3 to 6 years) who are unable to read letters. The client is positioned 20 ft from the symbol chart and the child 15 ft from the symbol card held by the test administrator. As the tester indicates one of the E symbols, or turns the card to one of the four positions, the client indicates the direction of the E's fingers. The test is done first with one eye covered and then the other. The Snellen symbol chart is administered and scored the same as the conventional Snellen letter chart.

The preschool vision screening employs the use of one of three tests depending upon the age of the child. The symbol card is used as explained to test children ages 3 to 6 years of age. To pass, the child must identify three of five E directions correctly with each eye.

The picture card vision test is used for children $2\frac{1}{2}$ to $2\frac{11}{12}$ years of age. A set of four pictures, a plastic eye occluder, and a 15-ft string are used covered. Normally, the child will track the light or toy with both eyes. The child fails the test if he objects to having one eye covered (usually the better eye) or if he fails to track with either eye.

Between the ages of 4 and 8, children test out at approximately 20/30; at about the age of 9, visual perception is approximately 20/20. The chart line that is interpreted most readily and accurately (three out of four or four out of six items) is the line that is used in the recording. Other charts are available for testing vision but the Snellen letter and symbol charts are the ones that are standardized and most commonly used.

Near visual acuity can be tested; however, many variables affect the reliability of the test. Some examiners rely on the client's demonstrated ease of reading a newspaper at approximately 12 in. from the eyes. A standardized near-vision acuity test is administered after far-vision testing and before any pupillary dilatation or funduscopic exam. The test requires comfortable reading light. A small matted non-glare-finished test card, such as a Jaeger test card, is used from which the client reads. The test card is placed 14 in. from the client's eyes. The client reads the card with first one eye covered and then the other. Scoring of near-vision acuity is determined by the type of visual test card used.

Color vision may be assessed in several ways. Most Snellen eye charts have a red and a green color bar. When this method is used, the client is requested to state the perceived color of both bars. The standardized Ishihara test for color vision is composed of cards with a background of colored dots and a superimposed figure of colored dots. The client is asked to describe any perceived figures. Abnormally, the superimposed figure is not perceived as different from the back. Color blindness is uncommon in females, with an incidence of 0.3 to 0.5 percent; however, 4 to 8 percent of males are color blind because of an inherited, recessive sex-linked trait.

INSPECTION

Continued assessment of the eye then proceeds to a general inspection of the eye structure. In children, observe for slanting of the eye, as an upward slant can be a racial or genetic characteristic and is a common finding in certain chromosomal abnormalities (Figure 6-8).

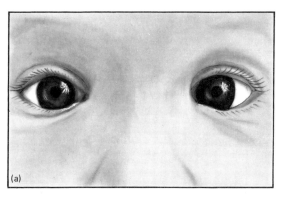

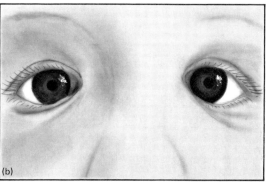

FIGURE 6-8
Normal and abnormal planes of the eye:
(a) normal plane of the eyes;
(b) abnormal downward slanting of the eyes.

Epicanthal folds, which are vertical folds of skin covering the inner canthus of the eye, may be seen in some children. They occur most often bilaterally and can give the appearance of crossed eyes (also termed strabismus). Epicanthal folds, although not always abnormal, are also associated with chromosomal abnormalities (Figure 6-9). These skin folds remain prominent until growth of the nasal bridge occurs.

In general, the eyes appear full and bright. Sunken eyes, which may have a dull appearance, can indicate the existence of a dehydrated and malnourished state. Pseudostrabismus is seen in newborns. It gives the appearance of crossed eyes, but can be differentiated from true strabismus by checking the bilateral symmetry of the corneal light reflex.

After the generalized inspection, observe the color, structure, and symmetry of the upper lid. The color generally blends with that of the face, but may be reddened in states of fever. The lower lid frequently blends into the facial skin, although with age it may assume a dusky color.

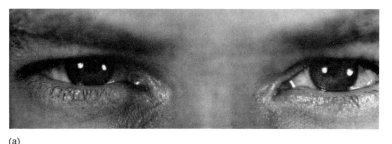
(a)

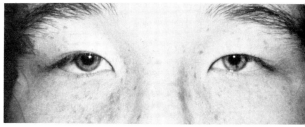
(b)

FIGURE 6-9

Epicanthal folds: (a) the normal eye without epicanthal folds;
(b) the normal eye with epicanthal folds.

The upper eyelids possess a fold that, when looking upward, disappears. In the elderly, atrophy and loss of elasticity in skin structures may increase the prominence of this fold.

While open, the lids should be in equal placement and cover the superior section of the limbus 1 to 3 mm, while the lower lid position is just below the inferior limbus margin. Abnormally, some lids may present ectropion, an outward eversion, or entropion, an inward turning of the lid. Observation of an eye in which the limbus and underlying sclera are visible is deviant from the normal and characteristic of lid retraction (Figure 6-10). While the lower lid generally reveals a margin of sclera, the marginal width increases with lower lid retraction. Epiphora, most frequently observed in the elderly, is the result of skin relaxation of the lower lid. It is characterized by the overflow of tears, which is most notable when the client is in a cold environment as the orbicularis muscle fails to compress and produce a siphoning effect for the nasolacrimal duct.

Lid lag may be demonstrated by observing associated eye and lid movements or specifically directing the client to follow the examiner's finger movements with the eyes. Lids that fail to follow in a downward direction, or demonstrate slowed movement when compared to the opposite lid, or close slowly in jerky movements, are described as lagging. Ptosis, a drooping of the eyelid, may be bilateral or unilateral (Figure 6-11). A true ptosis characteristically extends beyond 3 mm over the limbus of the eye and results in a narrowing of the palpebral fissure. Ptosis of the lid observed in the infant may be concomitant with epicanthal folds. Frequently, in this situation there is an abnormality with the levator muscles.

Slight edema may be present in the lid early in the morning upon awakening. This fluid infiltration subsides rapidly. Eyelid edema at other

FIGURE 6-10

Eyelid position: (a) normal positioning; (b) ectropion; (c) entropion;
(d) lid retraction. (Photos courtesy of University of Minnesota, Health
Sciences, Department of Ophthalmology.)

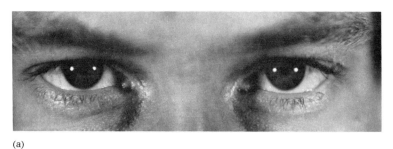
(a)

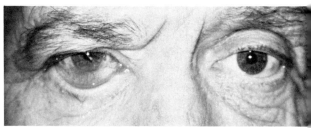
(b)

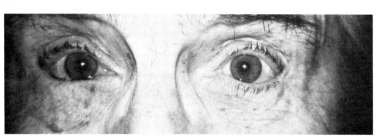
(c)

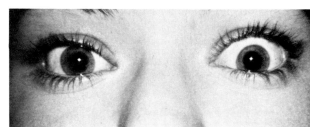
(d)

times or edema persisting over longer periods of time is abnormal and can occur with inflammation close to or in the lid, allergies, drug sensitivities, or with renal problems. In infants, this periorbital edema is associated with congestive heart failure.

The conjunctiva is divided into two parts. The palpebral conjunctiva lines the posterior surfaces of the superior and inferior lid. It contains vertical, yellow striations, which are the Meibomian glands and lymph follicles. Cyst formation in the Meibomian glands results in chalazions. When irritated, the lymph follicles enlarge and present fine whitish nodules. The palpebral conjunctiva is clear or translucent, and, therefore, the light pink color of the underlying tissue is seen.

Inspection of the palpebral conjunctiva is carried out through lid eversion. To inspect the lower palpebral conjunctiva, place the thumb or index finger on the exterior lid surface and gently pull in a downward direction (Figure 6-12). Inspect the presenting characteristics proceeding from the temporal to the nasal side.

Inspection of the upper lid conjunctiva involves several procedural steps and is not assessed as frequently as the lower lid conjunctiva. The client looks in a downward direction closing the eyelids loosely. The examiner applies downward pressure on the upper tarsal border with a small blunt object such as a cotton-tipped applicator. With the free hand, the examiner then grasps the upper eyelid margin or eyelashes, pulling downward and forward. The pressure of the blunt object is maintained until the lid is everted, exposing the palpebral conjunctiva. Replacement of the lid to its normal position is accomplished by gently pulling forward on the lid while the individual looks in an upward direction, or having the individual blink forcefully (Figure 6-13).

Extreme pallor of the upper or lower conjunctiva may indicate anemia. The bulbar conjunctiva, or second conjunctival division, covers the eye up to the limbus. It is transparent, revealing the whitish color of the underlying sclera. Inspection of the bulbar conjunctiva is accomplished by using a small pen light and having the individual look upward, downward, nasally, and temporally to maximally expose the conjunctival area. Normally, there are numerous small blood vessels present, especially toward the periphery of the eyeball. These vessels have a smooth appearance.

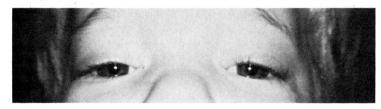
(a)

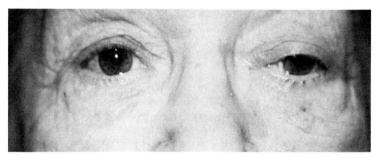
(b)

FIGURE 6-11
Ptosis of the eyelid: (a) bilateral; (b) unilateral. (Photos courtesy of University of Minnesota, Health Sciences, Department of Ophthalmology.)

FIGURE 6-12
Lower eyelid eversion.

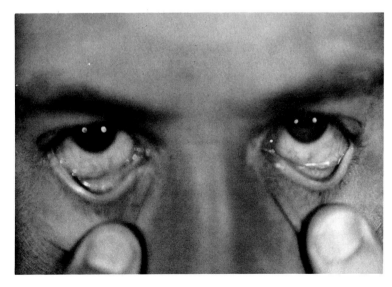

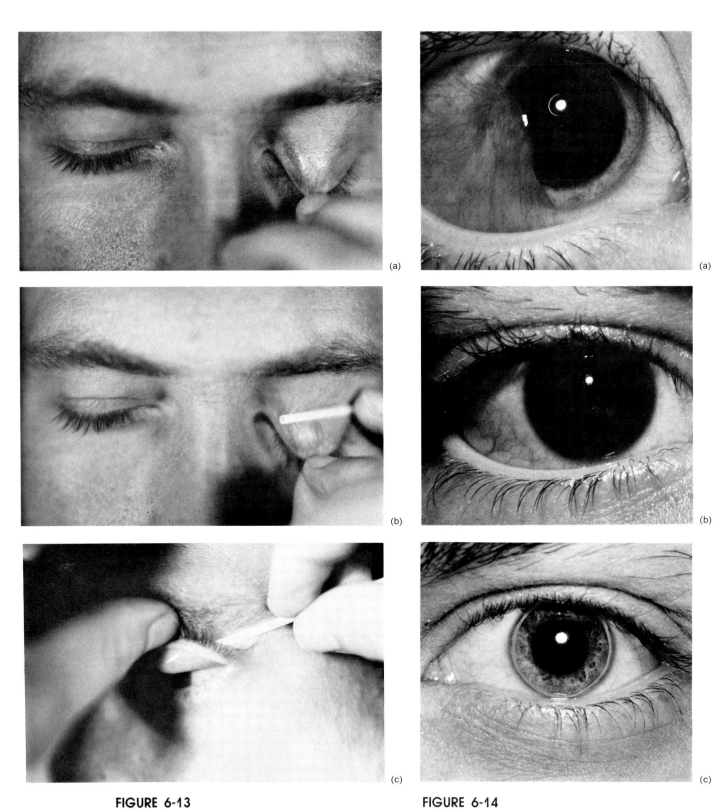

FIGURE 6-13
Eversion of the upper eyelid: (a) pull lid down; (b) place blunt object over tarsal border; (c) flip lid upward over object.

FIGURE 6-14
Changes of the eye frequently associated with aging: (a) pterygium; (b) pinguecula; (c) arcus senilis. (Photos courtesy of University of Minnesota, Health Sciences, Department of Ophthalmology.)

Several changes that are probably consistent with the aging process may be noted in the bulbar conjunctiva. The most frequently observed changes are pterygium, pinguecula, and arcus senilis (Figure 6-14(a), (b), and (c)). A pterygium is a triangular ingrowth of vascularized conjunctiva that extends from the nasal canthus toward or onto the cornea. Pterygiums are due to long-standing irritation and drying of the conjunctiva. They may interfere with visual acuity when the cornea is involved. A pinguecula is a triangular ingrowth originating on either side of the cornea, but most frequently on the nasal side. It is characterized by yellowish elastic tissue, which generally does not interfere with vision. Arcus senilis presents as a grayish ring at the border of the cornea. Between this grayish ring and the limbus is a clear zone. Arcus senilis is most easily visualized on darkly pigmented eyes.

The sclera generally appears opaque white. Occasionally, pigmented areas in the sclera may be seen in Caucasians, as well as in non-Caucasian races. Scleral thinning, a result of the aging process, may yield a bluish hue in the sclera of the elderly. Bluish-colored sclera, genetic in origin, are frequently associated with certain disease processes. Jaundice, a yellow pigment, can be observed in the sclera and is generally most prominent in the fornices.

The cornea is inspected for smoothness and transparency, characteristics that are essential for good vision. The corneal reflex can be tested by drawing a fine wisp of clean or sterile cotton across the surface of the cornea (Figure 6-15). The normal response to this stimulus is involuntary blinking. Abnormalities of the cornea include configuration irregularities and regions of dullness, lusterlessness, or absence of the corneal reflex.

From the cornea, the examiner proceeds to the pupils. In approximately 75 percent of the population the pupils are bilaterally, perfectly round and equal in size. The remaining 25 percent of the population may have slightly unequal pupils, which is a variation of normal. The size of the pupil varies from 3 to 7 mm in diameter (Figure 6-16).

In early infancy the pupils are small; in childhood they are larger than in adulthood. As aging continues, the pupils again decrease in size, becoming miotic in the elderly. Miotic pupils are seen more frequently in farsightedness or hyperopia.

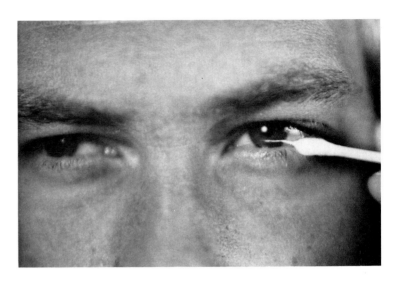

FIGURE 6-15
The corneal reflex elicited by touching the cornea with a fine wisp of cotton.

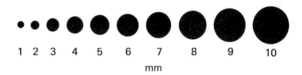

1 2 3 4 5 6 7 8 9 10
mm

FIGURE 6-16
Various diameters of the pupil in millimeters.

Pupil response is important in evaluating the central nervous system. To assess the direct and consensual pupillary response, ask the client to look straight ahead. Bring a bright light in from the side of the face as illustrated in Figure 6-17. The pupil into which the light is shone constricts (direct response) with the opposite pupil constricting simultaneously (indirect or consensual response). Determination of direct and indirect responses for both the right and left pupil is necessary. To ensure that each response is seen, stimulate the eye and observe for the direct response; then stimulate the same eye again noting the consensual response. The quality of the response is estimated.

Dilation of the pupil is the result of sympathetic activity and can be seen in some stages of anesthesia, hysteria, fright, glaucoma, blindness, and in dimly lighted or dark environments. Pupillary constriction is the result of parasympathetic activity and may be observed in morphine poisoning or excessive bright light stimulation.

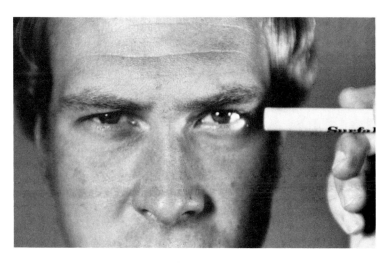

FIGURE 6-17
Direct and consensual pupillary reflex elicited by light.

FIGURE 6-18
Light-ray focus in myopia and hyperopia: (a) in myopia the eyeball is longer than normal, and light rays focus anterior to the retina; (b) in hyperopia the eyeball is shorter than normal; therefore, if light rays could pass through the retina, they would come to a focus posterior to the retina. In all the drawings the dot represents the focal point.

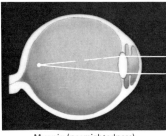
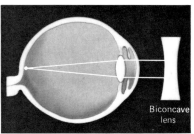

(a) Myopia (nearsightedness) — Correction — Biconcave lens

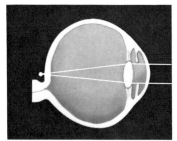
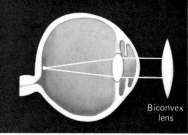

(b) Hyperopia (farsightedness) — Correction — Biconvex lens

The lens of the eye is a clear, smooth structure. In middle age, the lens begins to lose its elasticity. Near objects become more difficult to see since the point of accommodation is farther away. This condition or state, when occurring as a part of the aging process, is called **presbyopia.** This state frequently occurs by age 45. Irregularities in the curvature of the lens or cornea produce astigmatism. The lens adjusts its degree of convexity to accommodate for distance. Myopia, or nearsightedness, is the result of a persistent concavity that inhibits optimal focusing on distant objects and is frequently described as the eyeball being too long. This concavity results in the focus of light rays in front of the retina. On the other hand, hyperopia or farsightedness is a problem that presents as a difficulty in focusing on near objects. It is often described as light rays focusing behind the retina. Hyperopia is characteristic of infants. Heredity is the prime cause for myopia and hyperopia. Figure 6-18 illustrates light-ray focus in myopic and hyperopic states, with and without corrective lenses. Cataract formation is most common in the elderly and presents to the examiner a gray coloration of the lens. The presence of cataracts interferes with the client's visual perception.

Extraocular muscle movements are tested by requesting the individual to follow the examiner's finger through the six cardinal positions of gaze. The examiner begins with the index finger at the midpoint of the head at the level of the client's eyes, and then proceeds to the first position of gaze. The finger is then returned to midpoint before proceeding to the next position of gaze. The major movements assessed are illustrated in Figure 6-19.

If extraocular muscles are paralyzed or weak, strabismus can result. Nonparalytic strabismus, also termed noncomitant or nonconcomitant, is a defect in the position of the eyes relative to one another. The degree of relative positional deviation does not change with positional change of the eyes. Noncomitant strabismus occurs after trauma and is characterized by eye deviation dependent upon directional gaze. It generally subsides after 1 or 2 months without treatment. Comitant strabismus, a congenital defect in muscle insertion, will remain unless medical treatment is sought. It can progress to amblyopia, which is a suppression of the resulting double images and gradual loss of vision in the affected eye. When indicators of strabismus are present, prompt referral to an ophthalmologist is the proper course of action.

Near-point convergence is assessed at this time by placing the index finger at a central point between the eyes, approximately $1\frac{1}{2}$ ft from the face. The finger is then directed toward the face. The near point is determined by observing the distance from the face at which deviations of the eye occur. Normally, in the adult the near-point is between 50 and 75 mm in front of the eyes.

During the first month of life, the normal infant may reveal limited horizontal nystagmus from rotational eye movement. Spontaneous nystagmus is always abnormal. During the second month of life, an infant generally will look at objects with his eyes, but does not intentionally turn his head to see an object. The accuracy of the infant's sight is questionable at this time. In the third month, an infant looks at and follows objects with the head, unless the object is quickly moved past the visual field. Eye coordination has increased greatly when convergence of the eyes occurs as an object is brought toward the nose.

Muscle strength and position of the eye can also be determined by the Hirschberg test. In a dark room, with the client looking straight ahead, the examiner shines a light into the eyes from a distance of 1 to 2 ft. A small light reflex should be observed centrally on the convex surface of the cornea. This light reflex should be in the same position bilaterally. If one eye has loss of muscle strength, resulting in a positional deviation of the eye, the position of the light reflex will be asymmetrical. Figure 6-20 illustrates a centrally located light reflex and a displaced light reflex.

Another method of checking eye position in a child over 6 months of age is the cover test. This test is accomplished by placing an object approximately 1 ft in front of the eyes. After the eyes have focused on the object, cover one eye for several seconds, making sure not to touch the skin or the lash. Quickly remove the eye cover, observing the previously covered eye for any jerking or drifting from the focused position. This can be an indication of strabismus. Deviations toward the nose are called **esophoria.**

The peripheral visual fields are assessed grossly. Have the client look straight ahead and cover the eye not being examined. Use a small object such as a pencil, and move the object from a point well out of the normal peripheral visual fields in an arc toward the midline or the nose. Ask the client to say "now" when the object is

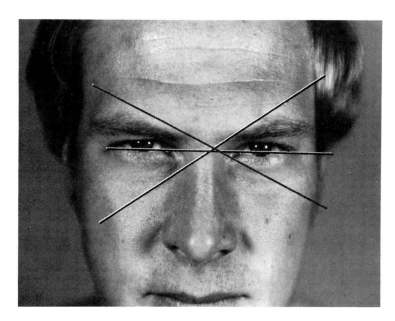

FIGURE 6-19
The six cardinal positions of gaze.

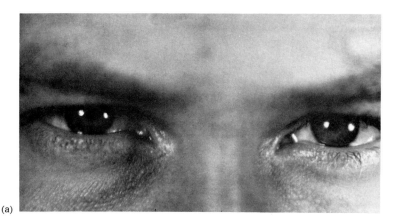

(a)

(b)

FIGURE 6-20
Comparative location of the corneal light reflex: (a) symmetrical; (b) asymmetrical. (Photos courtesy of University of Minnesota, Health Sciences, Department of Ophthalmology.)

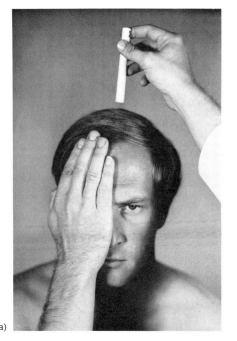

(a)

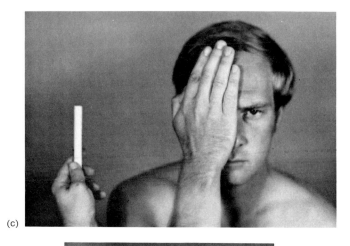

(c)

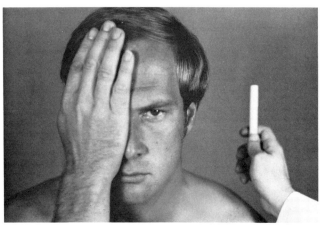

(b)

FIGURE 6-21
Assessment of peripheral visual fields: (d)
(a) superior; (b) temporal; (c) nasal; (d) downward.

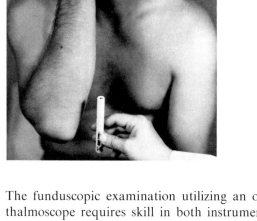

first sighted. The examiner must remember to proceed slowly or the approximated visual fields will be greatly incorrect (Figure 6-21). The normal peripheral visual fields are as follows:

1. Sixty degrees nasally.
2. Fifty degrees upward.
3. Ninety degrees temporally.
4. Seventy degrees downward.

OPHTHALMOSCOPIC EXAMINATION

The ophthalmoscope magnifies 14 times that which can be seen by the naked eye, and thus allows visualization of the internal eye structures along with any pathology or foreign material.

The funduscopic examination utilizing an ophthalmoscope requires skill in both instrumentation and interpretation, and is generally deferred as a tool used by the beginning-level practitioner.

A brief discussion of the use of the ophthalmoscope and interpretation of the findings is included to familiarize the student with the skill, examination process, and appropriate integration into the systematic assessment of the eye.

Many ophthalmoscopes are equipped with the following accessories:

1. Two different sized round light beams. The small light beam is used for the small or undilated pupil; the larger light beam is used for dilated or larger pupils.
2. A vertical slit that is used for gauging the

106

convexity, concavity, or smoothness of retinal lesions. Elevated or convex lesions yield a steplike appearance. Concave or indentations demonstrate a bowing away of the light; nondimensional shaped lesions appear flat.

3. A grid that consists of graphing lines is used to calibrate vessel or lesion size. These calibrations then allow the examiner to draw the lesion or vessel on a similar piece of graph paper. The grid, however, is rarely used.

4. The green beam is a red-free light. The green light is employed to assist in the determination of whether a black retinal spot is due to melanin or hemorrhage. Old hemorrhages, then viewed with the green light, take on a coal-black appearance; melanin deposits are more grayish in color.

When performing a funduscopic examination, ask the client to pick a spot and focus on it, even though the examiner's head may get in the way. To examine the left eye, the examiner uses his or her own left eye and left hand to manipulate the ophthalmoscope, and, while viewing the right eye, the examiner uses his or her own right eye and right hand. This prevents the nasal structures from interfering with the examination and prevents breathing directly into the client's face. The ophthalmoscope is rested upon the examiner's brow, and the procedure is initiated approximately $1\frac{1}{2}$ ft away from the subject with the appropriate-sized light beam focused on the pupil. The first finding upon visualization should be the red-light reflex, which originates from the sclera, choroid, retina, optic disc, and vessels. The red reflex normally presents itself as a fully round red reflection of the light beam without opacities. If the lens has subluxated, it is not centralized in the pupillary space, and the disc edge is visible as a change from a red reflex to a dark contour. When cataracts are present, dependent upon their size, the red reflex may be partially or totally absent. As the examiner moves closer, the red reflex is passed and the fundus of the eye is viewed. In the infant, the red reflex is often the only portion of the funduscopic examination performed, owing to the lack of cooperation and small pupil size.

The optic disc is visualized as a whitish, creamy-pink structure in which the temporal quadrant appears light in color. It is round or vertically oval in shape. A physiologic cup or depression is contained within the disc. It appears pale white, sometimes with almost a grayish hue, and its borders are never aligned with the peripheral disc border. The optic disc is approximately 1.5 mm in diameter and generally well defined (Figure 6-22). This diameter is referred to as the disc diameter (DD) and is used to describe visible structures in the eye as well as lesions. In the hyperopic individual, the disc may appear to be smaller with poorly defined borders. Frequently, the examiner may visualize a pigmented area of melanin at the disc margin that appears brownish gray in color. Also, a white scleral crescent or ring is visualized when there is exposure of the choroid at the opening or junction of the globe and optic disc.

The fundus of the eye varies in color, depending upon the client's pigmentation. Blond-haired, blue-eyed individuals present a bright-orange-colored fundus, whereas the fundus of blacks ranges from brownish gray to slate gray. The change in color presentation is due to light reflection off the pigmented epithelial layer.

The vessels of the internal eye are invisible to the examiner. The vessel wall structure, which lacks pigment, allows visualization of the blood column. The retinal arteries are 25 percent narrower than the veins and reflect an arterial light reflex, which is a narrow band of light in the center of the convex blood column. The veins are darker in color than the arteries, and those near the disc generally display slight pulsations as venous blood is forced out of the eye during arterial systole. Occasionally, a light reflex may be seen on the veins, but it is not a continuous band as it is on the artery. The veins and arteries intertwine with each other, but normally do not displace one another. At the site of arterial-venous crossing, or AV crossing, the adventitia of each joins to form a sheath that surrounds both vessels. AV crossing sites are important for the examiner to assess, as displacement or AV nicking may indicate the occurrence of arteriosclerotic process.

The macula, which lies to the temporal side of the disc approximately 2 disc diameters away, is avascular and the area of the best vision owing to the high concentration of cones. The diameter of the macula is approximately one disc diameter. Located in the center of the macula is the fovea centralis, a central depression appearing as a small, bright light reflection. After the age of 50, this structure may not be visible. When visualized, it is inspected carefully for any lesions or neovascularization.

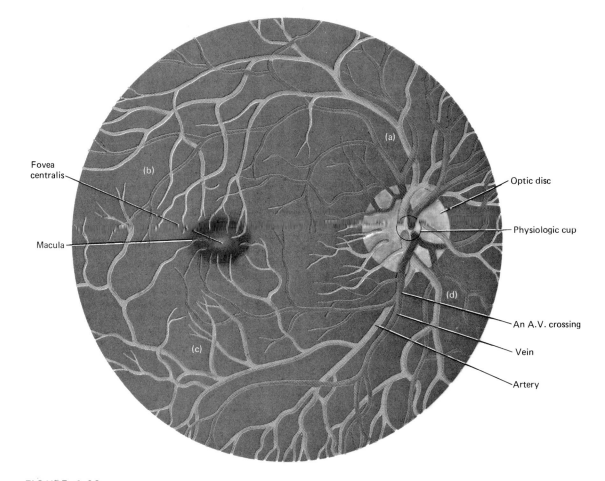

FIGURE 6-22
The structure and quadrants of the fundus of the eye: (a) superior nasal quadrant; (b) superior temporal quadrant; (c) inferior temporal quadrant; (d) inferior nasal quadrant.

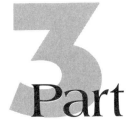

Part 3

STUDY GUIDE QUESTIONS

In the following client situations, identify and describe the subjective and objective data to be collected, the specific tools and procedures to be utilized in the collection of those data, and the rationale for the nursing assessment.

1. You are the community health nurse making the first visit to Mr. Jerold Daily's home. Mr. Daily, a 75-year-old widowed male, is experiencing difficulty caring for himself owing to visual problems.
2. Mrs. Sue Montae is concerned for her 1-year-old daughter Merilee's vision. She presents in your well-child clinic setting, complaining about Merilee's apparent ''cross-eyedness.''
3. You are functioning as a school nurse, and it is time to initiate eye screening for grades K, 1, 3, and 5.

SAMPLE FORMAT TO BE USED IN RESPONDING TO THE STUDY GUIDE QUESTIONS

SUBJECTIVE DATA TO BE COLLECTED	OBJECTIVE DATA TO BE COLLECTED	SPECIFIC TOOLS AND PROCEDURES TO BE UTILIZED	RATIONALE FOR NURSING ASSESSMENT

BIBLIOGRAPHY

ADLER, FRANCIS H., *Textbook of Ophthalmology.* Philadelphia: W. B. Saunders Company, 1962.

ALEXANDER, MARY M., and MARIE S. BROWN, *Pediatric Physical Diagnosis for Nursing,* pp. 48–70. New York: McGraw-Hill Book Company, 1974.

——, "Physical Examination, Part 5: Examining the Eye," *Nursing 73,* December 1973, pp. 41–46.

BROWN, MARIE S., and MARY A. MURPHY, *Ambulatory Pediatrics for Nurses,* pp. 201–214. New York: McGraw-Hill Book Company, 1975.

CAMPBELL, MILTON F., and others, "Funduscopy for the Office Clinician," *Patient Care,* December 1, 1976, pp. 84–92.

CERASOLI, JAMES R., and JAMES A. KIMBLE, "Common Eye Problems," *Primary Care,* pp. 137–160. Philadelphia: W. B. Saunders Company, March 1977.

CHINN, PEGGY L., and CYNTHIA J. LEITCH, *Handbook for Nursing Assessment of the Child.* Salt Lake City, Utah: University of Utah Printing Service, 1973.

DEGOWIN, ELMER L., and RICHARD L. DEGOWIN, *Bedside Diagnostic Examination* (3rd ed.), pp. 77–126. New York: Macmillan Publishing Co., Inc., 1970.

EVANS, WILLIAM F., *Anatomy and Physiology* (2nd ed.), pp. 207–225. Englewood Cliffs, N.J.: Prentice-Hall, Inc., 1976.

GORDON, DAN M., *The Fundamentals of Ophthalmoscopy.* Kalamazoo, Mich.: Upjohn Company, 1971.

HAVENER, WILLIAM H., *Synopsia of Ophthalmology* (4th ed.). St. Louis, Mo.: The C. V. Mosby Company, 1975.

HOLLINSHEAD, W. HENRY, *Textbook of Anatomy* (2nd ed.), pp. 901–921. New York: Harper & Row, Inc., 1967.

JUDGE, RICHARD, and GEORGE D. ZUIDEMA, *Physical Diagnosis: A Physiologic Approach to the Clinical Examination* (2nd ed.), pp. 75–100. Boston: Little, Brown and Company, 1968.

PRIOR, JOHN A., and JACK S. SILBERSTEIN, *Physical Diagnosis* (4th ed.), pp. 78–127. St. Louis, Mo.: The C. V. Mosby Company, 1973.

SPALTER, HAROLD F., and FREDERICK A. JAKOBIEC, "Macular Disorders Can Destroy the Eye's Area of Sharpest Vision," *Geriatrics,* April 1975, pp. 105–113.

STOCKER, FREDERICK W., and LAWRENCE W. MOORE, JR., "Detecting Changes in the Cornea That Come with Age," *Geriatrics,* May 1975, pp. 57–69.

THEODORE, FREDERICK H., "External Eye Problems in the Elderly," *Geriatrics,* April 1975, pp. 69–80.

7

The Nose

OBJECTIVES

1. Describe the structure of the nose.
2. Identify the functions of the nose.
3. Differentiate between and describe...
4. Identify the...
5. Discuss the...structures of the nose.
6. Internal...
7. Frontal and maxillary sinus...

REVIEW OF STRUCTURE AND FUNCTION

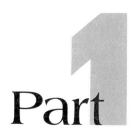

Part 1

STRUCTURE OF THE NOSE

The nose is composed of bone and cartilage. The frontal and maxillary facial bones are a part of the formation of the nasal bridge. Internally, the nose is divided into two passages by the septum, the medial wall of the internal nose. The anterior portion of the septum is cartilage; the posterior portion is composed of bone. The floor of the nose is formed by the palatine process of the maxilla; the roof is composed anteriorly by the frontal bone and posteriorly by the sphenoid bone. On the roof of the nose is the cribriform plate, which houses the olfactory nerve endings. Respiratory mucosa, a specialized tissue, lines the respiratory passages from the nasal vestibules to the bronchioles.

Arising from the lateral walls are the nasal turbinates, which run horizontally and appear as projecting elevations. The inferior turbinate has a thick mucosal membrane. It is composed of numerous venous plexuses and cavernous erectile tissue. The middle turbinate has a thick mucosal lining and is composed of the ethmoid bone; the superior turbinate is a thin mucosal projection

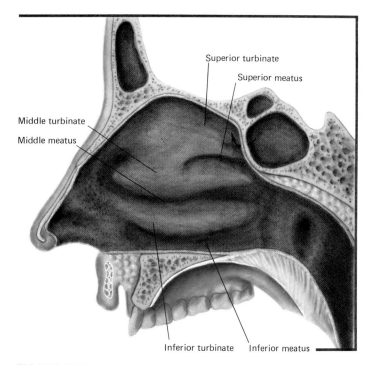

FIGURE 7-1
Anatomical location of the nasal turbinates.

from the ethmoid bone. The turbinates are bulbous anteriorly and diminish in size posteriorly (Figure 7-1).

FUNCTION OF THE NOSE

The major functions of the nose are the following:

1. Humidify air as it passes through the moist surfaces of the nasal mucous membrane. Some authorities state that the humidity of the air reaches up to 75 percent.

2. Elevate the temperature of the inflowing air up to 98.6°F as it passes over the extremely vascular surfaces of the turbinates.

3. Decontaminate the air by filtering out particles through the screening action of the hair and the mucous, which lines the mucous membrane.

4. Sense odors through the olfactory nerve endings, which protrude through the cribriform plate.

5. Resonate sound by amplifying and changing the timbre of the larynx sounds.

HEALTH ASSESSMENT OF THE NOSE

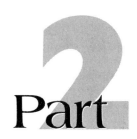
Part 2

INSPECTION

Inspection of the nose is initiated by close observation of the external structure. Note the facial appearance, color of the skin, presence or absence of swelling, and any external expression of pain or apprehension by the client. The nostrils are generally oval in shape and symmetrically positioned. The external nasal structures of the neonate appear less protruding than the adult, although the neonate has relatively wide nares. As growth ensues, protrusion and angulation become more prominent. The columna should be directly in the midline and should not exceed the diameter of each nostril in width. Fractures of the nasal bones can flatten or depress the bridge of the nose. Midline defects of the face or oral structures may present as marked deformities involving the nose (as in cleft lip and palate) or subtle deformities affecting only the nasal structure. These abnormalities can be readily identified by inspection of the nose in the immediate newborn period. Nasal flaring, a sign of respiratory distress in the infant, can be observed without difficulty. This sign is of little functional sig-

nificance but rather a primitive reflex in the newborn.

Observed or reported discharge is described in terms of its character, amount, duration, and location. The character of discharge may be watery, mucoid, purulent, crusty, or bloody. The amount is either slight, moderate, or profuse, and the duration is defined in specific terms of days, weeks, months, or years. The primary location of secretory drainage is from the nose (unilateral or bilateral nares) or from the nasopharynx into the pharynx. Nasal mucosa is described as deep pink, pale, congested, dry, hypertrophied, atrophied, or injected.

PALPATION

Palpate the external structure to determine any loss of support or presence of underlying lesions. To accomplish nasal palpation, the proper procedure is for the examiner to place one finger on each side of the nasal arch and gently palpate, moving the fingers from the bridge of the nose to the tip (Figure 7-2).

INSTRUMENTATION

Upon reaching the tip of the nose, the patency of the right and left nares can be determined by digital compression of one nostril at a time. Patency of the nares in the newborn is essential, because most newborns are obligatory nose breathers. Instrumentation is therefore recommended to rule out choanal atresia (a surgical emergency) in the newborn. The passage of a size 5 to 10 Fr. catheter down both nares confirms their patency. If partial occlusion of one nostril exists, the sound produced by forced expiration through the nose has a higher pitch in the adult and child when compared to forced expiration in a nonoccluded nose. If total obstruction of one nostril is present, the client will not be able to inspire or expire through the noncompressed naris (Figure 7-3).

Examination of the internal nares can be accomplished with the use of a light and a special nasal speculum, or with the otoscope head and the short, wide speculum attachment. Place your right hand on the client's forehead. This allows the examiner to control the tilt of the head for adequate visualization. If using the otoscope head, visualization may be facilitated if the thumb of the right hand can be placed on the nose tip with gentle upward pulling pressure (Figure 7-4). Internal nares inspection is generally not performed in the neonate.

Landmarks of the nares that should be noted during inspection are the vestibule, nasal septum, Kiesselbach's plexus, the inferior turbinate, and the middle turbinate (Figure 7-5).

1. The **vestibule** is the segment of the nose that contains hair follicles. Hair is generally more prominent in males and appears to thicken with age. The most common abnormality in the vestibule is inflammation of the hair follicles. The mucous membrane covering the vestibule should be deep pink in color and glistening.

2. The **nasal septum** is composed of bone and cartilage, which is covered by deep pink mucosa. The septum is not always straight, is never uniform in size, and is usually not exactly in the midline. It is thicker anteriorly than posteriorly. Deviations of the nasal septum are of no significance unless they occlude the nasal airway or, although not totally occluding the airway, create clinical problems. Two examples from an acute-care setting are when oxygen catheters or nasogastric tubes are being inserted. Septal lesions or

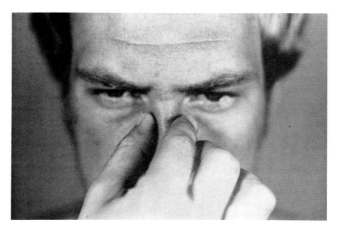

FIGURE 7-2
Palpation of the nose.

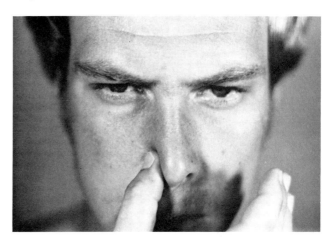

FIGURE 7-3
Assessment of the patency of the nares.

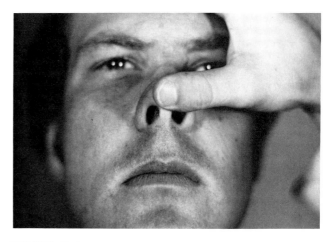

FIGURE 7-4
Placement of the examiner's hand in assessment of the internal nasal structures.

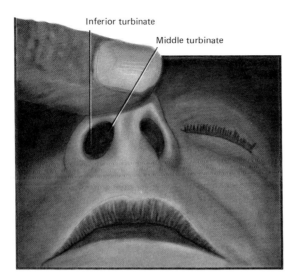

FIGURE 7-5
Anterior view of the nasal turbinates.

perforations can be caused by nose "picking," a nervous habit, or by sniffing drugs.

3. **Kiesselbach's plexus** is the convergence area of small, fragile arteries and veins located superficially on the anterior superior portion of the septum. It is commonly the site of many nose bleeds.

4. The **inferior turbinate** is a separate structure from the middle or superior turbinate. It is composed of erectile tissue and swells with irritation. Bilaterally, the inferior turbinates are generally not the same size. In individuals with pronounced allergies, the color of the inferior turbinates is bluish gray or pale pink, and its consistency is that of being swollen and boggy. Normally, its color is deep pink and its consistency appears firm.

5. The **middle turbinate** and the **superior turbinate** are rarely seen upon inspection of the internal nose from the anterior position.

The sinuses serve as resonating chambers and decrease the weight of the skull. The sinuses are lined with mucous membrane and possess cilia that mobilize secretions and move them along excretory pathways (Figure 7-6). Direct percussion of the frontal and maxillary sinuses will elicit any existing tenderness. Direct percussion is instituted utilizing the middle finger to strike the sinus area (Figure 7-7).

Wrist action should produce the force behind the finger and not the finger itself. The sinuses can be transilluminated with a special instrument if consolidation of mucus in the sinus is suspected. This examination is performed in a darkened room. The sinus cavities should illuminate clearly unless filled with exudate.

FIGURE 7-6

Anatomical location of the nasal sinuses from infancy to adulthood.

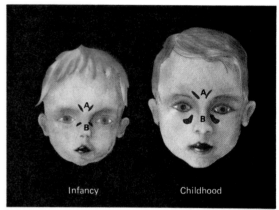

Infancy   Childhood

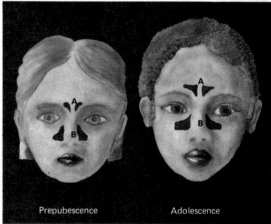

Prepubescence   Adolescence

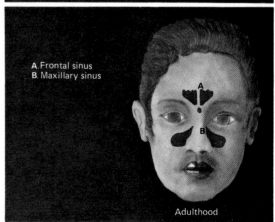

A. Frontal sinus
B. Maxillary sinus

Adulthood

114

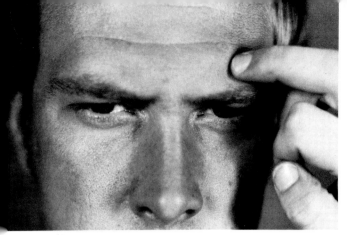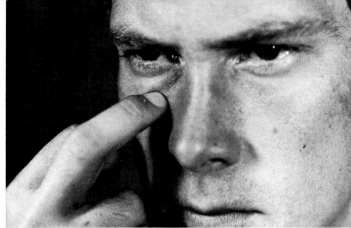

(a)   (b)

FIGURE 7-7
Direct percussion of the facial sinuses: (a) frontal; (b) maxillary.

STUDY GUIDE QUESTIONS

Part 3

In the following client situations, identify and describe the subjective and objective data to be collected, the specific tools and procedures to be utilized in the collection of those data, and the rationale for the nursing assessment.

1. John Kennedy, a 16-year-old male, enters the school clinic for the routine physical assessment to participate in sports. He reports that he broke his nose 1 year ago but received no medical intervention.
2. Marvin Jones is a 6-year-old male who is brought to the clinic by his father, who states that the child has a stuffy nose, nasal discharge, and a cough.
3. You are evaluating the nasal patency in Susan Rite, a 3-day-old infant.

SAMPLE FORMAT TO BE USED IN RESPONDING TO THE STUDY GUIDE QUESTIONS

SUBJECTIVE DATA TO BE COLLECTED	OBJECTIVE DATA TO BE COLLECTED	SPECIFIC TOOLS AND PROCEDURES TO BE UTILIZED	RATIONALE FOR NURSING ASSESSMENT

BIBLIOGRAPHY

ALEXANDER, MARY M., and MARIE S. BROWN, *Pediatric Physical Diagnosis for Nurses,* pp. 86–93. New York: McGraw-Hill Book Company, 1974.

BROWN, MARIE S., and MARY M. ALEXANDER, "Physical Examination, Part Nine: Examining the Nose," *Nursing 74,* July 1974, pp. 35–38.

DEGOWIN, ELMER L., and RICHARD L. DEGOWIN, *Bedside Diagnostic Examination* (3rd ed.), pp. 126–139. New York: Macmillan Publishing Co., Inc., 1976.

HOLLINSHEAD, W. HENRY, *Textbook of Anatomy* (2nd ed.), pp. 921–931. New York: Harper & Row, Inc., 1967.

PRIOR, JOHN A., and JACK S. SILBERSTEIN, *Physical Diagnosis* (4th ed.), pp. 161–168. St. Louis, Mo.: The C. V. Mosby Company, 1973.

8

The Mouth and Oropharynx

OBJECTIVES

1. Identify the structures of the mouth and oropharynx.
2. Identify additional landmarks of the mouth and oropharynx.
3. Describe the examination of the structures within the mouth.
4. Evaluate the integrity of the oral cavity.
   (a) Gum movement.
5. Characteristics of the oral mucosa.
6. Number, shape, and color of the teeth and integrity of both mouth and gum.
7. Characteristics and movement of the tongue.
8. Characteristics of the hard and soft palate.
9. Integrity of the cavity, mouth and teeth of the mouth.
10. Structures of the posterior oropharynx.

The primary function of the mouth or oral cavity is the reception of foodstuffs into the body. However, the oral cavity houses many structures with equally important functions. The external boundaries of the mouth include the cheeks (buccae) and lips (labia). The cheeks are normally symmetrical and rounded somewhat, but the shape of the cheeks varies with inherited genetic factors, the body structure, and nutritional and hydration states of each individual. The coloring of the cheek's integument is dependent upon genetic factors and sun exposure. The texture of the surface of the cheeks varies with age and sex. In the young child, the cheeks are smooth and soft, a characteristic that is also common to the female until postmenopause. The postpubertal male has a visible hair growth pattern on the cheeks, which is not true of the female. The extendability of the cheeks allows for interim storage of received foodstuff awaiting mastication and swallowing.

The lips aid in removing food from eating and drinking utensils, in holding foods in place for the incisor teeth to bite, and in the formation of sounds. The upper lip generally protrudes over the lower lip; however, its shape and position is directly affected by the bony structures beneath, that is, the mandible, maxilla, and teeth. The lips are attached to the facial structure by the frenula, which are located midline on the internal surface of the upper and lower lips (Figure 8-1).

The oral cavity is divided into two components, the vestibule and the mouth cavity proper. These components are separated by the teeth and gums. The vestibule is distal to the teeth and gums and is that area which comprises the internal surface of the cheeks and lips. The mouth cavity proper is that portion which houses the tongue and is proximal to the teeth and gums (Figure 8-2).

The oral mucosa is an extension of the skin but, because of its thinness, is more susceptible to trauma than the external integument. It is highly vascular, however, and therefore has a rapid healing capacity.

The purpose of the vestibule is to store food and maintain food on occlusive surfaces when mastication and initial lubrication of food with saliva are occurring. Two-thirds of the way back on the inner surface of the cheeks (in approximate alignment with the second upper molars) are Stensen's ducts. These ducts are the openings

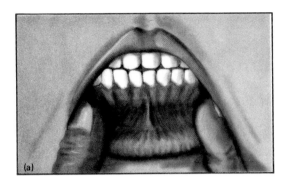

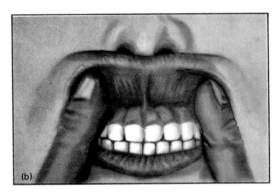

FIGURE 8-1

The oral frenula that secure the lips to the facial structures: (a) the inferior frenulum; (b) the superior frenulum.

FIGURE 8-2

The vestibule and mouth cavity proper.

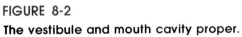

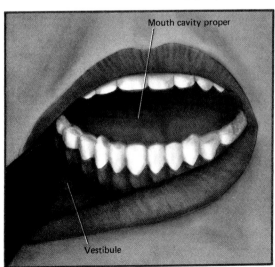

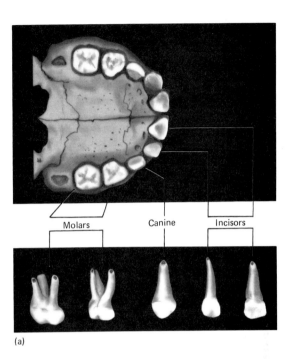

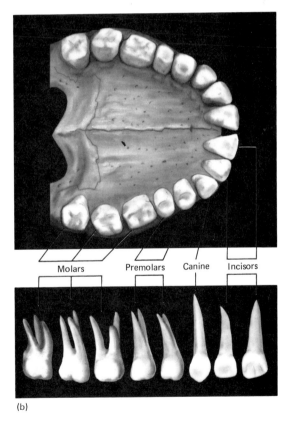

FIGURE 8-3

The teeth: (a) deciduous; (b) permanent; (c, next page) chronologic development of deciduous (primary) and permanent teeth.

Primary Dentition (chart)

Maxillary Teeth — columns: Central Incisor, Lateral Incisor, Cuspid, First Molar, Second Molar
Rows: 56 mos, 52 mos, 4 yrs., 44 mos, 40 mos, 3 yrs, 32 mos, 28 mos, 2 yrs, 20 mos, 16 mos, 1 yr, 8 mos, Birth, Conception

Mandibular teeth — rows: Conception, Birth, 4 mos, 8 mos, 1 yr, 16 mos, 20 mos, 2 yrs, 28 mos, 32 mos, 3 yrs, 40 mos, 44 mos, 4 yrs, 52 mos, 56 mos

Permanent Dentition (chart)

columns: Central Incisor, Lateral Incisor, Cuspid, First Biscuspid, Second Biscuspid, First Molar, Second Molar

Maxillary rows: 14 yrs, 13 yrs, 12 yrs, 11 yrs, 10 yrs, 9 yrs, 8 yrs, 7 yrs, 6 yrs, 5 yrs, 4 yrs, 3 yrs, 2 yrs, 1 yr, Birth, Conception

Mandibular rows: Conception, Birth, 1 yr, 2 yrs, 3 yrs, 4 yrs, 5 yrs, 6 yrs, 7 yrs, 8 yrs, 9 yrs, 10 yrs, 11 yrs, 12 yrs, 13 yrs, 14 yrs

How image corresponds to norms

Age root completed
Age tooth erupts into mouth
Age calcification of crown completed
Age organic matrix formation and calcification of crown begins

FIGURE 8-3 (continued)

(c) chronologic development of deciduous (primary) and permanent teeth.

120

for the secretions of the parotid glands. The secretions produced by the parotid glands and the other excretory glands in the mouth are called saliva. Saliva serves to moisten and lubricate foods, as well as to initiate starch and fat digestion. It further dilutes ingested liquids and foodstuffs that are acetic or alkaline, and cleanses the mouth after eating. Saliva also provides a lenitive and malacic effect to protect the mucosa and maintain a moist and softened surface within the mouth.

The teeth are primarily responsible for biting and mastication of solid foods. However, they also function as follows:

1. Prepare food for the swallowing process and increase the amount of surface exposure of ingested food to digestive secretions of the mouth and stomach.
2. Release chemical taste substances (which stimulate salivation) by means of the crushing action of the teeth.
3. Release volatile food components that in turn stimulate the olfactory nerve endings, thus resulting in palatability of food.
4. Detect hard or sharp materials that have the potential to cause trauma to the digestive tract.

Mastication, the act of chewing, generally ends in swallowing. Swallowing promotes removal of bacteria from the nasopharynx and pharynx. Bacteria is deposited by the nose, paranasal sinuses, middle ear, and through the action of the cilia, which pushes lung secretions up through the larynx into the oropharynx. In this manner, mastication serves as a protective as well as a preparatory digestive function.

Eruption of deciduous teeth begins at approximately 6 months of age and is complete at approximately 3 years of age. There are 20 deciduous teeth, including four incisors, two canine, and four bicuspids, on both the upper and lower jaws (Figure 8-3). The incisors are for biting, the canines for tearing, and the bicuspids for chewing or masticating foods. The deciduous teeth are replaced by 32 permanent teeth beginning at about 6 years of age. The permanent teeth include central incisors, lateral incisors, canines or cuspids, first and second premolars, and the first, second, and third molars on each side of the upper and lower jaws (Figure 8-3). The spacing

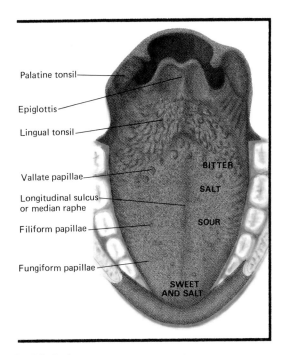

FIGURE 8-4

The anterior tongue, its papilla, areas of taste, longitudinal sulcus, and associated structures.

and alignment of teeth are dependent upon the size and shape of the jaw, as well as possible sucking habits of the individual during infancy. The teeth erupt from the gums. The gums provide integumentary protection for the roots of permanent teeth and the bony jaw.

The tongue is a muscular structure composed of striated muscle fibers. It aids in mastication of food, houses the taste receptors, and modifies voice sounds. Its anterior portion is called the **body,** the tip is termed the **apex,** and the posterior attached section is called the **base** or **root.** The medium sulcus divides the tongue longitudinally into the right and left halves. This sulcus is incomplete as it does not extend through the apex. The tongue is anchored to the back of the oral cavity at its base and to the floor of the mouth by the frenulum (Figure 8-4).

The anterior two-thirds of the tongue is covered with a thick mucosal membrane that protects the tongue during mastication and supports the multiple filiform and scattered fungiform papillae. The undersurface of the tongue is covered by a thin mucous membrane with ridges known as fimbriated folds. During mastication, the tongue serves to confine, shift, and return

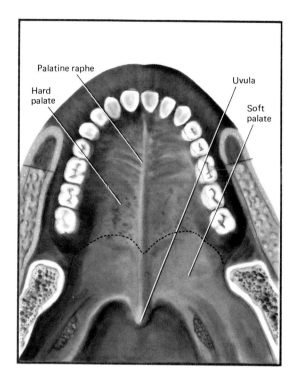

Palatine raphe

Hard palate

Uvula

Soft palate

FIGURE 8-5
The hard and soft palates.

food to the chewing surfaces of the teeth. It further carries food through the mouth for swallowing, mixes food with saliva, and aids in the removal of food particles from the teeth.

The roof of the mouth is made up of the hard and soft palates. Although the soft palate is composed of fibrous tissue, it is continuous with the bony hard palate (Figure 8-5). The soft palate rises during phonation and swallowing. Behind the palate lies the oropharynx. The uvula lies midline within the oropharynx and the tonsils. The pharyngeal lymph nodes or tonsils lie between the anterior and posterior pillars of the fauces. The oropharynx serves as a passageway for food, liquid, and saliva that is swallowed, as well as air inhaled via the mouth. It is likewise a passageway for air emitted from the body during vocalization or nonnasal expiration and for rejected foodstuffs emitted from the gastrointestinal tract. The middle ear communicates with the external atmosphere via the Eustachian tube, which opens into the oropharynx. The nasopharynx terminates at the base of the oropharynx at which point they both communicate with the larynx and esophagus.

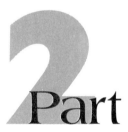

Part

HEALTH ASSESSMENT OF THE MOUTH AND OROPHARYNX

INSPECTION

A systematic assessment of the mouth and oropharynx begins with inspection of the external boundaries of the mouth, the cheeks, and the lips. The cheeks are normally symmetrical, although their shape and contour vary with each individual; for example, an obese individual has rounded cheeks owing to fat deposits, whereas the emaciated individual presents an in-drawn look. In the adult male, the number of hair follicles and color of the hairs varies with each person. The adult female has skin of smoother con-

sistency than the male, and has, generally, some extremely light hair, although variations of the amount and color exist dependent upon genetic factors. An excess amount of facial hair in the female is known as **hirsutism.** Blood vessels are generally not visualized through the surface of the external cheek.

The teeth play an important role in the appearance and position of the lips. In the absence of teeth, the labial structures may appear shrunken or concave, thus giving the mandible a more protruding appearance. The skin of the lips is thin, and thus the numerous underlying vascular structures give the lips their reddish appearance. When the oxygen-carrying power of the blood or oxygen delivery via the blood is decreased, the reddish hue of the lips takes on a bluish color. This is called **cyanosis**. The surface characteristics of the lips should be smooth and free of any lesions (Figure 8-6). Dehydration or wind chapping can cause peeling of the tissue, which results in the appearance of dry and cracked lips. This scaling of tissue predisposes the lips to infections as the first line of defense is interrupted.

In the newborn, sucking calluses (Figure 8-7) are frequently observed as crust or plaques on the outer epithelial layer of the upper lip. They are the result of friction created by sucking activity. These calluses generally persist for the few first weeks of life.

To inspect the oral mucosa of the vestibule, use a tongue blade to separate the internal cheek from the teeth and gums. A small pen light will serve to illuminate the cavity so that adequate visualization can be obtained. In the infant, visualization is best achieved when the child is crying. The mucous membrane of the vestibule is differentiated from the skin of the lips at the general curvature of the lips. The appearance of the mucous membrane is normally pinkish-red in color, smooth, and moist. Oral mucosa that is darkly pigmented may be indicative of endocrine pathology. Frequently, beginning with school-age children, scars that may be whitish or pinkish and appear to protrude above the buccal surface can be seen on the buccal membrane in a line that is parallel to the occlusal line. Scarring can be due to convulsions, poor tooth alignment, accidental biting, or from biting on the cheeks out of nervous habit. In the newborn, sucking pads can be observed and palpated within the cheek structure bilaterally. Stensen's duct, a small whitish-yellow or whitish-pink protrusion in approximate alignment with the second upper molar, is generally visible on inspection. In a person with mumps, the orifice of the duct becomes reddened.

Inspect the teeth for wear, notching, cavities, and missing members. Any of these conditions may lead to disruption of the occlusive surfaces, thereby lessening the grinding action of the teeth. With the tongue blade, probe the teeth to determine if they are firmly anchored. Loose teeth can be indicative of an inflammatory process or trauma. In the newborn, tooth buds may be visible; however, neonatal tooth eruption in the first

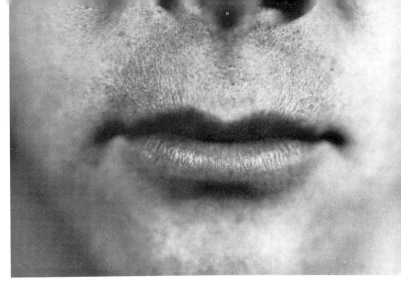

FIGURE 8-6
Surface characteristics of normal lips.

few weeks of life is infrequent. Often, if predeciduous neonatal teeth are present, they are removed prior to discharge from the hospital. This is done to prevent aspiration of the tooth by the neonate, as these teeth often loosen and dislodge without warning.

The color of the teeth is generally ivory, but variations exist. Yellow teeth can be the result of tobacco use; brownish-black tartar deposits can be due to calcium salts contained in the saliva. If the client has artificial dentures, they should be removed to completely assess the mouth. In clients who have lost or had all teeth extracted, the alveolar process is resorbed, and the angle of the jaw changes.

FIGURE 8-7
Sucking calluses in the infant.
(Photo courtesy of Mead Johnson.)

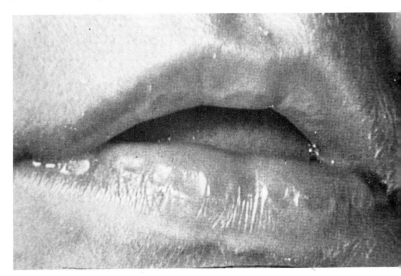

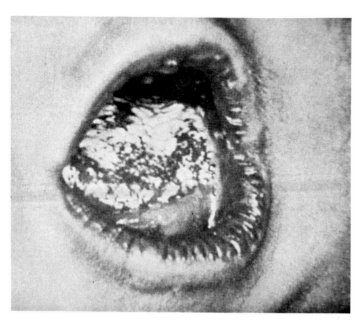

FIGURE 8-8
The appearance of thrush in the newborn.
(Photo courtesy of Mead Johnson.)

The normal color of Caucasian gums is pink. In blacks, gums are bluish in color and may contain brown pigmented areas. The gums should be solid in turgor, nonpainful when probed with the tongue blade, and with edges that are tightly approximated to the teeth. If the gums bleed easily upon brushing or upon gentle probing with the tongue blade, the integrity of the gums is questionable.

The anterior two-thirds of the tongue presents a smooth, yet roughened surface to the observer.

FIGURE 8-9
Assessment of the neuromuscular integrity of the tongue by observing protrusion of the tongue: (a) normal —midline; (b) abnormal—lateral deviation.

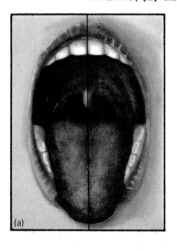
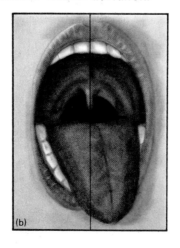

(a)   (b)

The posterior one-third presents itself as a smooth, slightly uneven or rugated surface with a mucosa that is thin in comparison to the anterior two-thirds. The anterior and posterior thirds of the tongue are separated by a V-shaped sulcus called the **sulcus terminalis.** The general color of the tongue is dull red, although frequently a thin white coating distorts the color. This is especially noticeable after a night's sleep, as the activity level of the tongue has decreased. This whitish coating should not be confused with thrush in the newborn, which presents as a cheesy white coating and cannot be displaced by gentle scraping with a tongue blade (Figure 8-8).

Movement of the tongue is enhanced when it is well lubricated by saliva. If the mouth is dry, as occurs in states of dehydration or anxiety, tongue movements become clumsy and slow. This can be noted in the client's poorly articulated speech.

Upon the examiner's request, the client protrudes the tongue out of the oral cavity. The tongue is assessed for (1) maintaining a midline position, (2) deviations to either the right or left, (3) fasciculations, and (4) atrophy. In the elderly, minute tremors may be observed on the apex of the tongue during its protrusion (Figure 8-9).

Inspect the horizontal plane and lateral margins of the tongue. Any white or bright red areas should be scraped with a tongue blade to determine if they are food particles or fixed abnormalities. If abnormalities are present, they should be described and recorded accurately. In the newborn, note the size of the tongue. It should fit the floor of the mouth appropriately. A tongue too large may indicate slowed mental development. A tongue of normal size, which rhythmically protrudes from the mouth, may indicate increased intracranial pressure.

Ask the client to place the tongue on the roof of the mouth. If able to demonstrate this action, the twelfth cranial nerve (hypoglossal) is intact. When the client has the tongue touching the roof of the mouth, inspect the visible portions of the floor of the mouth. Note the lingual ducts on each side of the frenulum, a structure that anchors the tongue to the floor of the mouth. Cancerous lesions are frequently seen in this area. Congenitally, the frenulum may be shorter than normal, producing a condition called tongue-tie or **ankyloglossia.** This condition affects the mobility of the tongue and may be reflected in the client's speech patterns. Figure 8-10 illustrates the anatomical location of the sublingual ducts.

The undersurface of the tongue appears smooth, pink, and moist. Because of the thin surface membrane of the posterior tongue, vessels may be visible between the frenulum and fimbriated folds.

Examination of the oropharynx requires the examiner to place the tongue blade two-thirds of the way onto the tongue, near the V-shaped sulcus. Push down and pull forward with the tongue blade. This action prevents the tongue from obstructing the view of the posterior oropharynx. The hard palate is a bony plate covered by mucous membrane and presents a pale pink, almost whitish color. It gives the appearance of being irregular as it possesses transverse rugae. The hard palate may also have a bony palatine protuberance called the **torus,** which is observed in the midline of the hard palate.

The soft palate is continuous with the hard palate and is much pinker in color. Upon observation, fine vessels are frequently prominent through the mucosa. In the neonate, Epstein's pearls may be visualized at the juncture of the hard and soft palate and appear as small whitish-yellow masses. Bohn's nodules may appear on the alveolar surface of the gums. These superficial lesions are keratin-containing cysts and appear as sperm or white or grayish nodules. These lesions are spontaneously shed in a few weeks and are of no pathological significance.

Evaluate the movement of the soft palate by having the client vocalize the syllable "ah." The soft palate normally rises during vocalization. If problems exist with the ninth and tenth cranial nerves, the palate sags on the affected side and movement is lacking during phonation (Figure 8-11). To assess the newborn's palate, palpate the hard and soft palate to ensure intactness and thereby establish the absence of a cleft.

Normally, the uvula remains in midline position during phonation. If it deviates laterally during phonation, pathology of the ninth and tenth cranial nerves is again indicated. The direction in which deviation occurs demonstrates which side is unaffected by problematic processes.

Last, inspect the tonsils, which lie deep in the oropharynx (Figure 8-12). They are normally pink and blend into the coloring of the pharynx. The tonsils enlarge in size until puberty and then diminish in size. The tonsils may have crypts in which whitish material collects. This material can be cell debris or food particles. If the tonsils are

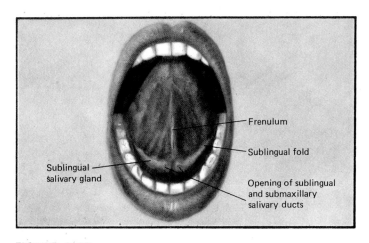

FIGURE 8-10
Location of the sublingual and submaxillary duct openings within the oral cavity.

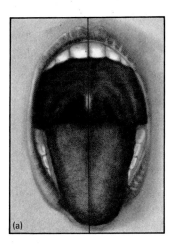 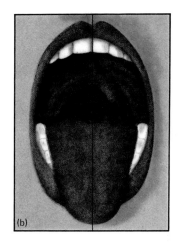

FIGURE 8-11
Assessment of soft-palate movement during phonation: (a) symmetrical; (b) asymmetrical.

inflamed, they become reddened and may accumulate patches of exudate. Edema, which occurs during inflammatory processes, results in tonsil enlargement of varying degrees. This can be unilateral or bilateral. The oropharynx should be an unobstructed passage, and webs or other membranous lesions should be noted.

Stimulate the gag reflex by placing the tongue blade at the base of the posterior oropharynx. Gagging demonstrates that the ninth and tenth cranial nerves are intact. Diminished or absent gag reflex indicates needed evaluation for nutritional intake via routes other than oral, as well as referral for medical diagnosis and therapy.

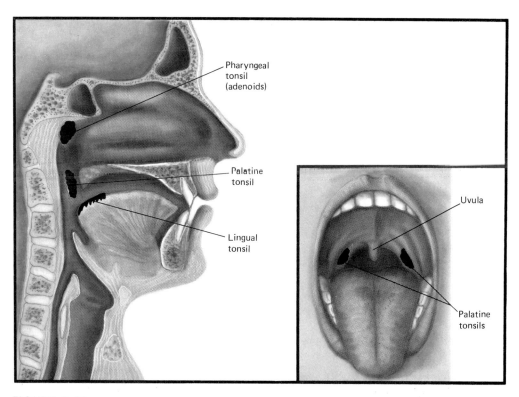

FIGURE 8-12
Anatomical location and assessment of the palatine tonsils.

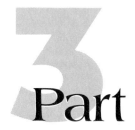

Part

STUDY GUIDE QUESTIONS

In the following client situations, identify and describe the subjective and objective data to be collected, the specific tools and procedures to be utilized in the collection of those data, and the rationale for the nursing assessment.

1. Lucy, a 2-week-old infant, presents in clinic with her 18-year-old mother, Linda Smith, for routine well-baby care. As you proceed through your assessment of the infant, you note, upon inspection of the mouth, grayish-white nodules at the junction of the hard and soft palate and a whitish material coating the tongue.

2. At your initial home visit of Mrs. Emma Kelsy, a 66-year-old widow, she complains to you of painful gums that bleed easily.

3. Bob Johnson, a 22-year-old male, complains to you, the company nurse, of a severe sore throat that is interfering with his eating and drinking.

SAMPLE FORMAT TO BE USED IN RESPONDING TO THE STUDY GUIDE QUESTIONS

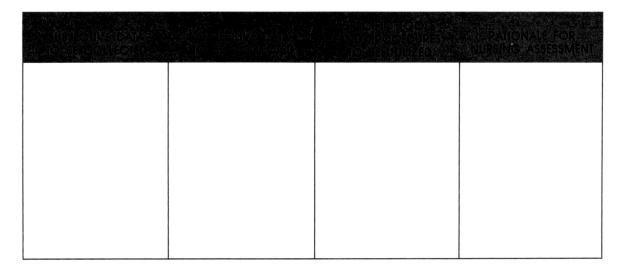

SUBJECTIVE DATA TO BE COLLECTED	OBJECTIVE DATA TO BE COLLECTED	EXAMINATION TOOLS AND PROCEDURES TO BE UTILIZED	RATIONALE FOR NURSING ASSESSMENT

BIBLIOGRAPHY

ALEXANDER, MARY M., and MARIE S. BROWN, *Pediatric Physical Diagnosis for Nurses,* pp. 95–109. New York: McGraw-Hill Book Company, 1974.

BROWN, MARIE S., and MARY M. ALEXANDER, "Physical Examination, Part 10: Mouth and Throat," *Nursing 74,* August 1974, pp. 57–61.

BURNSIDE, JOHN W., *Adam's Physical Diagnosis* (15th ed.), pp. 74–80. Baltimore, Md.: The Williams & Wilkins Company, 1974.

HOLLINSHEAD, W. HENRY, *Textbook of Anatomy* (2nd ed.), pp. 802–851, 933–954. New York: Harper & Row, Inc., 1967.

JONES, H., "Oral Ulceration," *Nursing Times,* October 18, 1973, pp. 1361–1363.

KLOUGH, GERTRUDE, and HAROLD N. NIEBEL, "Oral Cancer Detection—A Nursing Responsibility," *American Journal of Nursing,* April 1973, pp. 684–686.

KRULL, EDWARD A., ARNOLD C. FELLMAN, and LOIS A. FABIAN, "White Lesions of the Mouth," reprint from *Clinical Symposium,* 25, no. 2, 1973.

PRIOR, JOHN A., and JACK S. SILBERSTEIN, *Physical Diagnosis* (4th ed.), pp. 145–161. St. Louis, Mo.: The C. V. Mosby Company, 1973.

9
The Neck

REVIEW OF STRUCTURE AND FUNCTION

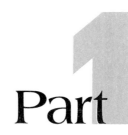

Part 1

Within the neck there are vital organs and structures that are essential to the well-being of the individual. The following is a list of the most important structures in the neck:

1. Thyroid gland
2. Trachea
3. Esophagus
4. Carotid arteries
5. Jugular veins
6. Lymph glands (nodes)
7. Sternocleidomastoid muscle
8. Trapezius muscle
9. Cervical vertebra surrounding the spinal cord

THYROID GLAND

The thyroid gland is composed of two lobes positioned on each side of the trachea and connected anteriorly by the thyroid isthmus (Figure 9-1). The thyroid gland is highly vascular, resulting in a rich blood supply to facilitate the uptake of iodine. Iodine is utilized in the production of

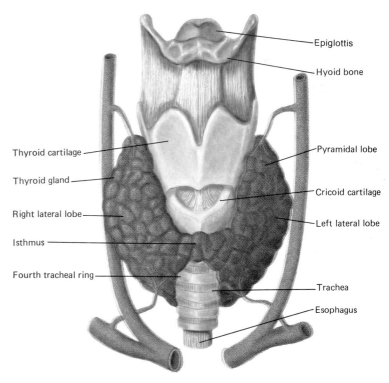

FIGURE 9-1

Anatomical location of the thyroid gland.

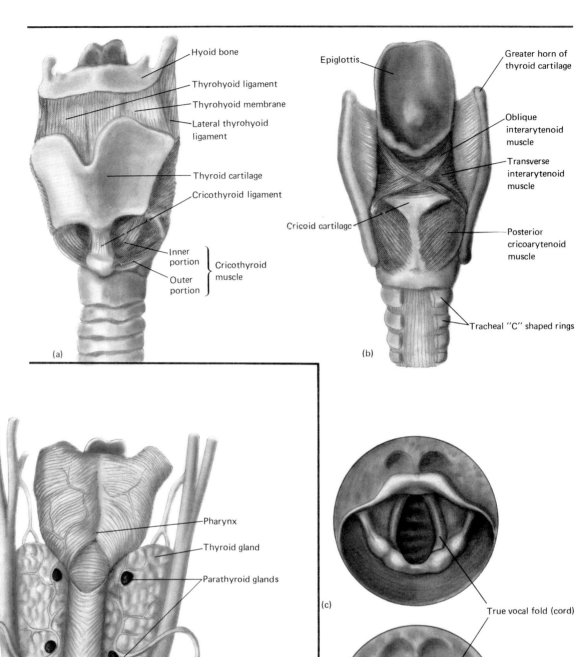

(a)

(b)

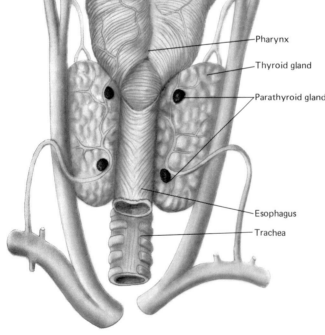

Pharynx

Thyroid gland

Parathyroid glands

Esophagus

Trachea

FIGURE 9-2

Anatomical location of the
parathyroid glands.

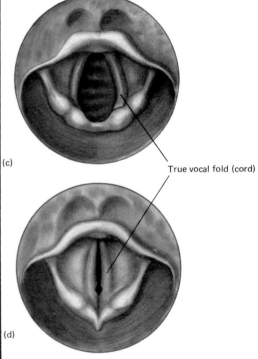

(c)

True vocal fold (cord)

(d)

FIGURE 9-3

The larynx: (a) anteriolateral view;
(b) posterior view; (c) true vocal
folds open; (d) true vocal folds closed.

thyroxin and triiodothyronine, the two thyroid hormones that regulate the rate of all basic cellular processes. An excess of thyroid hormone production (hyperthyroidism) yields a faster rate at which the system functions, resulting in an increased amount of energy utilized. An insufficient amount of thyroid hormone production (hypothyroidism) results in a decreased metabolic rate and a decreased need for energy intake.

The parathyroid glands are a group of four endocrine glands that either lie beneath or behind the upper and lower poles of the thyroid gland, or they may be embedded within the thyroid gland (Figure 9-2). The parathyroids control the levels of calcium and phosphorus circulating in the blood. If the circulating volume of calcium is low, this hormone activates a process through which calcium can be liberated from the bones, thereby increasing the amount in the blood.

The oropharynx is funnel shaped with its lower section leading to the esophagus and the larynx. The larynx contains the vocal cords (Figure 9-3). As air passes the cords while they are voluntarily approximated during exhalation, a sound is emitted. Immediately below and connected to the larynx is the trachea, which is cylindrical in shape and approximately 10 to 15 cm in length. Tracheal support, which is needed to prevent collapse of the structure, is derived from C-shaped cartilages (Figure 9-3) that are united by elastic ligaments. The incomplete section of the cartilage is on the posterior surface of the trachea. As the trachea descends, it disappears at the base of the neck behind the greater vessels and sternum. Between the levels of the sternal angle and the seventh thoracic vertebra, the trachea bifurcates into the right and left bronchi. The point of tracheal bifurcation is called the carina. Two of the main functions of the trachea are to provide an initial airway to the lungs and a route through which secretions from the lungs can be discharged.

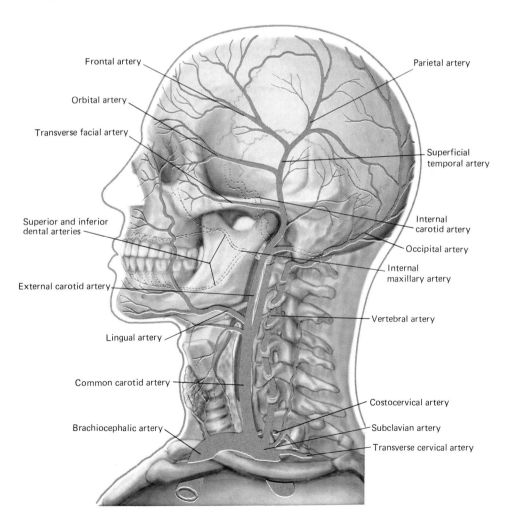

FIGURE 9-4

Major arteries of the head and neck.

Immediately posterior to the trachea is the esophagus, which extends from the pharynx to the stomach. The esophagus is a tubelike structure that passes through the diaphragm, a muscular barrier that prevents abdominal contents from entering into the chest cavity. The two main functions of the esophagus are to provide a route for ingested substances and to provide an outlet for materials offensive to the gastrointestinal system.

Bilateral to the anterior midline of the neck lie the carotid arteries. The common carotid artery on the right branches off from the brachiocephalic artery, while the left branches from the arch of the aorta. The common carotid arteries divide into the external and internal carotids and provide the blood supply to the head (Figure 9-4).

JUGULAR VEINS AND VENOUS PRESSURE

The jugular veins, the largest vessels in the neck, are located adjacent to the carotid arteries and provide a channel through which deoxygenated blood from the head returns to the heart. Bilaterally, the internal jugular vein terminates approximately 2.5 cm lateral to the sternoclavicular junction. At this point, it forms the innominate vein as it joins with the subclavian vein. The internal jugular vein forms the jugular bulb 2 to 3 cm superior to the medial portion of the clavicle. This is approximately in the depression between the two insertion points of the sternocleidomastoid muscles. In some individuals, the internal jugular vein may be anatomically located behind the sternocleidomastoid muscle.

The external jugular vein descends from the skull in a pathway that overlies the sternocleidomastoid muscle. It passes through the muscle and terminates behind the clavicle, where it joins the subclavian vein. Interference with a steady flow of venous return causes variation in the flow volume, resulting in visible volume waves or venous pulses. These flow waves are reflective of pressure gradients within the venous system. In the healthy state the pressure is highest in the distant venules, such as those in the extremities, and lowest in the vena cavas. The factors influencing venous pressure gradients are the volume of venous return flow entering the venous

system, vessel compliance and resistance, the patency or occlusive state of the venous system, and the competency of venous valves. The ability of the heart's right chamber to eject the volume of blood it receives and the tricuspid valve competence, which prevents backflow of blood, also affect venous pressure gradients.

Venous volume waves may consist of three or four vein pulsations, or positive deflections and two volume falls or negative deflections (Figure 9-5). The first positive deflection or pulsation is

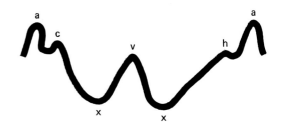

FIGURE 9-5
Venous volume waves.

the a wave, the largest venous wave, and occurs prior to atrial systole (atrial contraction). The second positive deflection is the c wave, which occurs during ventricular systole. The third positive deflection or wave is termed the v wave, and it occurs during late systole or early diastole. The negative deflections consist of the x and y depressions. The x depression occurs during atrial diastole; the y depression occurs during early ventricular diastole.

LYMPH NODES

The positions of the major lymph glands (nodes) of the neck are illustrated in Figure 9-6. The lymph glands are small bodies of lymphatic tissue enclosed by a fibrous connective tissue sac. They are found along the pathway of lymphatic vessels. Lymph is plasmalike fluid that contains white blood cells, especially lymphocytes. It is generally clear, although after a meal, lymph from the intestine contains fat globules that give it a milky appearance. Lymph passes through several nodes or glands prior to emptying into the venous blood. Lymph glands facilitate the filtering of red blood cells and bacteria, while adding lymph, globulin, and antibodies to the blood. The lymph glands are essentially ineffective in filtering out and destroying viruses.

CERVICAL MUSCLES AND VERTEBRAE

The sternocleidomastoid muscles originate from the sternoclavicular junctions and insert into the mastoid portion of the temporal bone bilaterally (Figure 9-7). This pair of muscles functions in the following manner:

1. The right sternocleidomastoid muscle draws the head to the right side.
2. The left sternocleidomastoid muscle draws the head to the left side.
3. The right and left sternocleidomastoid muscles together move the head forward.

The origin of the trapezius muscle begins at the base of the occipital bone and extends to the twelfth thoracic vertebra (Figure 9-8). Its insertion point is in the acromial process of the clavicle. Its function is to pull the head to the side and rotate the scapula.

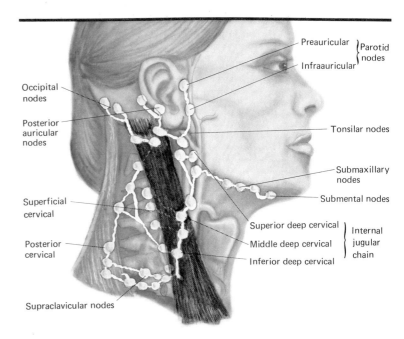

FIGURE 9-6
Anatomical location of the lymph glands in the neck.

FIGURE 9-8
Anatomical location of the trapezius muscle.

FIGURE 9-7
Anatomical location of the sternocleidomastoid muscle.

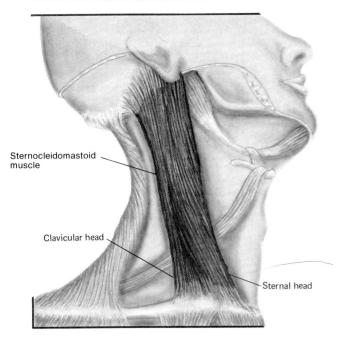

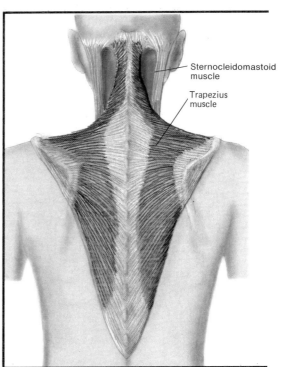

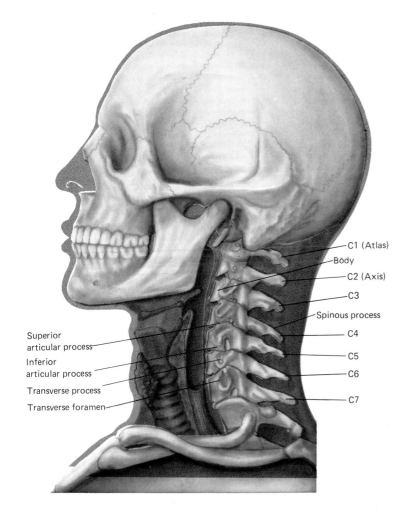

C1 (Atlas)
Body
C2 (Axis)
C3
Spinous process
C4
C5
C6
C7

Superior articular process
Inferior articular process
Transverse process
Transverse foramen

The vertebrae provide a protective enclosure for the spinal cord. Between each vertebra, nerve branches exit and extend toward the periphery. The vertebral bodies also provide structural support to the body, enabling the erect position to be maintained. The cervical vertebrae (Figure 9-9) are the smallest vertebral bodies of the spinal column. They are movable, allowing the head to change position. The seven cervical vertebrae are identified by number, beginning at the base of the skull: C1 (also called the atlas), C2 (also called the axis), C3, C4, C5, C6, and C7. Figure 9-9 identifies each of these vertebrae as well as examples of the main features of most vertebrae (body, spinous process, superior articular process, inferior articular process, and transverse process) and also the most outstanding feature of the cervical vertebrae, the transverse foramen.

FIGURE 9-9
The cervical vertebrae.

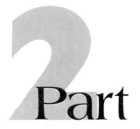
Part

HEALTH ASSESSMENT OF THE NECK

Systematic assessment is performed using the skills of inspection, palpation, and auscultation. The examiner first identifies key landmarks and regions that assist in the systematization of data collection. The muscular landmarks of the neck are the sternocleidomastoid and trapezius muscles. Subdivisions of the nuchal region consist of the anterior, lateral, and posterior regions.

INSPECTION

Inspect the integument of the neck for color, tone, and presence or absence of lesions. The size, shape, and symmetry of the neck are observed by comparing the anterior, lateral, and posterior triangles of the neck and the submandibular area (Figure 9-10). In the obese individual, the neck may appear asymmetrical owing to the fatty deposits. In the newborn, the neck appears short with multiple skin folds. The skin within these folds frequently remains moist and is prone to inflammation and tissue breakdown.

Inspect the supraclavicular area, including the suprasternal notch (Figure 9-11), which is immediately in front of the trachea. Retraction of the skin of the suprasternal notch on inspiration may indicate air hunger. At times, pulsation may be seen in this area. This can be due to an elongated aorta, which is considered a variation of normal.

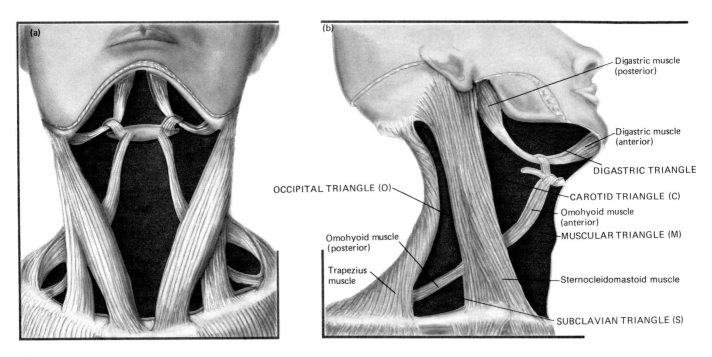

(a)

(b)

Digastric muscle (posterior)

Digastric muscle (anterior)

DIGASTRIC TRIANGLE

OCCIPITAL TRIANGLE (O)

CAROTID TRIANGLE (C)

Omohyoid muscle (anterior)

MUSCULAR TRIANGLE (M)

Omohyoid muscle (posterior)

Trapezius muscle

Sternocleidomastoid muscle

SUBCLAVIAN TRIANGLE (S)

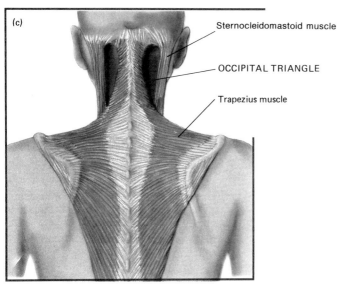

(c)

Sternocleidomastoid muscle

OCCIPITAL TRIANGLE

Trapezius muscle

FIGURE 9-10

The triangles of the neck:
(a) anterior region;
(b) left lateral region;
(c) posterior region.

Assessment of the venous pressure can be accomplished in several ways. Increased venous pressure may be the result of congestive heart failure, hypervolemia, and other pathological states. With the client supine, relaxed, and neck in neutral alignment with the body, determine the level of distention of the external jugular veins bilaterally. Normally, in this position, these veins are fully distended from the base of the neck to the angle of the jaw. Visualization of this distention is facilitated by viewing the right and left lateral neck regions obliquely (Figure 9-12).

FIGURE 9-11

The supraclavicular area and the suprasternal notch.

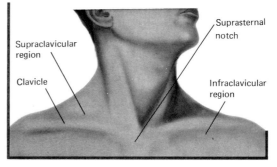

Supraclavicular region

Clavicle

Suprasternal notch

Infraclavicular region

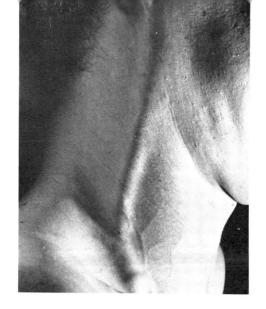

FIGURE 9-12
Oblique view of distended cervical veins.

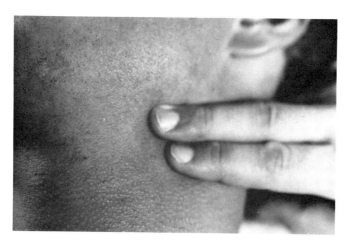

FIGURE 9-13
Occlusion of the external jugular vein immediately below the jaw to assess the direction of venous filling.

FIGURE 9-14
Occlusion of the external jugular vein immediately above the clavicle to assess the height of venous distension.

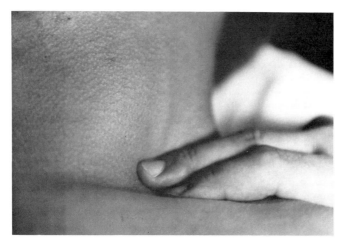

With the client supine and hips semiflexed to an angle of 15 to 35 degrees, the examiner may proceed with one of the several procedures to assess venous pressure.

1. Occlude the external jugular vein immediately below the jaw (Figure 9-13). In this maneuver, the direction of venous filling is determined. Normally, the proximal segment of the vein will collapse, resulting in distention at a lower level. The level of distention may fluctuate with respiration. When compression of the jugular vein fails to result in collapse, the segment proximal to the occlusion may be milked with digital compression in a downward direction. This process should result in collapse of the vein. Upon collapse, veins that fill from the lower segment result in a jugular distention level indicative of high venous pressure.

2. Occlude the external jugular vein immediately above the clavicle for 30 seconds (Figure 9-14). This time period allows the vein to fill and become distended. With the release of venous occlusion, observe the height of vein distention by the fluid column. Normally, this distension is several millimeters above the clavicle.

3. Place the client in a supine position at a 45 degree angle. It is important that flexion occur only at the hips, and that the neck remain in a neutral position. Next, identify the level of the manubrium sterni and then observe the height of venous distention bilaterally. The level of distention above the manubrium sterni may vary between 1 and 2 cm. Cervical vein distention over 2 cm is abnormal. An extremely elevated venous pressure may cause the cervical veins to distend up to the level of the jaw angle. Unilateral venous distention may indicate abnormalities such as kinking of the left innominate vein, aortic arch aneurysm, or the presence of arteriosclerotic processes.

4. Observe the internal jugular vein for venous pulse waves. Normally, they appear as slow undulating movements. Abnormal waves may be large and are easily recognized. Pulsations observed need to be differentiated from arterial pulses prior to assessing the undulating movements.

5. Manual pressure applied over the abdomen

in the region of the liver for approximately 1 minute may result in a minimally increased or decreased level of venous distention. If a rise in the jugular distention level occurs and remains continuous while abdominal pressure is applied, it is indicative of increased venous pressure. This maneuver is called the *hepatojugular reflux.*

INSPECTION AND PALPATION

Following the assessment of venous pressure, the carotid arteries are inspected for pulsations. Generally, this pulsation, if visible, is located near the anterior edge of the sternocleidomastoid muscle. Palpation is initiated by locating the right carotid artery with the index finger and second and third digit, and noting the regularity, rate, rhythm, and quality of the pulsation. Second, in the same manner, palpate the left carotid artery for regularity, rate, rhythm, and quality. Third, bilateral comparison is made by palpating the right and left carotid arteries simultaneously. Normally, the pulsation rate, regularity, rhythm, and quality are the same. Light palpation is used to assess the carotids, as deep palpation may occlude the carotid arteries, especially if pathology is present. It is important not to rub the carotid arteries, as this may result in reflex slowing the heart, or bradycardia.

AUSCULTATION

Auscultation of the vascular structures in the neck is performed to assess the presence or absence of bruits and venous hums. Bruits are murmurs in the peripheral arteries. They are medium- to high-pitched, and best auscultated with the bell of the stethoscope. Bruits are described by their pitch, intensity of sound, and point of occurrence within the cardiac cycle. The carotid artery is auscultated beginning at the base of the neck and moving gradually toward the skull. Bruits that increase in intensity as the skull is approached generally originate intracranially; bruits that increase in intensity toward the base of the neck frequently originate from the greater vessels or the heart. Venous hums are continuous, low- to medium-pitched humming sounds that occur in the cervical veins of many children and young adults, and are of greatest intensity when the client is sitting and inspiring. Venous hums can be readily stopped by occluding the jugular veins at the base of the neck. They are generally considered to have little significance, but must be discriminated from a bruit.

PALPATION

Lymph Nodes

In assessing the lymph nodes the neck is palpated anteriorly, laterally, and posteriorly. Several methods may be used to accomplish this procedure. The examiner may place the left hand on the client's head, enabling control of head movements in any direction, and thereby making the major nodal areas more accessible (Figure 9-15). The right hand is then used to palpate the areas overlying the nodes. A second method is to palpate the bilateral neck regions with the right and left hand simultaneously (Figure 9-16). Palpation of the lymph nodes is performed with the palmar surface of the fingers moving in a gentle circular motion, exerting only light pressure.

Examine in sequence the sites of lymph nodes (Figure 9-17), as identified in the following listing.

1. Postauricular nodes: lie bilaterally behind the auricle, overlying the mastoid process.
2. Superficial cervical nodes: lie bilaterally behind the posterior border of the upper half of the sternocleidomastoid muscle.
3. Supraclavicular nodes: lie bilaterally superior to the clavicle in the region of the clavicular sternocleidomastoid muscle origin.
4. Jugular nodes: lie bilaterally along the anterior border of the sternocleidomastoid muscle.
5. Preauricular nodes: lie bilaterally in front of the auricle.
6. Submaxillary nodes: lie beneath the angle of the jaw bilaterally.
7. Submental nodes: lie under the chin on either side of the midline.
8. Suboccipital nodes: lie in the apex of the cervical triangle in the posterior neck.
9. Posterior cervical nodes: lie bilaterally in front of the upper margin of the trapezius muscle.

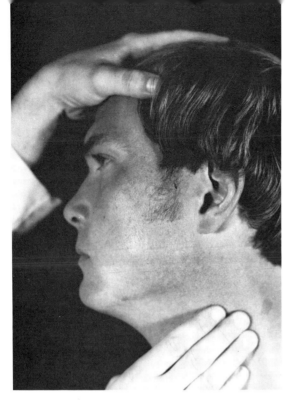

FIGURE 9-15

Unilateral palpation of the cervical lymph nodes, using one hand to control and support the position of the head.

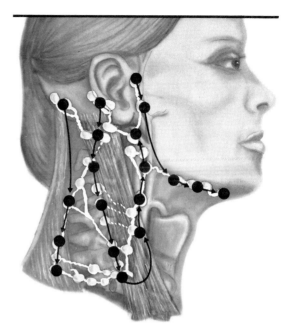

FIGURE 9-17

A systematic and sequential method of palpating the lymph nodes.

Generally, most lymph nodes are not palpable, although an occasional node is found to be enlarged, firm, nontender, and mobile. This is generally of the submental or submandibular nodes. Frequently, these nodes are enlarged owing to inflammatory processes such as tonsillitis or pharyngitis. Shotty nodes are characterized by small and firm nodes that are clustered. This finding is most frequently within normal limits. Abnormal lymph glands are those which may be swollen, hard, tender, bunched, or matted and adherent to the skin or underlying structures.

FIGURE 9-16

Bilateral palpation of the cervical lymph nodes.

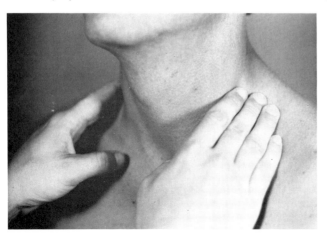

Thyroid Gland

Palpation of the thyroid gland requires care and gentleness, as well as considerable practice with validation. Palpation of the thyroid gland by the beginning-level practitioner may be inappropriate, depending upon the nurse's role and use of collected data, and is presented here only to encourage awareness and understanding of the process.

Palpation of the thyroid gland for surface characteristics, consistency, size, and shape may be accomplished by one or several maneuvers.

1. Anterior palpation is accomplished with the examiner in front of the client. The client is requested to tilt the head laterally, or the examiner may inform the individual of what is going to transpire and proceed to gently grasp the head and tilt it in an optimal lateral flexed position. This position reduces the tension of the sternocleidomastoid muscle, thus facilitating palpation of the gland. The examiner displaces the thyroid cartilage from the side on which the sternocleidomastoid muscle is tense. Dis-

placement may be accomplished with the thumb while the fingers rest on the neck or with three fingers closely approximated. With the fingers of the opposite hand, on the side of the relaxed sternocleidomastoid muscle, grasp the thyroid on the medial or medial posterior portion of the lateral lobe while the thumb is on the anterior aspect of the lateral lobe. Frequently, the thumb is also palpating a section of the thyroid isthmus. Once the thyroid gland is grasped, the client is requested to swallow. It is during the movement produced by swallowing that the characteristics of the thyroid gland are assessed (Figure 9-18). This process is repeated for assessment of the opposite lateral lobe.

2. Posterior palpation is accomplished with the examiner facing the client's back. The client is requested to tilt the head to the right or left side, or the examiner may explain to the client what is about to transpire and tilt the head in a lateral flexed position. Displacement of the thyroid in the direction of the side that is to be palpated is best accomplished with three fingers while the thumb rests on the posterior neck region (Figure 9-19). The opposite hand then grasps the thyroid. The fingers palpate the anterior portion of the lateral lobe while the thumb palpates the medial or medial–posterior section of the thyroid's lateral lobe. The client is again requested to swallow and, during this movement, the thyroid is assessed. This process is repeated for the opposite lateral thyroid lobe.

3. Simultaneous palpation of the anterior right and left lateral thyroid lobes is accomplished by placing the fingers of the right and left hand anterior to the sternocleidomastoid muscle and slightly displacing it posteriorly while the client's neck is slightly flexed (Figure 9-20). The client is requested to swallow, and the anterior and medial portion of the right and left lobes can be assessed.

4. Anterior palpation of the thyroid isthmus may be performed by direct, gentle, forward pressure applied immediately above the cricoid cartilage. While the client swallows, the isthmus is assessed.

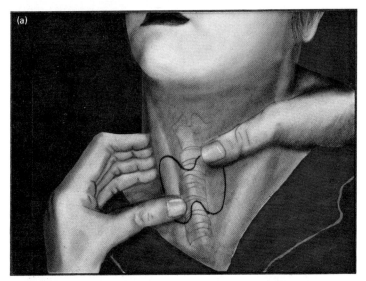

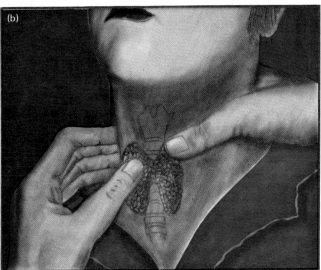

FIGURE 9-18

Anterior palpation of the thyroid:
(a) displacement of the trachea;
(b) palpation of the thyroid with the examiner facing the client.

FIGURE 9-19

Posterior palpation of the thyroid with the examiner behind the client.

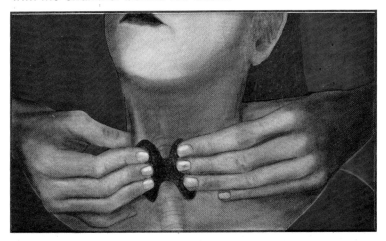

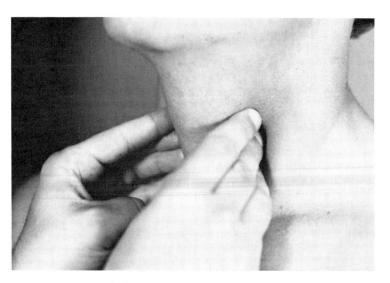

FIGURE 9-20
Bilateral palpation of the lateral lobes of the thyroid gland.

FIGURE 9-21
Range of motion of the neck:
(a) flexion; (b) extension;
(c) hyperextension;
(d) lateral bending;
(e) lateral rotation.

5. The presence or absence of thyroid enlargement of the lower lobe can be assessed by placing a finger on each side of the trachea in the suprasternal notch. The client is requested to swallow, and the presence or absence of lower lobe enlargement is determined.

6. Enlargement of the thyroid that creates compression of the trachea may be assessed by applying gentle compression of the lateral lobes of the thyroid. If tracheal compression is present from an enlarged thyroid, the increase in compression may cause stridor as the client inspires deeply. This process is called **Kocher's test.**

The normal characteristics of the thyroid gland include a smooth surface, firm consistency, nontender to gentle pressure, and weight of approximately 15 to 20 g. Nodules, asymmetrical lobe enlargement or bilateral enlargement, and hardness are abnormal findings and require fur-

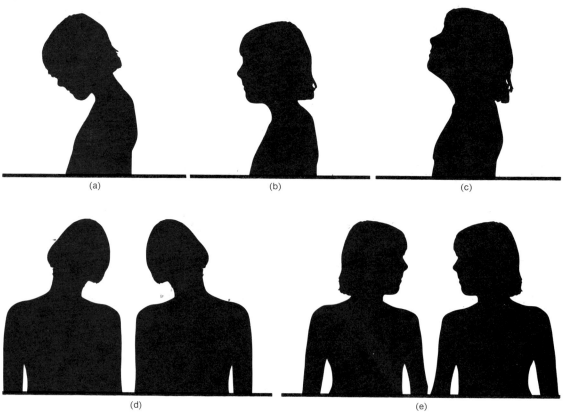

(a)   (b)   (c)

(d)   (e)

ther expert follow-up and referral. The thyroid gland is enlarged when it is 25 g or larger.

The final step of assessing the thyroid gland is accomplished through auscultation. The diaphragm is utilized to ascertain the presence of bruits. Bruits may arise when the highly vascular gland becomes hyperplastic and velocity of blood flow is increased. Normally, bruits are not present in the thyroid gland.

RANGE OF MOTION

Mobility of the cervical spine is evaluated through active and passive range of motion. Active range of motion is assessed by requesting the client to demonstrate neck mobility by following the examiner's demonstration of moving the head forward, right, left, back, and then circular. When passive range of motion is utilized to assess mobility, the examiner is able to ascertain any clicks or grating sensations in the cervical spine

area. When assessing the infant, passively turn the head from side to side to determine mobility. The normal ranges of motion are flexion of 45 degrees, extension of 0 degrees, hyperextension of 45 degrees, rotation to the right and left of 45 degrees, and lateral bending to the right and left of 45 degrees (Figure 9-21).

From middle age on, the most common problem causing limited cervical spinal mobility is arthritis. Limitation of movement is varied depending upon the degree of affliction. Arthritis may produce a grating sound on passive movement owing to fibrotic tissue changes and cartilaginous degeneration. Reflex muscle spasm or protective splinting may be present in the trapezius and sternocleidomastoid muscles unilaterally or bilaterally. The degree of muscle spasm may affect the position in which the head is held. On palpation these muscles feel taut and hard in consistency. Decreased ranges of motion in the newborn may indicate a congenital vertebral anomaly or trauma to muscle, bone, or nerves.

STUDY GUIDE QUESTIONS

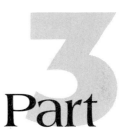

Part 3

In the following client situations, identify and describe the subjective and objective data to be collected, the specific tools and procedures to be utilized in the collection of those data, and the rationale for the nursing assessment.

1. Carolyn Krimp, an obese 25-year-old female, states her neck feels full and tight.

2. Mr. John Bohem, a 55-year-old male, is hospitalized with a medical diagnosis of congestive heart failure. You are to determine the level of venous distention of the external jugular veins.

3. Mrs. Peggy Quinn is a 40-year-old single female, 5 ft 8 in. tall and weighing 160 lb, who presents for a physical examination. You have computed the assessment of the head and are ready to initiate the assessment of the neck in the apparently well client.

4. Mrs. Pamela Guthrie and her 6-week-old daughter have returned for a 6-week well-baby check. Mrs. Guthrie's concern about the baby's status is that she refuses to breast feed on the right side and does not actively turn her head to the left.

SAMPLE FORMAT TO BE USED IN RESPONDING TO THE STUDY GUIDE QUESTIONS

SUBJECTIVE DATA TO BE COLLECTED	OBJECTIVE DATA TO BE COLLECTED	SPECIFIC TOOLS AND PROCEDURES TO BE UTILIZED	RATIONALE FOR NURSING ASSESSMENT

BIBLIOGRAPHY

BUCKINGHAM, WILLIAM R., MARSHALL SPORBERG, and MARTIN BRANDFONBRENER, *A Primer of Clinical Diagnosis*, pp. 32–42. New York: Harper & Row, Inc., 1971.

COLMAN, ARNOLD L., *Clinical Examination of the Jugular Venous Pulse*. Springfield, Ill.: Charles C Thomas Publisher, 1966.

GORDON, EVERETT J., *Diagnosis and Treatment of Common Neck Disorders*. Northridge, California: Riker Laboratories, Inc., 1976.

HOCHSTEIN, ELLIOT, and ALBERT L. RUBIN, *Physical Diagnosis*, pp. 72–84. New York: McGraw-Hill Book Company, 1964.

HOLLINSHEAD, W. HENRY, *Textbook of Anatomy* (2nd ed.), pp. 758–790. New York: Harper & Row, Inc., 1967.

HOPPENFELD, STANLEY, *Physical Examination of the Spine and Extremities*, pp. 105–132. New York: Appleton-Century-Crofts, 1976.

PRIOR, JOHN A., and JACK S. SILBERSTEIN, *Physical Diagnosis*, pp. 71–77. St. Louis, Mo.: The C. V. Mosby Company, 1973.

SCHLANT, ROBERT C., and J. WILLIS HURST, "Assessment of Cardiac Function at the Bedside," *Geriatrics*, June 1975, pp. 49–53.

The Chest and Pulmonary System

10

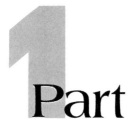

Part 1

REVIEW OF STRUCTURE AND FUNCTION

CHEST

The right and left sides of the chest can be seen as separate but interdependent components of the chest. Each side of the anterior and posterior chest has major landmarks. The landmarks of the anterior chest are as follows:

1. Suprasternal notch
2. Right and left supraclavicular area
3. Right and left clavicular area
4. Right and left mid-clavicular area
5. Right and left infraclavicular area
6. Right and left mammary area
7. Right and left hypochondriac area

Figure 10-1 illustrates the location of the anterior landmarks as numbered.

The landmarks of the posterior chest wall are as follows:

1. Seventh cervical vertebra (it is normally the protruding vertebra in the cervical column)
2. Right and left suprascapular area
3. Right and left scapulae

4. Right and left inferior scapular tip
5. Right and left infrascapular area
6. Interscapular area
7. Mid-vertebral column

Figure 10-2 illustrates by number the location of the landmarks of the posterior chest wall.

The axillary area is also divided for descriptive purposes. Figure 10-3 illustrates the anterior, mid, and posterior division of the axillary chest wall.

Anatomical sites on the anterior chest wall can be used to approximate locations on the posterior chest wall. The suprasternal notch is located immediately superior to the sternum, with the angle of Louis in alignment with the second rib anteriorly and the fifth thoracic vertebra posteriorly. The xiphisternal articulation is in approximate alignment with thoracic vertebrae nine to eleven.

The skin of the chest is generally lighter in color than the face, except in sun exposure, and is characteristic of the individual's main complexion. The skin should present a smooth appearance without nodules or flakiness. In the male, when sexual maturation has occurred, the secondary sex characteristic of chest hair appears,

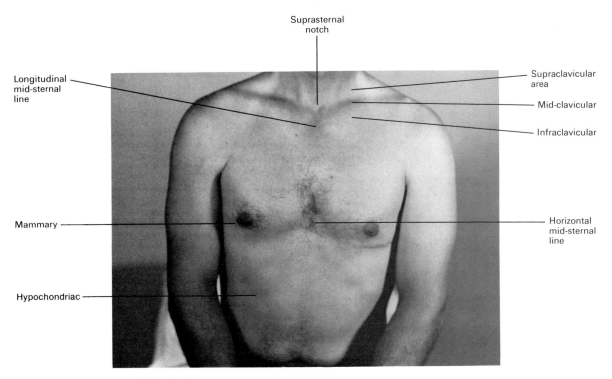

FIGURE 10-1
Landmarks of the anterior chest.

FIGURE 10-2
Landmarks of the posterior chest.

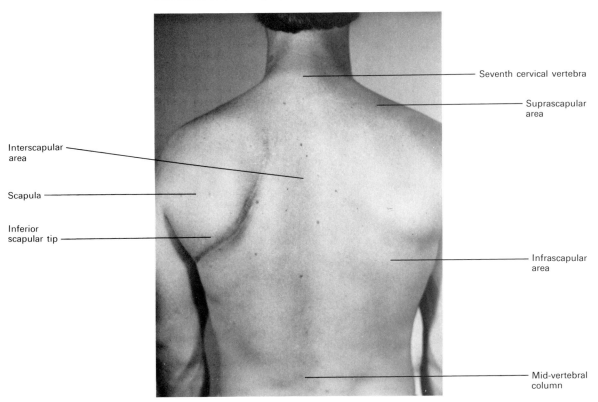

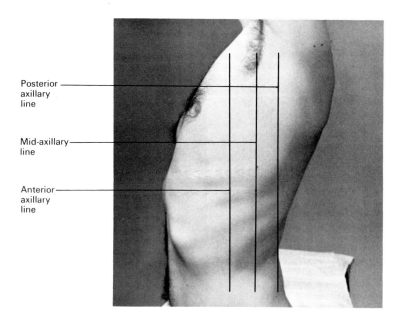

Posterior
axillary
line

Mid-axillary
line

Anterior
axillary
line

FIGURE 10-3
Divisions of the axillary region of the thoracic wall.

and varies in amount and color with the individual. Frequently, in the elderly male, the hair thins and looses its coarse characteristic. Females may present with little if any hair on the chest; however, if present, it is generally sparse, fuzzy, and light in color. Development of the mammary glands occurs with sexual maturation of the female. A more thorough discussion of the breast has been deferred to Chapter 12.

RESPIRATORY SYSTEM

The respiratory system begins with the nose, progresses to the trachea, then into the left and right bronchi at approximately the second rib anteriorly and the fifth thoracic vertebra posteriorly. These bronchi further bifurcate many times, leading to the air sacs of the lungs, called the **alveoli.** It is within the alveoli where gas exchange between the lungs and blood occurs.

The process of respiration can be divided into internal and external respiration. Internal respiration is carried out by exchange of oxygen (O_2) and carbon dioxide (CO_2) at the cellular level in the alveoli. Carbon dioxide is diffused from the

blood, and oxygen is consumed by the blood. The level of circulating carbon dioxide in the blood stimulates the respiratory center in the brain to activate the external component of respiration. External respiration is demonstrated by the active muscular process of inspiration and passive expiration, and it is observed as the rise and fall of the chest. The normal resting rates of external respiration for various age groups are as follows:

1. Newborn: generally 30 to 60 per minute.
2. Infant: 20 to 40 per minute.
3. Young child: 15 to 25 per minute.
4. Preadolescent and adult: 10 to 24 per minute.

The movement of the chest during the respiratory cycle is created by active muscular contraction. Costal respirations, also known as thoracic, are often shallow to medium in depth and are observed as an upward and outward expansion of the chest. Abdominal respirations are frequently of a medium to increased depth. They are observed as abdominal movement, which is created by the descent of the diaphragm. Thoracic respirations are more characteristic of women; men tend to be abdominal breathers. During sleep, most individuals breathe with the diaphragm muscle only. Newborns and children up to the approximate age of 7 are abdominal breathers.

The respiratory system possesses several protective mechanisms. Coughing is a forced expiratory volume of air that can clear obstructive materials such as mucus from the airways. Sneezing, similar to the cough, also serves to clear the airways. Yawning is a mechanism that forces the individual to inspire deeply, thereby creating greater expansion of the lungs, particularly in those alveoli that are not fully expanded during normal inspiration.

Several of the basic functions of the pulmonary system can be summarized into the following three categories:

1. Maintain adequate gas exchange.
2. Assist in maintaining an appropriate acid–base balance.
3. Assist in regulating the secretion of water from the body.

HEALTH ASSESSMENT OF THE CHEST AND PULMONARY SYSTEM

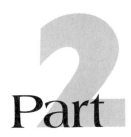

INSPECTION

Assessment of the chest begins with identification of landmarks. These prominent locations are used to describe more accurately where an abnormality or area of concern is found. The mammary area is appropriate to use only when describing the breast. The anatomical location, size, and shape of the breast vary so greatly among individuals that description becomes inaccurate when attempting to record or report thoracic findings to other health-care team members. Figure 10-4 illustrates an area of concern that may be hypothetically described as a circular lesion, 1 cm in diameter, located in the right mid-clavicular, mid-sternal intersection.

After identifying the landmarks, observe the shape of the chest. In the infant, the chest presents a very rounded, almost barrel appearance (Figure 10-5). As the child progresses toward adulthood, the lateral chest becomes broader than the anterior–posterior chest (Figure 10-6).

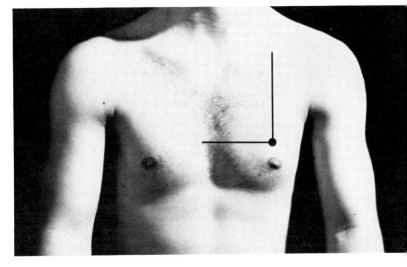

FIGURE 10-4
Using landmarks of the anterior chest, this lesion's location would be described as being "at the point of right midclavicular-midsternal intersection."

FIGURE 10-5
Chest contours of the young child: (a) an infant; (b) a toddler.

(a)

(b)

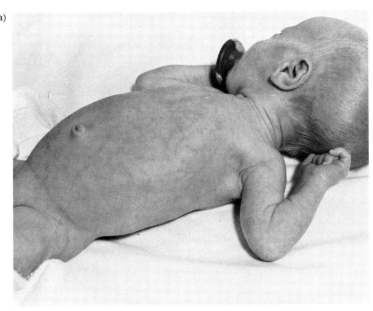

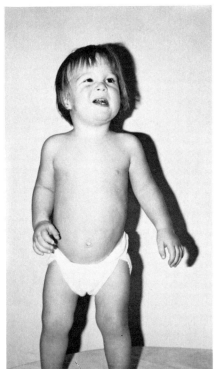

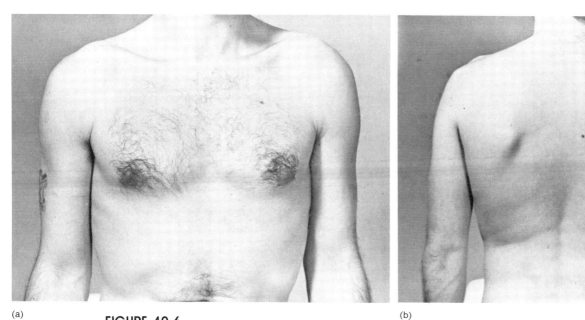

(a) (b)

FIGURE 10-6
Chest contours of an adult: (a) anterior; (b) posterior.

FIGURE 10-7
Abnormal concavity of the lower sternum:
pectus excavatum. Courtesy of William
Brennom, M.D., St. Paul, Minnesota.

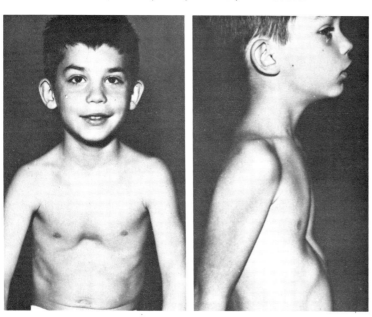

FIGURE 10-8
Abnormal convexity of the lower sternum:
pectus carinatum, or pigeon chest.

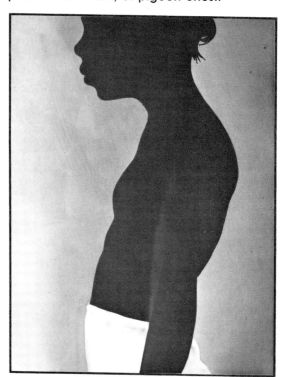

This growth results in an anteroposterior to lateral ratio of 1:2 or 5:7. Frequently, in the elderly, without an underlying disease process, the ratio diminishes as the anteroposterior diameter increases. Pectus excavatum, or funnel chest (Figure 10-7), presents as a concavity of the lower segment of the sternum. A severe degree of sternal depression may affect the anteroposterior to lateral diameter ratio. Pectus carinatum, or pigeon chest (Figure 10-8), presents an increased anteroposterior diameter and the anterior chest is accentuated in a forward direction. Deviations of the spinal column, such as kyphosis, may also affect the shape and diameter of the thoracic wall.

Inspect the skin for color, dimpling, and presence of lesions. If lesions, such as nevi, are found, inquire as to the duration of their existence and changes in size and color. Carefully observe for areas of skin irritation, such as the bra line, especially in obese women. In males, note the pattern, type, and amount of chest hair. A common occurrence in men is folliculitis, an inflammation of the hair follicle. Muscles of the chest, especially in the region of the neck and shoulders, are inspected for evidence of hypertrophy. Hypertrophy in this region can be associated with emphysema; however, this finding is not uncommon in athletes.

Following inspection of the skin on the anterior and posterior chest walls assess the respiratory pattern. This assessment should include observation of rate and pattern, type and depth, symmetry of chest expansion, and position assumed by the individual to facilitate respiration.

The type of respiratory movement is determined by the primary motion associated with inspiration and expiration. An upward and outward movement of the chest is called **thoracic respiration;** movement of the abdominal wall is called **abdominal respiration.** Respirations are then recorded as thoracic or abdominal. Depth of respiration is assessed by observing the excursion of thoracic structures and diaphragm. In the adult male, deep inspiration produces an excursion of 5 to 7.5 cm. Depth of respirations is more readily assessed through observation of the abdomen in the neonate, since they are obligatory diaphragmatic breathers.

Symmetry of chest expansion is assessed by comparing the right and left sides of the thoracic wall while the individual inspires and expires.

Normally, the thoracic wall should expand evenly and equally. If there is any asymmetry in chest wall expansion, it is described and recorded. Asymmetrical expansion can occur if one lung is functioning normally, but the other is congested, as in pneumonia. If this is the case, the chest wall of the involved side may not expand as much as the uninvolved side. The normal, healthy individual does not assume any specific supportive position to facilitate the respiratory process.

In infants and children, inspection of the thoracic structures, especially the interspaces, is most important. In the infant, there is an increased amount of soft tissue and cartilage, resulting in a smaller amount of bony structure and more flexibility. Respiratory distress can frequently be observed by retraction of the intercostal spaces during inspiration. Bulging of the intercostal spaces may indicate abnormal changes in intrathoracic pressures, and is associated with the expiratory phase of respiration in the adult or child. Retraction and bulging of the intercostal spaces may be seen in the same client.

Inspiration and expiration equal one complete respiratory cycle. To calculate the respiratory rate for 1 minute, observe and count the number of respiratory cycles for 30 seconds. The total is then multiplied by 2 to ascertain the rate for 1 minute. If an individual presents with any degree of respiratory distress, the respiratory cycles should be counted for a full minute.

The normal respiratory pattern is described as one of ease, without excessive exertion to inhale or exhale, with inhalation being active, whereas expiration is passive. In adults, the observed ratio of inspiration expiration is 2:3; in children the ratio is 1:3. Abnormally, the expiratory phase may be prolonged, as in emphysema. When prolonged expiration occurs, the client will frequently purse the lips during the expiratory phase, thereby increasing expiratory pressure. The major types of respirations observed in a clinical setting are presented in Table 10-1.

PALPATION

After assessing the thoracic cage and pulmonary system through inspection, palpation is implemented. Place your finger pads on the skin surface, and use a gentle circular motion to

TABLE 10-1

Some of the Major Types of Respirations

TYPE OF RESPIRATIONS	RATE	RHYTHM	DEPTH	RESPIRATORY CYCLE
EUPNEA	Adult: 10 to 25 Child: 15 to 25 Infant: 30 to 60	Smooth Even	Variable	Inspiration active; expiration passive
TACHYPNEA OR POLYPNEA	Increased	Regular or irregular	Within normal range or decreased	Inspiration active; expiration passive
BRADYPNEA	Decreased	Regular or irregular	Normal to increased	Inspiration active; expiration passive
APNEA	Variable	Irregular	Variable	Inspiration active; temporary cessation in the resting expiratory phase
HYPERPNEA	Normal or increased	Regular	Increased	Inspiration active, usually prolonged; expiration passive
CHEYNE–STOKES	Variable	Rhythmic increases and decreases in regularity	Sequential changes from increased to decreased depth	Inspiration active; expiration passive with recurring periods of apnea
HYPERVENTILATION	Increased	Regular or irregular	May be of increased depth	Inspiration active; expiration passive; respiratory cycle shortened
HYPOVENTILATION	Decreased	Regular or irregular	Decreased	Inspiration active; expiration passive; respiratory cycle lengthened
KUSSMAUL BREATHING; AIR HUNGER; GASPING	Variable generally	Regular or irregular	Increased	Inspiration active; expiration passive
APNEUSIS	Decreased	Regular or irregular	Variable	Inspiration active; cessation during inspiration; expiration passive
DYSPNEA 1. Inspiratory	Increased or decreased	Irregular	Variable	Inspiration active, stridor may be present; expiration passive
2. Expiratory	Increased or decreased	Irregular	Variable	Inspiration active; expiration active and prolonged
3. Orthopnea	Increased or decreased	Irregular	Variable	Inspiration active; expiration passive (occurs in supine position)
4. Paroxysmal	Increased or decreased	Irregular	Variable	Inspiration active; expiration passive

determine the characteristics of the skin and underlying muscle tone. Palpate the large muscle masses, intercostal spaces, and costochondral junctions near the sternum. On palpation, the muscles should feel firm and smooth. In infants, palpation may be electively limited to the area of the axillary nodes, suprasternal notch, and some areas of the skin. The suprasternal notch is palpated to determine the presence and intensity of aortic arch pulsations and to assess tracheal positioning in all age groups. Due to the small chest circumference of the infant, inspection frequently yields as much information as palpation.

If tenderness of the chest wall is present, it can be elicited by palpation. As a general rule, tenderness localized in a pinpoint area is superficial. In other words, it originates within the skin or subcutaneous tissue. Palpation is performed in a systematic method, using one hand to assess half of the chest first, followed by the second half, or with both hands assessing each half at the same time. Palpation with one hand has the advantage of placing the opposite hand on the client's shoulder for support. Whichever method is used, begin in the lateral shoulder region and progress in the infraclavicular area to the sternum, down its lateral margins, and finally cover the remainder of the thoracic cage, including the axillary region.

Palpation is also used to evaluate vocal or tactile fremitus when the nurse anticipates the presence of pulmonary congestion or consolidation. The client speaks a resonant phrase, such as "ninety-nine," with consistent pitch and intensity, while the examiner palpates with the ball of the same hand symmetrical sites on the anterior and posterior chest. Vocal fremitus is not generally palpated for in infants and children, as it is intense due to the high frequency and number of sound waves transmitted to the chest wall. In adults, tactile fremitus is normally present. Palpable vibrations have the greatest intensity near the origin of the sound and decrease in intensity toward the periphery. Experience guides the examiner in making determination of normal and abnormal tactile vibrations. Increased fremitus frequently indicates lung consolidation, as liquefied or solid substances transmit vibrations readily; diminished or absent fremitus may indicate a pleural fluid, air, or mass, as these will decrease the transmission of vibrations.

Anterior chest wall expansion is determined by placing the fingers toward the axilla and approximating the thumbs on the sternum an equal distance apart. Posterior chest expansion is determined by placing the fingers toward the axilla and approximating the thumbs near the spinal column. Ask the individual to inspire deeply and observe the divergence of the thumbs. If the distance is asymmetrical, one section of the lung may not be expanding as fully as the other. Figure 10-9(a) through (e) illustrates the locations used to determine expansion on the anterior and posterior thoracic wall.

PERCUSSION

Normally, over the lung fields the density is minimal owing to the air-filled structures of the pulmonary system. Bony structures and soft tissues such as heart, liver, and diaphragm have greater density because of the increased cell mass. Determination of density is accomplished through mediated percussion. The terminal digit of the left middle finger is applied to an interspace of the thoracic wall. The distal joint of the placed finger is struck sharply with the middle finger of the opposite hand. The fingers of the right hand are partially flexed, and the hand moves loosely from the wrist. The right hand is withdrawn rapidly after it strikes the mediating finger to avoid muting the sound obtained (Figure 10-10). In infants, percussion is not utilized because of its low yield of significant data.

When the examiner percusses over the lung-filled portions of the chest, a resonant sound is received and presents the characteristics of loud intensity, low pitch, and long duration. In states of overinflation of the lungs, such as emphysema, a hyperresonant sound is returned. It possesses loud intensity and deep pitch of prolonged duration. Increased cell mass structures, such as the liver, heart, and bones, transmit a dull sound upon percussion. Dull sounds are transmitted as a noise with medium intensity, pitch, and duration. Another sound that generally indicates gross abnormality of the thoracic cavity is flatness. This sound presents with a soft intensity, high pitch, and very short duration, and may be elicited when normal lung tissue is replaced by a solid tissue or fluid mass.

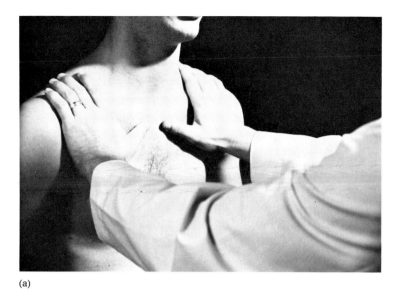

(a)

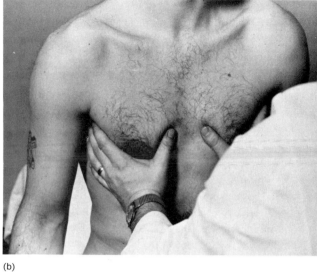

(b)

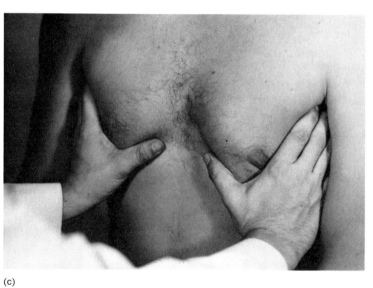

(c)

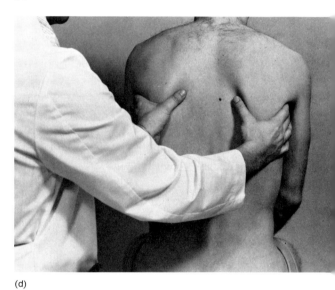

(d)

FIGURE 10-9
Placement of the examiner's hands to assess
thoracic expansion: (a) apical expansion;
(b) anterior mid-thoracic; (c) anterior low
thoracic; (d) posterior mid-thoracic;
(e) posterior, base of thorax.

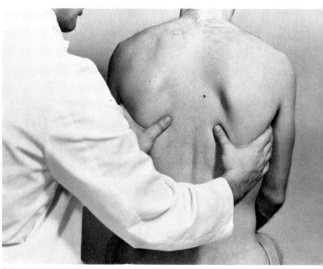

(e)

Percussion is carried out in a systematic manner, beginning at the apex of the lung fields as bilateral comparisons are made. Comparison permits the examiner to use one area as a control in assessing the other (Figure 10-11(a) and (b)).

AUSCULTATION

Auscultation follows percussion of the chest wall. Ongoing auscultatory assessment of the lung fields can assist in the determination of normalcy or alterations in the client's status; for example, pulmonary edema, consolidation, atelectasis or displacement of an endotracheal tube.

Sound in the lungs originates from two primary sources. Alveolar separation, called the **vesicular element,** produces the local noise during the inspiratory phase. The **glottic hiss** or laryngeal component is produced from air passing through the larynx. This air movement sets up vibrations that in turn are transmitted as noises.

The four characteristics important in auscultation of sound are pitch, intensity, quality, and duration. Frequency or pitch refers to the number of wave cycles generated each second. The number of wave cycles per second determines the pitch of a sound. A high-pitched or high-frequency sound has a greater number of wave cycles per second than a low-pitched or low-frequency sound. Amplitude or intensity determines the range of loudness or softness of the sound. The greater the amplitude or intensity, the louder the sound, and vice versa. Quality refers to the character of the sound, and descriptive terminology is used to promote the communication of this aspect to others. Breezy, swishy, tubular, harsh, fine, bubbling, and creaking are some commonly used terms. Duration or longevity describes the phase or phases of the respiratory cycle in which the sound is heard. It can also be used to describe the originating and terminating points of the sound. To present these characteristics, lung sounds are graphically illustrated, as in Figure 10-12.

The line directed upward indicates inspiration, and the line directed downward indicates expiration. The pitch is the degree of the angle between the baseline and the inspiration line. In Figure 10-12, inspiration has greater amplitude than expiration. Duration or longevity is depicted as inspiration being two times longer than expiration during auscultation.

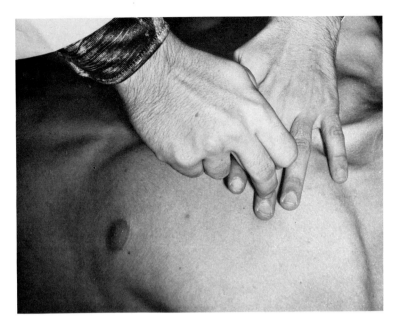

FIGURE 10-10
Mediated percussion.

FIGURE 10-11
Symmetrical percussion sites of the chest wall: (a) anterior; (b) posterior.

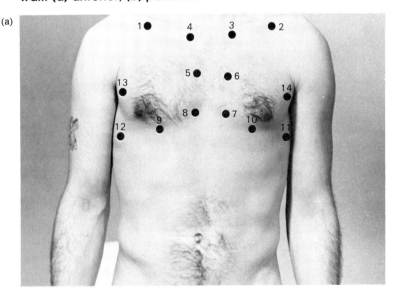

(a)

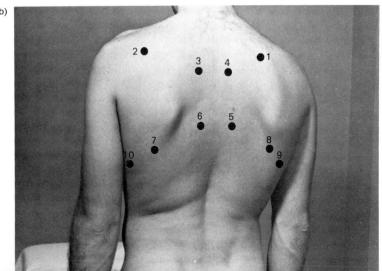

(b)

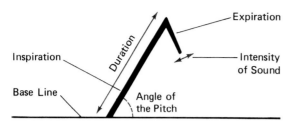

FIGURE 10-12

Graphic illustration of breath sounds,
consisting of a base line,
an inspiratory upswing line, and
an expiratory downswing line.
The length of the inspiratory and
expiratory lines indicate duration,
while the width of the line
indicates intensity of the sound.
The angle created by the inspiratory
upswing line and the base line
indicates the pitch of the sound.
The greater the angle,
the higher the pitch.

Variations of the frequency or pitch of the sound are elicited through the use of the two chest pieces, the bell and the diaphragm. The bell chest piece transmits sounds, especially those of a low frequency or pitch, and should be placed on the skin firmly enough to form a seal, but gently enough so that wave-cycle transmission is not impaired. The diaphragm chest piece transmits only high-frequency or high-pitched sound well, and is placed upon the skin with firm pressure. It does not, however, necessarily need to form a seal to transmit the sound. The diaphragm is most frequently used to assess the lung sounds.

The most favorable position for the client to assume during the process of auscultation is sitting with the shoulders slightly relaxed. When the sitting position is not possible for the client to assume, auscultation of the lung field should be performed with the client supine. In the supine position, auscultation of the posterior lung fields is achieved by turning the client to the lateral positions.

Instruct the client to mouth breathe, taking fairly deep breaths, but avoiding hyperventilation. Respirations should be of normal effort. Forced or maximal respiration is used only if certain abnormal sounds are suspected, or if a need exists to accentuate diminished breath sounds.

Interference and false impressions of lung sounds may develop if the following occur:

1. The examiner breathes on the stethoscope tubing.
2. The tubing rubs on sheets or side rails.
3. The stethoscope tubing is cracked.
4. Excessive hair on the chest is present (sometimes lightly wetting the hair decreases hair-friction sounds).
5. The diaphragm is cracked or has been replaced with an inadequate substitute, such as X-ray film.
6. Muscle movements are created by a tense or shivering client.

The lung fields are auscultated in a systematic manner, comparing bilateral sites. In this manner, one lung field serves as a control for the other. Generally, auscultation is initiated begin-

FIGURE 10-13
Pulmonary auscultatory sites in the adult: (a) anterior chest; (b) posterior chest.

(a)

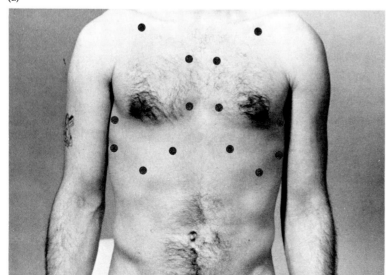

(b)

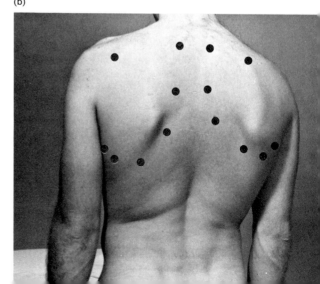

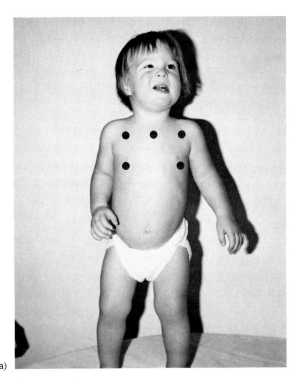

(a)

FIGURE 10-14
Pulmonary auscultatory sites in the
young child: (a) anterior chest;
(b) posterior chest.

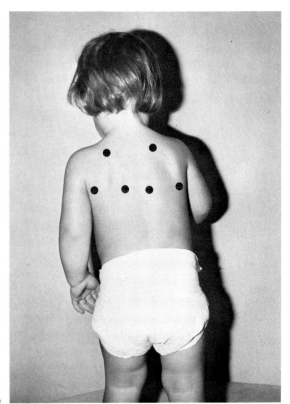

(b)

ning in the upper thorax and proceeds centrally and downward, and finally upward to the axillary region. This method is deviated from when auscultation is performed on the elderly. In this instance, auscultation begins in the periphery to determine the presence of atelectatic rales, which disappear after the first few deep breaths.

The areas for anterior and posterior auscultation for the adult are illustrated in Figure 10-13(a) and (b). Figure 10-14 (a) and (b) illustrates anterior and posterior auscultatory sites in the young infant.

Breath Sounds

Breath sounds are divided into normal, adventitious, voice, and abnormal voice sounds.

Normal breath sounds are tracheal, bronchial, bronchovesicular, and vesicular. Tracheal breath sounds (Figure 10-15) originate from the glottic hiss. Tracheal breath sounds have a high pitch, are loud, and have the quality of being very tubular and harsh. The duration of inspiration is equal to expiration, and the two phases of the respiratory cycle are separated by a brief pause. Tracheal sounds are heard normally over the trachea.

FIGURE 10-15
Tracheal breath sounds.

Bronchial breath sounds (Figure 10-16) are auscultated over the manubrium. Their characteristics are high pitch, high intensity, and a loud tubular and harsh quality. The duration of expiration is twice as long as inspiration. The sounds produced in inspiration and expiration are separated by a brief pause.

FIGURE 10-16
Bronchial breath sounds.

Bronchovesicular breath sounds (Figure 10-17) are normally auscultated over the upper one third of the sternum, beginning on a level below the manubrium and in the interscapular region. They originate from the glottic hiss and are a combination of bronchial and vesicular sounds. The characteristics of bronchovesicular sounds are medium to high pitch, moderate amplitude, and the quality of a blowing muffled sound. The duration of inspiration is equal to expiration, and the sounds produced by each respiratory phase are not separated.

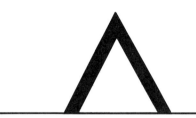

FIGURE 10-17
Bronchovesicular breath sounds.

Vesicular sounds (Figure 10-18) originate from local noise or alveoli opening on inspiration and the glottic hiss during expiration. They are auscultated in the periphery of the lung fields. The characteristics of vesicular sounds are medium to low pitch, low amplitude, and the quality of being breezy, swishing, or rustling. Inspiration is three times the duration of expiration, and the sounds of each phase are not separated.

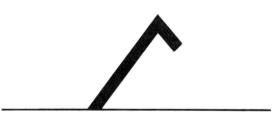

FIGURE 10-18
Vesicular breath sounds.

In summary, the location of normal breath sounds in the adult is illustrated in Figure 10-19(a) and (b). Tracheal, bronchial, bronchovesicular, and vesicular breath sounds are normal only when auscultated in the described areas; otherwise they are abnormal. For example, a bronchial sound located in the left lower lobe, a peripheral area of the lung fields, would be abnormal. Variations in the amplitude of the sound exist. In obese or muscular individuals, breath sounds may be distant, whereas in the very thin individual or child, sounds may be harsher.

There are characteristic differences in the infant's and especially the neonate's pulmonary system, as compared to the older child and the adult, that demand variation in the method of assessment. The primary characteristic of the infant's chest is its small size, which decreases the value of palpation and usually negates the value of percussion. However, because of the infant's small size, inspection and observation become highly valuable methods of data collection and are much more reliable and valid sources of objective data in the infant.

Specifically, the infant has much smaller effective tidal volumes of approximately 6 to 10 cc/kg. The compliance of the infant's lung is decreased, whereas the compliance of the chest wall is increased due to its decreased muscular adequacy and cartilaginous skeletal structures. Diaphragmatic breathing is the primary mode of respiratory movement in the infant, but effectiveness of this mode can be decreased by the characteristic recumbent position of the infant. Furthermore, the infant's respiratory excursion is markedly affected by positional changes. Most infants are obligatory nose breathers and will exhibit distress if the nasal passages are occluded.

The depth and rhythm of the infant's respirations, as well as the I:E ratio, vary, and premature infants may normally exhibit periodic breathing with marked pauses between respiratory cycles. Through inspection, the examiner can obtain data regarding coughing; labored breathing; the noise of breathing, such as wheezing, grunting, and stridors; cyanosis; rate of respiration; amount of mucus; presence of nasal flaring; retractions, head bobbing; and thoracic configuration and movement.

Auscultation is the other method employed to assess the infant's pulmonary status. This method also differs in the infant, primarily because of the chest size, as well as the decreased ratio of alveoli to airways. Therefore, there are fewer sites of auscultation in the infant, as seen in Figure 10-14(a) and (b). The sounds normally transmitted have a more tubular or bronchial quality even at the periphery. As a result, bronchovesicular breath sounds are the primary sounds transmitted, rather than vesicular sounds.

Although auscultation is helpful in the infant's pulmonary assessment, marked deviations in

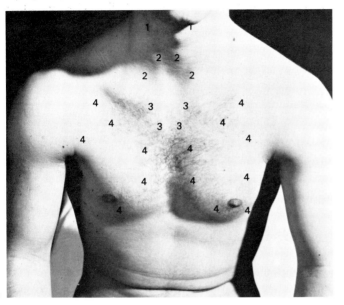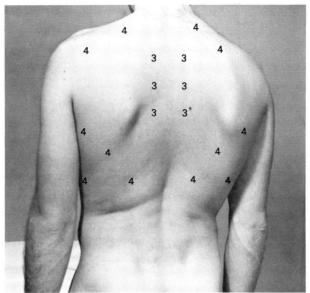

FIGURE 10-19
Locations of breath sounds: (a) anterior chest; (b) posterior chest.
(1) denotes tracheal sounds, (2) bronchial sounds,
(3) bronchovesicular sounds, and (4) vesicular sounds.

respiratory status are best identified by careful inspection and frequent observation. A few additional adventitious sounds are characteristic of the infant, aside from rales, rhonchi, and wheezes:

1. Delayed air entry, which is barely audible breath sounds in the periphery upon deep inspiration, as with crying.
2. Expiratory grunting, which is the sound produced by closing the glottis upon expiration, thus retarding the expiratory phase and creating a back pressure to combat atelectasis.
3. Stridor, which is an inspiratory crowing sound due to upper airway obstruction.

Two scoring systems are available for objectively integrating the physical signs of respiratory distress to establish its clinical severity. The Downes' scoring system is specific for assessing the severity of newborn respiratory distress. This system looks at five clinical parameters of neonatal respiratory distress: cyanosis, retractions, grunting, air entry during deep inspiration, and

Cyanosis	None	In air	In 40% O_2
Retractions	None	Mild	Severe
Grunting	None	Audible with stethoscope	Audible without stethoscope
Air Entry (crying)	Clear	Delayed or decreased	Barely audible
Respiratory Rate	< 60	60-80	> 80 or apneic episodes

FIGURE 10-20
The Downes' RDS scoring system, used to assess respiratory distress in the newborn. This is an index designed to assess objectively the clinical severity of hyaline membrane disease. The scoring index uses five separate clinical observations and scores them on a basis of 0, 1, or 2 points. The more abnormal the observation is, the higher the score. Allow the infant to stabilize for at least five minutes at a constant FiO_2 before scoring. Used with permission from Downes, Vidyasagar, Morrow, and Boggs, "Respiratory Distress Syndrome of Newborn Infants," Clinical Pediatrics, 9:6, p. 326.

0	Synchronized with abdominal movement	No retractions	No retraction	None	None
1	Lag of upper chest on inspiration	Retractions barely visible	Retraction barely visible	Minimal	Heard with stethoscope only
2	See-saw respirations (marked asynchrony of upper and lower chest on inspiration)	Retractions marked	Retraction marked	Marked	Heard without stethoscope

FIGURE 10-21

The Silverman and Andersen index, used to assess an infant's respiratory status. The scoring index uses five separate clinical observations and scores them on a basis of 0, 1, or 2 points. The score of respiratory status is obtained by totaling the values assigned to each clinical sign that best indicates the infant's observed appearance. A total score of 0 indicates no respiratory distress; a total score of 10 indicates severe respiratory distress. Used with permission from W. A. Silverman and D. H. Andersen, Pediatrics, 17:1, 1956. Copyright American Academy of Pediatrics 1956.

respiratory rate. The assessment is made after the infant has been in a stable environment for at least 5 minutes. A score of 4 or above for more than 2 hours indicates clinical respiratory distress (Figure 10-20). Likewise, the Silverman and Andersen index is a tool for evaluating an infant's respiratory status. The rated observations include chest lag, intercostal retractions, xiphoid retractions, nasal flaring, and expiratory grunting. This index is scored the same as the Downes' system, but is not necessarily specific for newborn respiratory distress. It has also been found useful for evaluating older infants (Figure 10-21).

Adventitious breath sounds in the older child and adult are abnormal sounds superimposed over the normal breath sounds, and include rales, rhonchi, wheezes, and friction rubs. Rales and rhonchi are further subdivided according to the characteristics of pitch, amplitude, quality, and duration. There are multiple ways to classify the subdivisions of the adventitious sounds, but only one will be presented.

Rales result from the passage of air through secretions present in alveoli and tubular air passageways. There are multiple ways to subdivide these sounds. The subdivision of rales are fine, medium, and coarse. Fine or crepitant rales (Figure 10-22) are heard at the end of inspiration as high-pitched, soft, cracking, or popping noises. Fine rale noises are the vibrations generated by the separation of alveolar walls, which have

mildly adhered to each other owing to the presence of pus or abnormal amounts of fluids within the alveoli. Fine rales are auscultated in the periphery, as opposed to the central chest area.

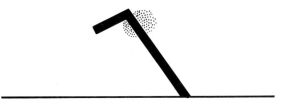

FIGURE 10-22
Fine or crepitant rales.

Medium or subcrepitant rales (Figure 10-23) arise from fluid or mucus-filled bronchial walls that are separated by the passage of air. The sound has low pitch, high amplitude, and a wet-moist quality, occurring in early or mid-inspiration.

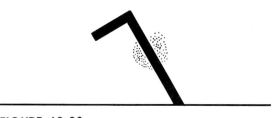

FIGURE 10-23
Medium or subcrepitant rales.

Coarse or bubbling rales (Figure 10-24) originate in the larger airways that contain fluid or mucous secretions. They possess the characteristics of low pitch and a loud bubbling quality, and occur most frequently during expiration, but can also be heard during inspiration.

FIGURE 10-24
Coarse or bubbling rales.

Rhonchi (Figure 10-25) are divided into the categories of (1) musical or sibilant and (2) sonorous, according to the pitch of the sound. Sibilant or musical rhonchi are of high pitch and possess a musical quality; sonorous are low pitched and are described as resembling someone snoring. Rhonchi are continuous sounds produced by the passage of air through edematous or spasmodic airways or through tubular structures laden with tenacious mucus. They are most frequently heard during expiration, although the greater the amounts of secretions or narrowing of structures, the more likely rhonchi will be heard during inspiration and expiration. The quality, pitch, intensity, and duration are variable with the degree of pulmonary abnormalities. The lower the pitch, the more likely that the origin is from the bronchi or trachea.

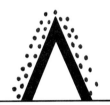

FIGURE 10-25
Rhonchi.

Wheezing (Figure 10-26) is a high-pitched, musical sound resulting from the decreased intraluminal size of airways owing to smooth muscle contraction, edema, or secretions. Wheezing can be heard on inspiration, but is more commonly heard during expiration.

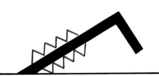

FIGURE 10-26
Wheezing.

Pleural friction rub (Figure 10-27) arises from irritated or inflamed pleura rubbing against each other without the normal lubricating substance. It occurs most frequently at the end of inspiration and possesses the characteristics of high pitch, moderate loudness, and a quality described as jerky and leathery.

FIGURE 10-27
Pleural friction rub.

Normal voice sounds originate from vocal-cord vibrations set up by the passage of air through the larynx. The vibrations or sounds are transmitted through the tubular and alveolar structures of the lung and finally to the chest wall. As the sounds travel through the anatomical structures, distinctness of the sound is lost; therefore, the closer the examiner auscultates near the origin of sound, the greater the resonance and intensity of the sound. The determination of voice sound clarity is generally not done while collecting data, unless other abnormal pulmonary signs present themselves.

The normal voice sound (Figure 10-28) may be elicited by requesting the client to say "ninety-nine" or "thirty-three" or "sixty-six." The lung fields are auscultated and the quality of the normal sound is muffled. The "ninety-nine" is used because of its resonant quality.

FIGURE 10-28
**A normal voice sound of "99"
to auscultation.**

Client Vocalizes	Examiner Auscultates a Muffled
99	

When the client is requested to say "ninety-nine" or "thirty-three" or "sixty-six," and auscultation yields a clear sound of the vocalized numeral, the results are termed **bronchophony** (Figure 10-29). The distinctness of sound transmission is created by mucus- or fluid-filled alveoli or by cellular mass replacing alveolar tissue.

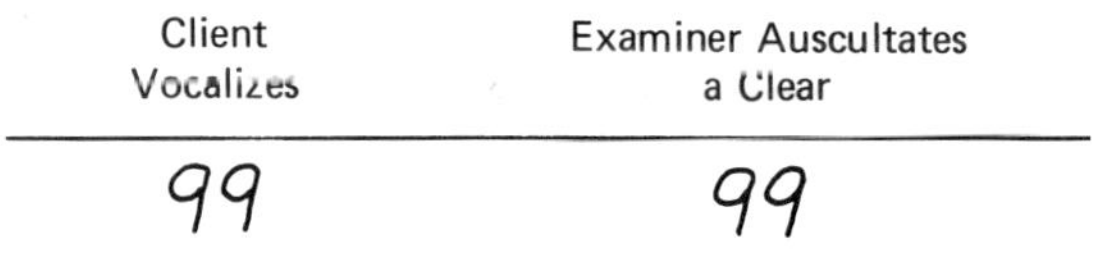

Client Vocalizes	Examiner Auscultates a Clear
99	99

FIGURE 10-29
Bronchophony.

Auscultation of voice sounds can also be accomplished by requesting the client to say the letter "e," a pure or nonresonant quality sound. The normal voice sound (Figure 10-30) is auscultated as a muffled, indistinct sound. Egophony

Client Vocalizes	Examiner Auscultates a Muffled
e	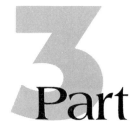

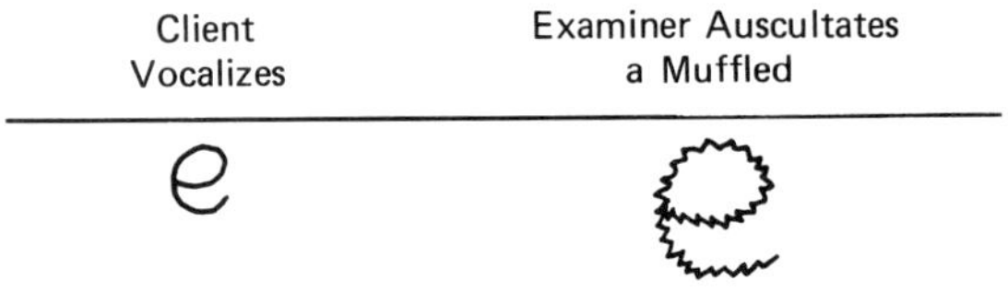

FIGURE 10-30
Normal voice of "e" to auscultation.

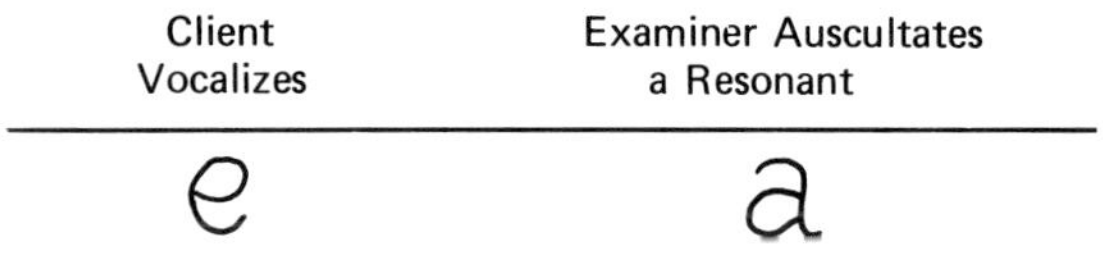

(Figure 10-31), an abnormal voice sound, is auscultated when the client vocalizes "e" and the examiner perceives a nasal sounding "a." This "e" to "a" change is heard primarily above a pleural effusion.

Client Vocalizes	Examiner Auscultates a Resonant
e	a

FIGURE 10-31
Egophony.

Another auscultatory process for differentiating normal and abnormal voice sounds is to have the client whisper numerals such as one, two, or three. The test is normal when these sounds are muffled upon auscultation, while clearly transmitted sounds indicate that consolidation is present. These sounds are termed **whispered pectoriloquy** (Figure 10-32).

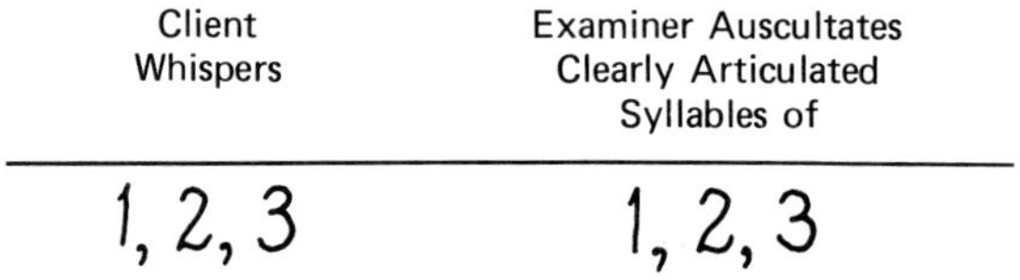

Client Whispers	Examiner Auscultates Clearly Articulated Syllables of
1, 2, 3	1, 2, 3

FIGURE 10-32
Whispered pectoriloquy.

Part 3

STUDY GUIDE QUESTIONS

In the following client situations, identify and describe the subjective and objective data to be collected, the specific tools and procedures to be utilized in the collection of those data, and the rationale for the nursing assessment.

1. Mr. Richard Brown, a 48-year-old male, complains to the industrial nurse about intermittent mid-thoracic pain of 2-week duration.

2. During your interview with 30-year-old Mr. Johnson, you notice that he has an intermittent, harsh, productive cough.

3. Baby girl Smith is an infant who was the product of a normal female with an uncomplicated pregnancy, labor, and delivery. At 2 hours of age, she begins to have intermittent cyanotic spells.

4. Mrs. Jolene Masser, a 69-year-old married female, 5 ft 5 in. tall and 190 lb presents for a yearly physical exam. You are ready to begin the chest and pulmonary assessment.

SAMPLE FORMAT TO BE USED IN RESPONDING TO THE STUDY GUIDE QUESTIONS

SUBJECTIVE DATA TO BE COLLECTED	OBJECTIVE DATA TO BE COLLECTED	SPECIFIC TOOLS AND PROCEDURES TO BE UTILIZED	RATIONALE FOR NURSING ASSESSMENT

BIBLIOGRAPHY

ALEXANDER, MARY M., and MARIE S. BROWN, *Pediatric Physical Diagnosis for Nurses,* pp. 112–130. New York: McGraw-Hill Book Company, 1974.

————, "Physical Examination, Part 12: Chest and Lungs," *Nursing 75,* January 1975, pp. 44–48.

BASTA, LOFTY L., PETRONIO T. LERONA, and LEWIS E. JANUARY, "Physical and Radiologic Examination of the Lung in the Evaluation of Cardiac Disease," *American Heart Journal,* August 1975, pp. 255–264.

DRUGER, GEORGE, *The Chest: Its Signs and Sounds.* n.p.: Humetrics Corporation, 1973.

HOCHSTEIN, ELLIOT, and ALBERT L. RUBIN, *Physical Diagnosis,* pp. 128–165. New York: McGraw-Hill Book Company, 1964.

HOLLENSHEAD, W. HENRY, *Textbook of Anatomy* (2nd ed.), pp. 495–525. New York: Harper & Row, Inc., 1967.

JUDGE, RICHARD D., and GEORGE D. ZUIDEMIA, eds., *Physical Diagnosis: A Physiological Approach to the Clinical Examination* (2nd ed.), pp. 131–164. Boston: Little, Brown and Company, 1968.

LAPP, N. L. and others, "Lung Volumes and Flow Rates in Black and White Subjects," *Thorax,* March 1974, pp. 185–188.

LITTMAN, DAVID, "Stethoscopes and Auscultation," *American Journal of Nursing,* July 1972, pp. 1238–1241.

PRIOR, JOHN A., and JACK S. SILBERSTEIN, *Physical Diagnosis* (4th ed.), pp. 169–208. St. Louis, Mo.: The C. V. Mosby Company, 1973.

SANTIS, MARTIN, "Examination of the Respiratory System," *Dental Clinics of North America,* January 1974, pp. 127–136.

11

The Heart

OBJECTIVES

- Describe the structure and function of the heart
- Identify the location of the heart and great vessels within the chest
- Identify the names of the heart valves and their locations within the heart
- Describe the direction of blood flow through the heart
- Describe the electrical conductivity pathway of the heart
- Systematically assess the heart
- Recognize rhythms that put a patient at risk for...
- Indicate blood pressure
- Take a pulse
- Visualize and palpate where to listen at the point of maximal impulse
- Identify movement through the use of palpation
- Note and identify often-missed pulses
- Auscultate heart sounds through the five cardiac auscultation areas
- Identify systolic and diastolic murmurs
- Identify configurations the heart that are abnormal
- Identify risk of heart infection

REVIEW OF STRUCTURE AND FUNCTION

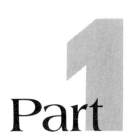

Part 1

The heart is one of the primary organs of the body. It is a four-chambered organ, and its walls consist of three layers, the epicardium (outer layer), myocardium (middle layer), and the endocardium (inner layer). It functions as a double pump that circulates the blood through the lungs for gas exchange and throughout the body for oxygen and nutrient transport at the systemic cellular level.

Surrounding the heart is a fibrous sac called the **pericardium.** This sac is composed of two basic layers, an external fibrous layer and an internal serous layer. The pericardial cavity, a potential space between these two layers, contains pericardial fluid, which maintains lubrication of the heart walls during contraction. This sac extends over the entire surface of the heart, as well as the immediate proximal portions of the aorta and pulmonary veins, after which it becomes continuous with the outer layer of these vessels.

The heart can be divided into the right and left sides and the upper and lower halves. The two sides of the heart are separated by the septum. The right side of the heart consists of the right atrium and the right ventricle. Its musculature is

less dense than that of the left side of the heart because, with ejection of its contents, minimal resistance to blood flow is encountered. The right ventricle is located near the anterior chest wall.

The left side of the heart consists of the left atrium and left ventricle. This half of the heart has a greater muscular mass than the right. This increased muscle density is required for ejection of blood into the systemic circulation, where greater resistance to blood flow is encountered. Anatomically, the left ventricle is positioned posteriorly, with its inferior surface in contact with the diaphragm. Figure 11-1(a) illustrates the positional relationship of the atria and ventricles.

The right atrium receives venous blood from the systemic and coronary circulation through the superior vena cava, the inferior vena cava, and the coronary sinus. From the right atrium, blood flows through the tricuspid valve into the right ventricle. The tricuspid valve serves as a barrier to prevent blood from returning into the right atrium from the right ventricle. It is composed of three leaflets connected to the endocardium by the chordae tendineae, which, in turn, are attached to the papillary muscle. The chordae tendineae prevent inversion of the valve during high

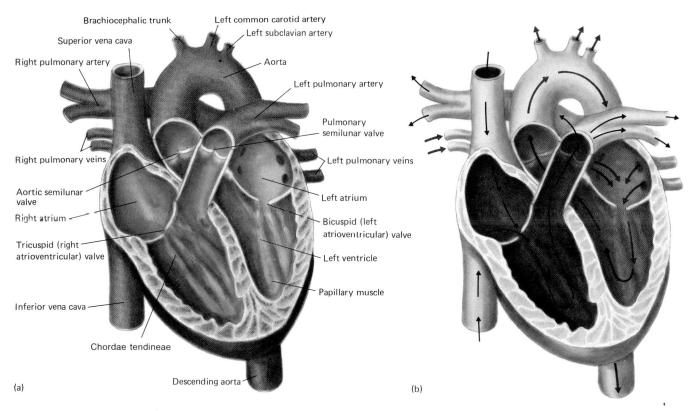

FIGURE 11-1

Positional relationship of the atria, ventricles, and greater vessels (a), and direction of the blood flow (b). In (b) black arrows indicate pulmonary and venous flow; red arrows show arterial flow.

pressure states. Contraction of the right ventricle ejects blood into the pulmonary artery, which is the initial route to reoxygenation of venous blood. This is the only artery in the body that carries deoxygenated or venous blood. Return of the oxygenated blood to the heart is accomplished through the pulmonary veins, which empty into the left atrium. The pulmonary veins are the only veins in the body that carry arterial blood. From the left atrium, blood is channeled into the left ventricle through the bicuspid (mitral) valve. This valve also functions as a barrier, preventing backflow of blood from the left ventricle into the left atrium, and is composed of leaflets attached to the ventricular wall via the chordae tendineae and papillary muscle. Again, as with the mitral valve, the chordae tendineae prevent inversion of the valve. Finally, the blood is ejected from the left ventricle into the systemic circulation and coronary circulation via the aorta. Figure 11-1(b) illustrates the direction of blood flow through the heart.

The semilunar valves, or the aortic and pulmonic valves, also serve to prevent regurgitation or backflow of blood into their respective preced-

ing chambers, the right and left ventricles. The aortic valve is located at the entrance of the aorta; the pulmonic valve is located at the entrance of the pulmonary artery. The semilunar valves are composed of three symmetrical cusps. The opening and closing of these valves is thought to be due to pressure changes in the ventricles, pulmonary vein, and aorta.

The left ventricle of a healthy adult ejects approximately 70 ml of blood into the peripheral circulatory system with each contraction. This ejection volume is termed stroke volume. Stroke volume multiplied by the heart rate per minute yields what is known as the cardiac output. Minute volume or cardiac output varies with the degree of physical or emotional activity that is occurring. The neurological and endocrine systems also influence the cardiac output through regulation of heart rate. The sympathetic nervous system and cardiac nerves promote acceleration of the heart rate; the parasympathetic system, through the vagus nerve, acts as a decelerator. Epinephrine, a hormone secreted in increased quantities during periods of excitement, also increases the heart rate.

164

Contraction of cardiac muscle is the result of electrical activity of the muscle fibers. Normally, this electrical activity originates in the sinoatrial node (SA node), which is called the cardiac pacemaker. This node, located in the right atrium near the superior vena cava inlet, rhythmically stimulates the electrical activity of other cardiac muscle fibers. From the SA node, the electrical impulse travels to the atrioventricular node (AV node). As it proceeds toward the AV node, it stimulates contraction of the atrial muscle fibers. The AV node directs the impulse to the bundle of His, which distributes it to the Purkinje fibers, resulting in contraction of the ventricles. Figure 11-2 illustrates the electroconductive pathway of the heart.

Atrial contraction has a longer duration than ventricular contraction. While atrial contraction is occurring, the ventricular fibers are at rest and, likewise, while the ventricles are contracting, the atrial fibers are at rest. Just as the contracting phase of the heart is essential, so is the resting phase. The various phases of electroconductivity can be recorded through the use of the electrocardiograph.

The electrocardiographic tracing is composed of a P wave, QRS complex, and a T wave. The P wave represents depolarization of the atria. Ventricular depolarization is represented by the QRS complex. The T wave demonstrates repolarization of the ventricles.

The volume of blood ejected from the left ventricle encounters resistance from the walls of the blood vessels, at the same time exerting pressure against the walls of these vessels. This measurable pressure phenomenon is termed blood pressure, and is divided into systolic and diastolic phases. The systolic phase occurs when the left ventricle ejects blood into the systemic circulation, creating a maximal pressure. A minimal pressure state, or diastole, occurs when the ventricles are at rest or not ejecting blood into the aorta. The amount of pressure varies, dependent upon vessel and blood status. Vessel factors affecting the pressure exerted by the arteries are lumen size, elasticity of the walls, and the degree of dilation or constriction. Pressure factors originating from the blood include the velocity at which it travels, viscosity, and circulating volume.

Taking the aforementioned factors into consideration, the body may be likened to a check and balance system through the vasomotor centers in the medulla via the pressoreceptors and chemoreceptors. From the vasomotor center in the medulla impulses originate to maintain pressure states through vasodilation or constriction of the arteries. The pressoreceptors located in the carotid and aortic sinuses respond to decreased pressure states by relaying impulses to the medullary vasomotor center to initiate impulses for vasoconstriction. Chemoreceptors, responsive to variations in oxygen and blood pH levels also relay impulses to initiate the appropriate vasomotor response.

Many other factors affect the pressure status of the arteries, some of which are physical and emotional activity level, temperature of the environment and body, tension, pain, and irregular heart rhythms such as premature ventricular contractions.

The mathematical difference between the systolic pressure and the diastolic pressure is called the pulse pressure. This pressure is affected by the stroke volume and the distensibility of the arteries. The greater the volume of ejected blood and heart rate, the greater is the pulse pressure.

The pulsations produced by the stroke volume are palpable at the systemic arterial sites. The strength and pattern of this pulsatile distention of the vessels is called a pulse and is reflective of activity within the circulatory system.

FIGURE 11-2
Electroconductive pathway of the heart.

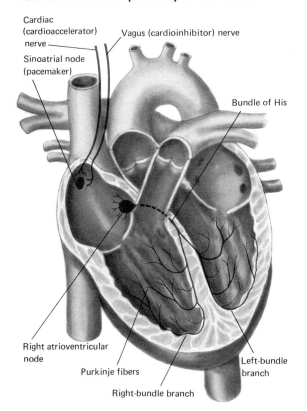

Cardiac (cardioaccelerator) nerve

Vagus (cardioinhibitor) nerve

Sinoatrial node (pacemaker)

Bundle of His

Right atrioventricular node

Purkinje fibers

Left-bundle branch

Right-bundle branch

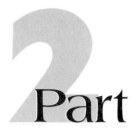

Part 2

HEALTH ASSESSMENT OF THE HEART

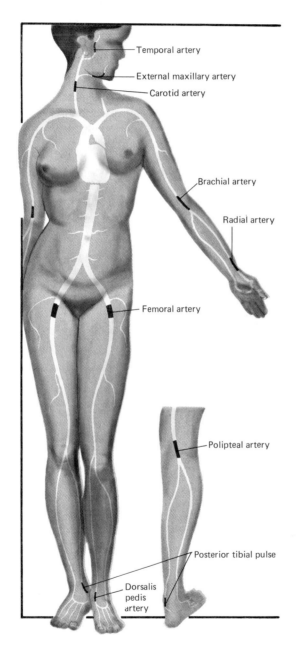

- Temporal artery
- External maxillary artery
- Carotid artery
- Brachial artery
- Radial artery
- Femoral artery
- Polipteal artery
- Posterior tibial pulse
- Dorsalis pedis artery

FIGURE 11-3
Major palpable locations of systemic pulsations.

The cardiac system evaluation is initiated through determination of pulse status and blood pressure, followed by a systematic pattern of inspection, palpation, and auscultation.

Palpation of the pulse yields more than just the rate within a unit of time. The pattern and intensity of the pulsation are also assessed. The characteristics of the pulse are interpreted through the sensory receptors in the fingertips as they compress the artery against a solid underlying structure. The amount of pressure applied depends on the size of the artery being palpated.

Generally, the radial pulse is palpated to ascertain the characteristics of pulsation, although other systemic locations may be used. Figure 11-3 illustrates the major locations of systemic pulsations that are readily accessible to palpation.

The pulse rate is calculated by counting the impulses for 30 seconds and then multiplying the figure by 2. This gives the rate per minute. Counting pulsations for 30 seconds is accurate only if a regular rhythm is present. If the rhythm is irregular, the pulse is counted for a full minute. Palpation of the brachial, femoral, and popliteal pulses is facilitated by encouraging semiflexion of the nearest joint. This relaxes the overlying muscle structures, enabling compression of the underlying artery. In the neonate and younger child, palpation of pulses located in joint areas is more readily obtained during a time when voluntary relaxation occurs.

When palpation of the carotid arteries occurs, do not rub the area, or reflex slowing of the heart may occur, resulting in bradycardia. This is especially important in the elderly and individuals with cardiac pathology. Table 11-1 illustrates the normal pulse ranges for various age groups.

The rhythm or pattern of a pulse is described as regular, irregular, or irregularly regular. A regular rhythm is one in which pulsations occur with methodical sequence. An irregular pulse is one with no descriptive pattern. An irregularly regular pulse has a describable pattern such as 1,

TABLE 11-1
Normal Pulse Ranges for Various Age Groups

AGE	TACHYCARDIA	NORMAL RATE*	BRADYCARDIA
Newborn	Above 180	120 to 140	Less than 90
Infancy 1 to 2 years	160 or above	80 to 140	Less than 80
Toddler 2 to 3.5 years	Above 140	80 to 130	Less than 80
Preschool 3.5 to 6 years	Above 125	70 to 115	Less than 70
School age 6 to 12 years	Above 120	60 to 110	Less than 60
Adolescent and adult	Above 110	60 to 100	Less than 60

*Variations may be within normal limits for individuals.

2, 3, —, 1, 2, 3, —. An irregularly regular pulse requires a pattern description to be recorded in order to facilitate its interpretation.

The normal pulse is described as regular in rhythm and consistent in intensity. It is characterized by attainment of maximal intensity quickly and a slower decrescendo of the impulse. A full or increased pulse may be regular in rhythm, but it has an obviously increased, consistent intensity. Bounding pulses are variable in rate and are forceful, with rapid attainment of maximal intensity followed by a rapid decline in intensity of pulsation. A weak pulse is one for which minimal pulsation is present. Palpable pulses that are rapid, weak, and of waxing and waning intensity are termed thready. In pulsus alternans, the pulsation is alternately strong and then weak. Pulsus alternans frequently occurs with digitalis toxicity. Pulsus paradoxus is present when pulsations are diminished during respiratory inspiration and strengthened during expiration. The changes in pulsation intensity associated with pulsus paradoxus are due to changes in intrathoracic pressure.

Frequently, the intensity of the pulse is recorded in numerical form. In this format, the top most figure of the employed scale is used as the denominator, while the examiner's perception of the intensity is recorded as the numerator. A commonly used scale is as follows:

0—absent
1—diminished
2—normal
3—full or increased
4—bounding

A normal pulse would then be recorded as 2/4. Use of the grading scale does not preclude describing the pattern of the pulse.

BILATERAL COMPARISON OF PULSES

Bilateral comparison of pulses is accomplished by palpating the right and left branches of the artery in its bilateral locations simultaneously with the fingers of the right and left hands (Figure 11-4). In doing so, one artery pulsation serves as a control for the other. Normally, bilaterally palpated pulses should feel equal in rate, pattern, and intensity. Differences between bilateral pulses may be due to the inexperienced examiner's compression pressure differences or to partial or complete obstruction of circulatory vessels or stenosis. Generally, bilateral comparison of rate, pattern, and intensity of vessels is made while the examiner is assessing the specific area, such as the carotids during the neck assessment, or the femoral pulses during the abdominal or extremity assessment.

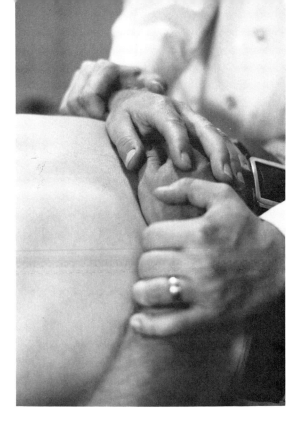

FIGURE 11-4
Bilateral palpation of the radial pulses.

INDIRECT BLOOD PRESSURE MEASUREMENT

Indirectly measured blood pressures that are most accurate are basal blood pressures. Basal or baseline pressures are not obtained from a single reading but from several readings, with the individual at the maximal comfort state such as sleep, upon first awakening, or after several hours of rest in a reclining position. Generally, to determine as accurately as possible what a client's blood pressure is, the client should be sitting, although it can be measured with the client lying or standing. The client's forearm must always be supported at the level of the heart. Generally, positions in which the pressure is taken are recorded as L (lying) or St (standing), while sitting receives no abbreviations. The extremity in which the pressure is obtained is also recorded as RA (right arm) or LA (left arm). Examples of recordings are as follows: L: RA 120/70/60; St: LA 130/80/72.

To obtain a measurement of the indirect blood pressure, a sphygmomanometer and stethoscope are used. The sphygmomanometer consists of a distensible bag, often called a compression bag or bladder; a cuff; a nonexpandable material in which the inflatable bag is housed, and which also serves to wrap around the individual's extremity; an air inflation bulb; and a manometer with a dial and a numerical scale from which the indirect blood-pressure reading is taken.

The manometer used in reading the pressure may be one of two types: the mercury or the aneroid. The mercury manometer (Figure 11-5(a)) functions by air pressure that forces the mercury from its reservoir up a numerically scaled glass tubing. Allowing the air to escape permits the mercury to return to the reservoir. During the mercury's descent, it bounces when pulsations are strong enough.

The aneroid is a round gauge that has an indicator or pointer attached centrally. The gauge ascends the numerical scale as air is forced into the distensible bag. As the air is released, the indicator descends the scale of numerals and will bounce when pulsations are strong enough. Figure 11-5(b) illustrates the aneroid manometer.

When measuring the indirect blood pressure, the cuff used should be approximately 20 percent wider than the diameter of the extremity around which it will be wrapped. A cuff that is too small yields a false high pressure; if too large, the cuff yields a pressure that is inaccurately low. The cuff size for an average adult is around 12 to 14 cm in width; for infants and children, generally the sizes are 2.5, 5, and 8 cm. For obese individuals, cuff sizes may range from 18 to 20 cm in width.

The appropriate-sized cuff is placed 2.5 cm above the antecubital space, with the distensible or compression bag on the medial or inner aspect of the arm. The examiner then palpates the brachial pulse, which is located medially on the antecubital space. The stethoscope is then placed over the brachial impulse. Next palpate the radial pulsation, and, while palpating it, inflate the cuff 30 or 40 mm of mercury above the mark where the radial pulsations disappeared. This means that the examiner must concentrate on three things at once:

1. Radial pulsations and their disappearance.
2. Manometer dial.
3. Insufflation of the cuff.

The cuff is then deflated at approximately 3 mm of mercury per second. The sounds heard are termed the sounds of Korotkoff and will be heard in five phases, as illustrated in Table 11-2.

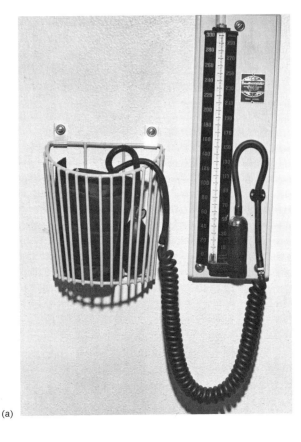

(a)

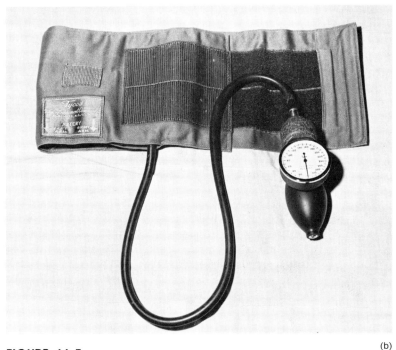

(b)

FIGURE 11-5
Manometers used for indirect measurement of systemic blood pressure: (a) mercury; (b) aneroid.

TABLE 11-2
Sounds of Korotkoff

I	Onset of a faint, but clear tapping sound; sound increases in intensity (systolic pressure)
II	Sound changes from distinct tapping to a murmur or swishing quality
III	Return to a loud, crisp, clear tapping sound; increase in intensity
IV	Sudden change to an abrupt muffled sound with a blowing quality and decreased intensity (index of diastolic pressure)
V	Cessation of sound (pressure that most closely approximates a directly measured pressure)

To take the blood pressure, the examiner listens to the Korotkoff sounds, notes the numerical points at which sound changes occur on the manometer scale, and records them; the phases recorded are I, IV, and V.

In infants, blood pressure is difficult to obtain by auscultation. The flush method is often employed to obtain a mean pressure in the neonate. The flush method requires the use of a small distensible cuff approximately 2.5 cm wide, which is wrapped about the forearm or foreleg just above the wrist or ankle, respectively. The cuff is connected to the aerometer and inflated to approximately 120 mm of mercury while the distal portion of the extremity (hand or foot) is compressed by either the examiner's hand or an ace bandage tightly wrapped around it. The compressing pressure, which serves to blanch the skin, is then released and the manometer is allowed to drop. The point at which the distal portion of the extremity flushes completely is noted and recorded as number/F. Flush blood pressures are most accurate if the child is not cold stressed and if the same extremity is used serially. Bounce or Doppler pressures are often used in the older infant or when flush pressures are of questionable accuracy.

PULSE PRESSURE

Pulse pressure is derived from the mathematical differences between the systolic and diastolic pressures. An example of its calculation is as follows:

Systolic (onset of sound)	130
Diastolic (cessation of sound)	-70
Pulse pressure	60 mm Hg

Abnormal increases in the pulse pressure are due to increased stroke volume, ejection velocity, and an increased vascular resistance to distensibility. An increase in stroke volume and ejection velocity can occur in healthy clients who have been physically active, or anxious over the impending examination or the situation or environment in which they are in. Pathological states that can lead to an increased pulse pressure are complete heart block, circulatory overload, anemia, atherosclerosis, and coarctation of the aorta.

A decrease in pulse pressure is due to a decrease in stroke volume, increased peripheral resistance, or hypovolemia of the vascular system. A decreased pulse pressure is generally not found in the healthy individual. Heart failure, shock, decreased intravascular volume, and aortic coarctation are some causes of decreased pulse pressure.

INSPECTION

The heart lies at an angle within the chest. If one draws an imaginary line from the right mid-clavicular area to the left mid-hypochondriac region, an approximation of the heart's angle is obtained. The extreme right border of the heart, which is primarily the right atrial border, is located approximately at the right side of the sternum between the third and fifth intercostal spaces. The apex of the heart is formed by the ventricles, primarily the left ventricle. During ventricular contraction, the apex rotates forward and to the right, coming closer to the chest wall. This positional change often produces a palpable and sometimes visible thrust, called the apical impulse or point of maximal intensity (PMI). The PMI is well localized, approximately 2 to 3 cm in diameter or smaller, and can be seen for a brief

duration, in the fifth interspace, approximately 8 cm from the left mid-sternal line (Figure 11-6). Visualization of this impulse can be accomplished by inspecting the chest directly and obliquely with the client in a sitting, supine, or left lateral recumbent position.

The PMI can increase in amplitude, shift further to the left, and remain somewhat localized (3 to 5 cm) in left ventricular hypertrophy with dilation and left-sided heart failure. In right sided heart failure with hypertrophy, the PMI may be displaced more toward the right sternal border. A right-sided shift can also occur if intrathoracic abnormalities exist in the left side of the chest. Emphysema that has progressed considerably can shift the heart downward to give an epigastric impulse. During pregnancy, the PMI may be displaced laterally to the mid-clavicular line.

The PMI is less likely to be visualized in obese and muscular individuals, owing to the increased density of the chest. Requesting the client to cease breathing at the end of expiration frequently enables visualization of the PMI. In the nonobese child, the PMI is readily visible, but located slightly further to the left than in the adult.

Epigastric impulses may be seen in young children and adults, especially those who are thin. If normal, these pulsations correspond to the timing of the arterial pulse. Abnormal epigastric pulsation in the infant may indicate cardiomegaly or a left pneumothorax.

PALPATION

Next, palpate the precordial area where the PMI was visualized, using the palmar surface of the fingers with the client in a sitting or supine position. When the PMI is not visualized, palpate the area in the mid-clavicular mid-sternal line intersection. If the client is unable to breathe adequately in a supine position, a semi-Fowler's position does not significantly alter thoracic movements. From middle age on, the perception of the PMI requires careful palpation, and it frequently cannot be felt, as the force of the heart's forward thrust diminishes with age. Normally, the PMI is palpated as a quick, brief, and forward projection against the chest wall. The thrust amplitude may be accentuated in clients with a thin chest wall, abnormally depressed sternum, and in hyperkinetic states. An impulse that is faint to palpation with the client in the supine position may be more readily palpable when the client's position is changed to the left lateral. A PMI that is easily palpable in the supine position and vigorously accentuated in the left lateral position may be indicative of pathology.

Following palpation of the PMI, the rest of the precordial region, especially the apical, midprecordial, parasternal, pulmonic, aortic, sternoclavicular, and epigastric areas (Figure 11-7) are palpated to determine the presence or absence of thrills, thrusts, heaves, retractions, bulges, and lifts. Thrills are palpable murmurs; in other words, they are the vibratory sensations projected from a site of turbulent blood flow. Thrills should be identified as systolic or diastolic by their relationship to the PMI. Thrills are generally associated with pathological states. A thrust is an outward chest movement of increased amplitude; a heave is an outward movement of prolonged duration with or without increased amplitude. Retraction is an inward movement. The word *lift* describes outward movement of the sternal or parasternal area.

PERCUSSION

Percussion of the precordial area yields few data and is therefore seldom utilized in the assessment of the heart. In the past, it was used to determine the size and position of the heart. Today, X rays of the chest provide those data with more accuracy.

AUSCULTATION

Auscultation of the chest for cardiac sounds enables determination of the apical pulse, as well as assessment of cardiac status. The apical rate is determined by counting the number of beats per minute. The apical pulse can be compared to the radial pulse. This is accomplished by auscultating the apical pulse while palpating the radial pulse. Normally, the pulse rates are equal or of minimal discrepancy. Obvious differences between the rates are abnormal. This difference is termed pulse deficit. If a pulse deficit exists, it is generally assessed by two examiners, one auscultating the apical rate and the other palpating the radial pulse during the same period of time.

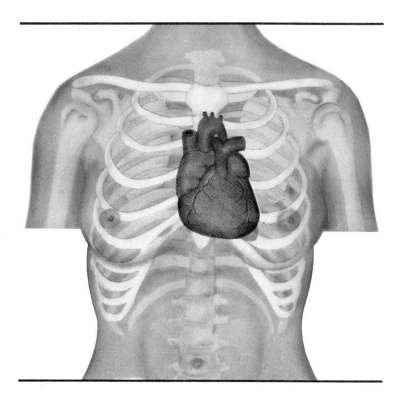

FIGURE 11-6

Anatomical location of the point of maximal intensity (PMI).

FIGURE 11-7

Precordial regions palpated to determine the presence of thrills, thrusts, heaves, retractions, bulges, and lifts.

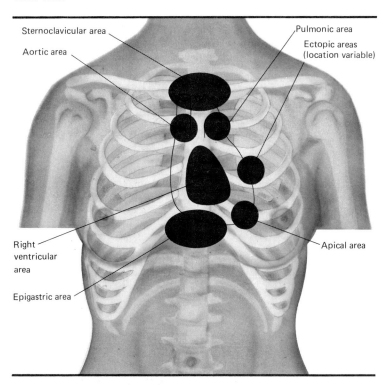

Sternoclavicular area

Aortic area

Pulmonic area

Ectopic areas (location variable)

Right ventricular area

Epigastric area

Apical area

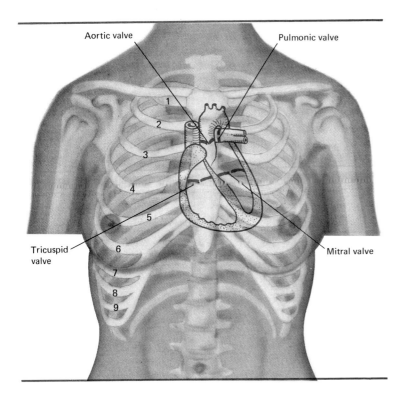

FIGURE 11-8
Anatomical locations of the heart valves.

FIGURE 11-9
Cardiac auscultatory sites.

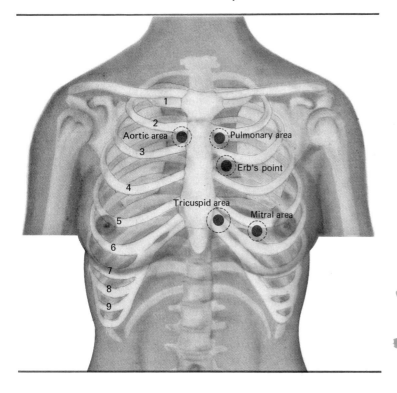

If heart sounds are difficult to distinguish during active respiration, ask the person to hold her or his breath. Clients with barrel chest and emphysema often render auscultation of heart sounds difficult owing to the presence of multiple adventitious breath sounds and the increased distance for sound transmission. Even in the face of structural deterrents, an apical pulse can be obtained by placing the stethoscope immediately below the xyphoid process. Obesity can preclude obtaining an apical pulse of any quality.

The heart sounds are auscultated at several locations. To identify the auscultatory sites, it is necessary to recognize the fact that the anatomical locations of the heart valves and the points of their respective maximal sound transmission are not the same. The aortic valve is located deep within the chest. The sound produced as the result of its closure is transmitted in the direction of blood flow (i.e., the ascending aorta and its greater curvature). The events involving the aortic valve are auscultated with the greatest clarity in the second intercostal space immediately to the right of the sternum. The pulmonic valve is located more proximal to the chest wall, and the resulting sounds of closure are most audible in the second intercostal space immediately to the left of the sternum. The tricuspid valve is located proximal to the surface of the chest wall. The sounds produced after its closure can be auscultated in the fourth and fifth intercostal spaces near the left sternal border. Like the aortic valve, the mitral valve is located distal to the anterior chest wall, and its sounds are transmitted in the direction of blood flow (i.e., toward the apex of the heart). Figure 11-8 illustrates anatomical locations of the valves; Figure 11-9 illustrates the anatomical location of auscultatory sites.

Contraction of the heart muscle produces two primary sounds. S_1, the first heart sound, is characteristically described as lubb. The sound generated in S_1 results from turbulent blood flow against the mitral and tricuspid valves following their closure. Normally, the mitral valve closes approximately 0.02 to 0.03 seconds before the tricuspid valve. S_1 is followed by a quiet period called **systole**, during which the ventricles are in a stage of contraction to eject blood from the ventricular chambers.

S_2, the second heart sound, is described as dupp and follows the systolic period. It is the result of turbulent blood flow against the closed

FIGURE 11-10 (right, above)
The cardiac cycle.

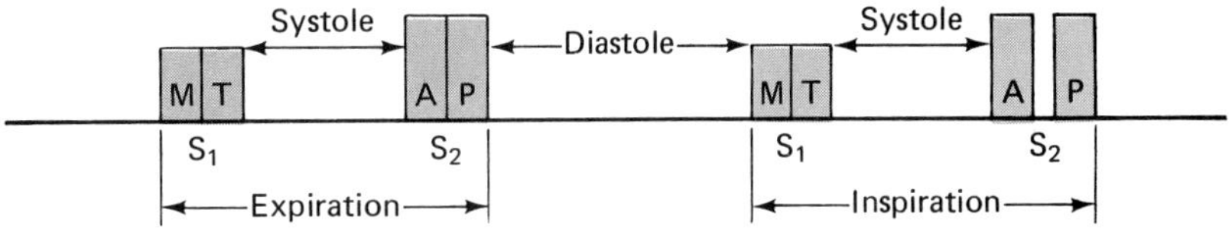

FIGURE 11-11 (right, below)
Graphic illustration of the relationship of heart sounds S_3 and S_4 to S_1 and S_2.

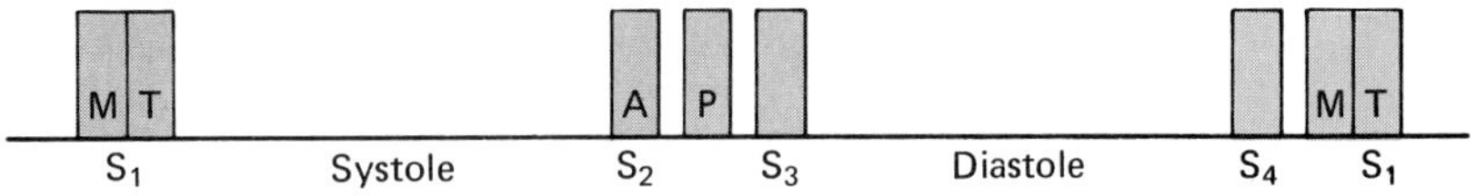

aortic and pulmonic valves. The aortic valve closes prior to the pulmonic valve, and the difference in closure timing is affected by the respiratory phase in which closure occurs. S_2 is followed by diastole, another quiet period like systole. During diastole, the right and left ventricles are filling with blood from the atria (Figure 11-10).

The heart may produce two more sounds, which are termed S_3 and S_4. S_3 generally occurs approximately 0.12 to 0.14 seconds after S_2. Its origin is thought to be due to the increased pressure needed to complete ventricular filling after the blood in the ventricles has reached a certain level. S_3 is common in the young, especially those with a slow ventricular rate, and it generally disappears around the age of 20. After 30 years of age, the presence of S_3 is rare and is associated with possible cardiac pathology.

S_4 occurs late in diastole, either just prior to S_1 or within the sound of S_1. S_4 is thought to be caused by late ventricular filling, the tensing of the atrioventricular valve structures, and atrial muscular contraction. S_4 is seldom differentiated from S_1 by auscultation except occasionally in young children. Discriminating S_3 and S_4 from a split first or second sound is difficult and requires much experience (Figure 11-11).

When auscultating over the aortic and pulmonic auscultatory sites, S_2 is heard with greater intensity than S_1. When auscultating over the mitral and tricuspid sites, S_1 has the greatest intensity. In the infant and toddler, the chest is smaller in circumference and thin walled compared to the adult. These characteristics increase the amplitude of sound transmission. The auscultatory sites in the child are similar to those of the adult, but less localized.

Auscultation of the heart can be done with the client in a sitting, supine, or left lateral recumbent position. More than one position may be assumed to facilitate validation of auscultatory findings. When auscultating the heart, first establish the rate. When establishing the apical rate, S_1 and S_2 equal one beat. It is important to discriminate the radial from the apical pulse rates when recording findings. This is accomplished by preceding the recorded rate with A or AP for apical. After the rate and rhythm have been established, the examiner listens only to S_1 or lubb, then to S_2 or dubb. Proceed to listen to systole and finally to diastole in the same manner. S_1 presents a low-pitched sound, whereas the transmitted sound of S_2 is of a higher pitch. During S_1, the closure of the mitral valve occurs prior to the closure of the tricuspid valve. Generally, S_1 is heard as one sound but can be transmitted as two sounds owing to the increased timing between the closure of the valves. The double sound is called a split S_1. S_2 is more commonly auscultated as a split sound. Splitting of S_2 normally varies with respirations. The split may be increased if the client takes a deep breath. Deep breathing changes intrathoracic pressure and increases venous return to the heart. To auscultate splitting of the heart sounds requires much practice, as this splitting can be abnormal.

Murmurs are sounds produced by turbulent blood flow within the heart and great vessels. Murmurs may or may not indicate heart disease as they may exist in direct cardiovascular pathology, such as stenotic or incompetent valves or sclerotic or aneurysmal arteries. Benign murmurs may exist in hyperkinetic states or anemic conditions. Pregnancy may result in a murmur called mammary souffle, which is due to an intensely dilated anastomosis between the aortic and internal mammary intercostal arteries. Generally, this murmur is not pathologic unless it continues beyond the sixth week postpartum.

If murmurs are auscultated, several characteristics should be described and communicated to other health-care personnel. The important char-

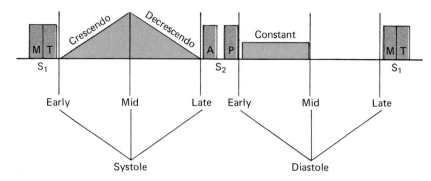

FIGURE 11-12

Graphic illustration of cardiac murmurs. Systole and diastole can be divided into three phases of early, mid, and late. Murmur duration is described using these phases, such as early-to-mid, mid-to-late, early-to-late, or pansystolic. Murmur intensity is described as crescending, decrescending, or of constant intensity.

acteristics include the location of the murmur in the cardiac cycle, the anatomical location and distribution of sound throughout the chest, the location of maximal intensity, and the pitch and amplitude of the murmur. Figure 11-12 illustrates location and amplitude of murmurs in systole and diastole. The intensity of murmurs is most frequently described by a grading system proposed by Freeman and Levine. This proposed system is used for systolic murmurs and ranges from grade I through grade VI. A grade I murmur is barely audible and generally determined present only after the examiner has perceived the normal sounds present. Grade II murmurs are faint, but more readily identified during the auscultatory process. Systolic murmurs that are graded III or IV possess a medium intensity and are at times the most difficult to distinguish. Some practitioners distinguish between grades III and IV by associating the presence of a vibratory thrill with a grade IV, V, or VI murmur. Grade V is described as a loud murmur; grade VI is intensely loud and can be frequently heard with the stethoscope partially or completely off the chest.

Innocent, benign, or functional murmurs are present in nonpathological states. Generally, an innocent murmur is low pitched, soft and blowing, and can therefore be perceived best with the bell chest piece. The intensity of this murmur ranges between grades I and III. The respiratory cycle may affect the intensity of the innocent murmur. A decrease in intensity occurs with inspiration, whereas expiration may increase its intensity. Usually, murmurs heard in the immediate newborn period (first week of life) are

within normal limits unless associated with tachycardia, tachypnea, hepatosplenomegaly, lethargy or extreme irritability, cyanosis of nonpulmonary origin, feeding intolerance, or failure to thrive. Murmurs persisting beyond the first week of life may or may not be pathologic and require further evaluation and follow up. In practice, a large number of elderly clients are found to present some type of systolic murmur, even when the presence of cardiac pathology is not confirmed.

The term click is used to describe an extra systolic sound. Clicks may occur in early, mid, or late systole, and are characterized by a clear, loud sound, which is most prominent when the client is in a sitting position and may be accentuated by forced expiration. Clicks arising from the aortic valve are generally most intense at the apex of the heart. Pulmonic clicks are auscultated most clearly in the left second intercostal space, and change markedly in intensity with respiration. During inspiration, the intensity may decrease to below audible levels, and then accentuate during expiration.

An extra diastolic sound is termed a snap. The quality of this sound is described by its name. Diastolic snaps radiate toward the base of the heart. The snap can be accentuated by positioning the client in the recumbent or left lateral position. The respiratory phase of expiration can also increase the intensity of the snapping sound, as well as an increase in stroke volume through exercise or hyperkinetic states. Associated with the diastolic snap is a resultant thrill, which is palpable on the chest.

174

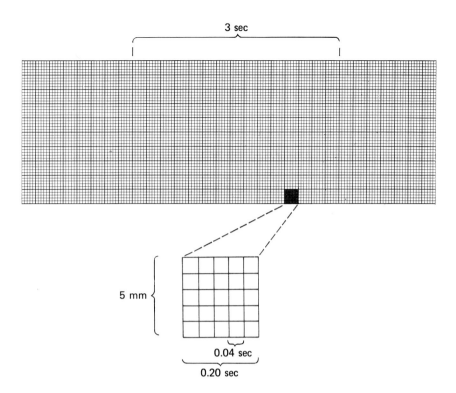

FIGURE 11-13
Electrocardiographic tracing
paper, illustrating the
space-time relationship.

3 sec

5 mm

0.04 sec

0.20 sec

ELECTROCARDIOGRAPH

Another mode commonly used in assessing the cardiac status is the electrocardiogram tracing (ECG). This graphic recording (Figure 11-13) is not a direct use of the tools of inspection, palpation, percussion, and auscultation, but is frequently analyzed by nurses to determine the status of the electroconductive system of the heart. Generally, most nurses are exposed to the lead II tracing, and, therefore, it will be discussed here. The following information is far from a complete presentation concerning the ECG, but is an introduction to its interpretation.

The width of one small square equals 0.04 second; a combination of five small squares represents 0.2 second. Superior to the graphic squares are vertical lines. These lines are fifteen 0.2-second squares apart or 3 seconds apart. The height of a single square is equivalent to 0.1 millivolt (mV); the height of five small squares is representative of 0.5 mV.

Basic Deflection of the ECG

The tracing produced by the stylograph needle when no electrical cardiac activity is present is called the isoelectric or baseline. Deflections of the stylus tracing above this line during electrical activity are called **positive deflections;** deflections below or in a downward direction from this line are termed **negative deflections.** The P wave (Figure 11-14) represents depolarization of the atria. In lead II, the P wave possesses an upward deflection of less than 2.5 mV. The duration of a

FIGURE 11-14
The normal electrocardiographic tracing.

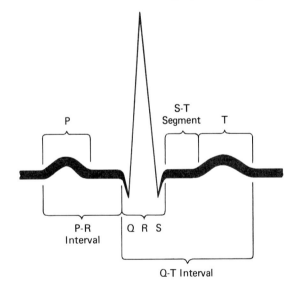

P

S-T
Segment

T

P-R
Interval

Q R S

Q-T Interval

normal P wave may be up to 0.11 second. This duration is calculated by determining the number of 0.04-second blocks that it encompasses and then multiplying 0.4 by this number. A P wave that is notched and of appropriate duration is generally normal and representative of electrical activity in the right and left atria.

The next major configuration assessed is the PR interval (Figure 11-14). This interval extends from the beginning of the P wave to the beginning of the R wave. The duration of the PR interval ranges from 0.12 to 0.20 second. This duration varies directly with the heart rate, as do all the deflections of the ECG. The PR segment of the PR interval begins at the end of the P wave and extends to the beginning of the R wave (Figure 11-14). It corresponds to the time it takes impulses to travel through the AV node and traverse the bundle of His, prior to its bifurcation. Therefore, any disruption in this pathway may be represented by an increase in the duration of the PR segment.

The QRS (Figure 11-14) represents ventricular depolarization. It follows the P wave and is initiated by a negative deflection, the Q wave, then a positive deflection, the R wave, and finally a negative deflection, the S wave. The time duration of the QRS complex ranges from 0.06 to 0.12 second. Generally, the complex has a narrow configuration. Although the Q wave may not always be present, the complex is always referred to as the QRS complex.

The ST segment (Figure 11-14) follows the QRS complex and includes the period of time from the end of the S wave to the beginning of the T wave. The ST segment corresponds to the depolarized state of all ventricular fibers.

The T wave (Figure 11-14) is normally a positive deflection (in lead II) following the QRS complex. This wave corresponds to the repolarization of the ventricles. T-wave duration and height are variable.

Finally, the U wave, a small positive deflection, may follow the T wave. Frequently, this wave is not seen on the ECG tracing. It is thought to be due to delayed polarization of some cells.

The heart rate may be calculated by several methods using the ECG tracing. It is important to remember which method can or cannot be used with a regular or irregular rhythm. One method is to obtain a 6-in. strip, count the number of complete cycles (the P, QRS, T waves) that occur within this strip, and multiply it by 10. The 6-in. strip is representative of 6 seconds. When multiplying by 10, the rate for 60 seconds or a 1-minute time period is obtained. For example, seven complete cycles in a 6-second strip is equivalent to a rate of 70 beats per minute. A 3-second strip may also be used. In this case, it is

TABLE 11-3

1	300
2	150
3	100
4	75
5	60
6	50
7	43
8	37
9	33

multiplied by 20. This method of rate calculation may be used whether the rhythm is regular or irregular.

A rate calculation that is appropriate only to a regular rhythm is to determine the number of large squares or 0.2-second intervals that exist between consecutive P waves or consecutive R waves. The number of squares is then divided into 300 to determine the rate. Table 11-3 presents time intervals or large squares occurring between each P or R wave and the resultant division into 300, or the rate.

Another method appropriate only when a regular rhythm is present is to count the interval spaces between two wave deflections (R–R) and divide this into 60 seconds.

Normal Sinus Rhythm

A normal sinus rhythm (Figure 11-15(a)) is always indicative of an impulse that originated in the SA node. A sinus rhythm exists when the P waves in a strip are of the same configuration and interval from each other throughout the strip, and are always followed by a QRS complex and a T wave. Normally, the SA node fires at a rate between 60 and 100 times per minute. If the originating impulse remains in the SA node, but falls below a rate of 60, and the rhythm remains constant, the rate is termed sinus bradycardia (Figure 11-15(b)). Sinus bradycardia is significant, as it may be a preceding factor to lethal tachyarrhythmias. The opposite is true if the rate exceeds 100. This state is termed sinus tachycardia (Figure 11-15(c)).

If the impulse originates in the SA node, but the rhythm at which it fires is erratic and all other variables remain constant, the term utilized is sinus arrhythmia. If the SA node fails to originate an impulse (sinus arrest) (Figure 11-15(d)), or fails to transmit the impulse (exit block), the atrial musculature is unable to respond and, consequently, the P wave is absent from the ECG tracing. Thus normal sinus rhythm is disrupted. To analyze an arrhythmia, the P wave, PR interval, and QRS complex are studied carefully as to direction of the deflection, width of the wave, PR interval, and QRS complex.

When impulses are initiated in atrial tissue other than the SA node, they are premature. Premature atrial contraction (Figure 11-15(e)) impulses originate prior to the SA node impulses and may be effective in depolarizing the cardiac muscle. This prematurity can result in a hidden or negatively deflected P wave. P waves may be hidden in the T wave, resulting in a slightly more peaked positive deflection. Premature atrial contractions may or may not be followed by a QRS complex, dependent upon the refractory state of the ventricles and the rapidity at which the originating impulses occur. Generally, the heart can respond with a full cycle up to 200 impulses per minute. Premature atrial contractions are also referred to as atrial premature contraction, atrial extrasystoles, or atrial ectopic beats.

An ectopic focus or site of an originating impulse other than the SA node creates changes in the P wave, however minimal. If the originating impulse arises in tissue other than the SA node and distal to this node, the PR interval is generally decreased in duration.

Atrial tachycardia (Figure 11-15(f)) occurs when the originating impulse is outside the SA node, and the impulse site becomes the cardiac pacemaker. The rate may vary from 160 to 240 cycles per minute. With a rate of such rapidity, the P waves are frequently hidden, while the QRS complex generally remains normal, although narrow, and the rhythm regular.

Premature atrial contractions that are consecutive, at least five in number, and appear and disappear suddenly are termed **paroxysmal atrial tachycardia** (Figure 11-15(g)). If the atrial rate at which impulses occur ranges between 250 and 350 beats per minute, the condition is termed atrial flutter (Figure 11-15(h)). Generally, the impulses are occurring so rapidly that conduction of all impulses through the AV node is not possible, and one impulse out of two is conducted through the heart's conductive system.

Atrial impulses occurring at a rate faster than 350 per minute establish the condition of **atrial fibrillation** (Figure 11-15(i)). In such a state, the impulses that are able to pass through the AV node are limited. This results in an irregular rhythm of ventricular depolarization, which is reflected on the tracing. Generally, the atrial rate cannot be calculated, and the QRS complex remains narrow and frequently within normal limits.

Arrhythmias Arising from Nodal Origin

Nodal arrhythmias originate when the atrioventricular (AV) junctional tissue becomes the pacemaker of the heart. When nodal arrhythmias exist, depolarization of the atrial tissue occurs in reverse of the normal atrial conduction pathway. This results in a negative deflection of the P wave, which may precede, follow, or be hidden within the QRS complex. The location of the P wave on the tracing indicates in which segment of the AV junctional tissue the impulse originated. When impulses arise in the superior portion of the AV junctional tissue, the P wave precedes the QRS complex, and the PR interval is less than 0.12 second. The decreased PR interval is due to the lessened distance necessary to pass through the AV node. When the atria and ventricles receive an impulse simultaneously for depolarization, the P wave is hidden within the QRS complex. An impulse with this origin is thought to arise from a midpoint in the AV junctional tissue. Impulses originating low in the AV junctional tissue result in a P wave following the QRS complex. In this case, the PR interval is measured by determining the time duration from the beginning of the QRS complex to the beginning of the P wave. Any of the nodal rhythms with different origins may exist. These are known as **multifocal nodal rhythms.** Nodal rhythms that are rapid or slow may compromise cardiac output. Figure 11-16 illustrates a nodal rhythm in which the impulse arises in the mid-portion of the AV junctional tissue.

Atrioventricular blocks can exist in various degrees and are the result of problems in the conduction of impulses from the atria to the ventricles. Conduction impairments are common with prolonged PR intervals. First-degree block (Figure 11-17(a)) is represented by a delay in

FIGURE 11-15

Electrocardiographic tracings of cardiac rhythms: (a) normal sinus rhythm; (b) sinus bradycardia; (c) sinus tachycardia; (d) sinus arrest; (e) premature atrial contraction and a wandering pacemaker; (f) atrial tachycardia; (g) paroxysmal atrial tachycardia; (h) atrial flutter; (i) atrial fibrillation.

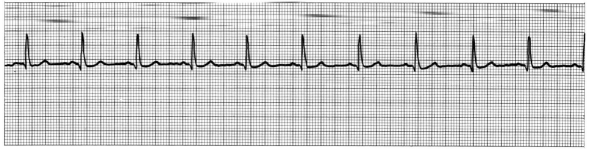

(a) Normal sinus rhythm

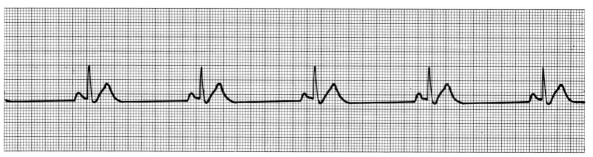

(b) Sinus bradycardia

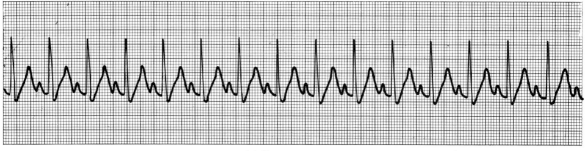

(c) Sinus tachycardia

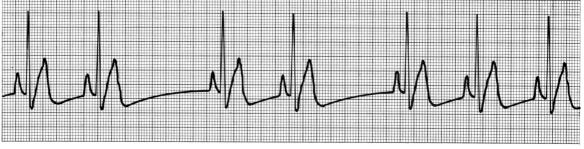

(d) Sinus arrest

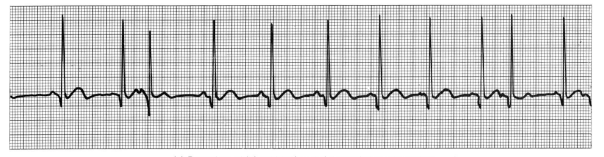

(e) Premature atrial contraction and a wandering pacemaker

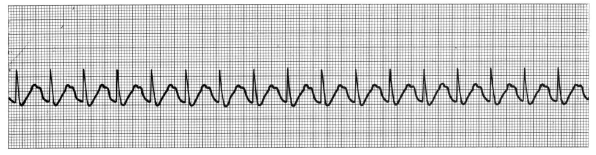

(f) Atrial tachycardia

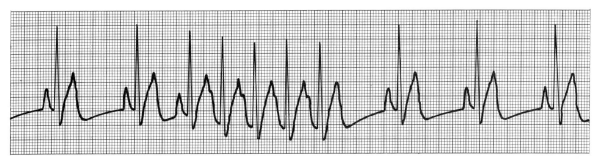

(g) Paroxysmal atrial tachycardia

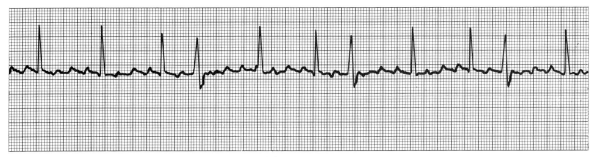

(h) Atrial flutter

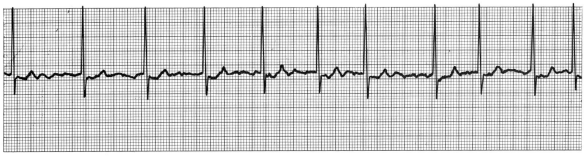

(i) Atrial fibrillation

179

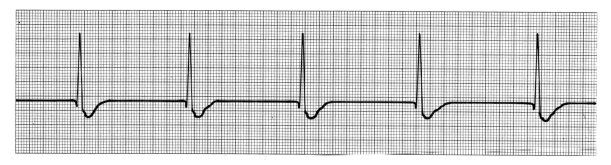

FIGURE 11 16
Nodal rhythm with impulse arising in the mid-portion of the AV junctional region.

FIGURE 11-17
Electrocardiographic tracings of heart block: (a) first-degree heart block; (b) second-degree heart block; (c) third-degree or complete heart block.

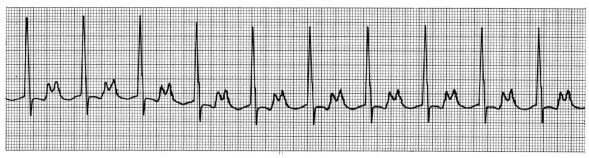

(a) First-degree heart block

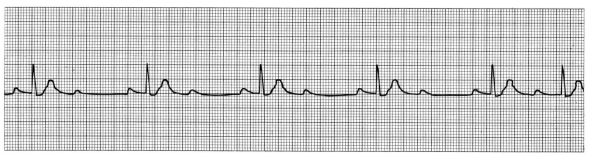

(b) Second-degree heart block

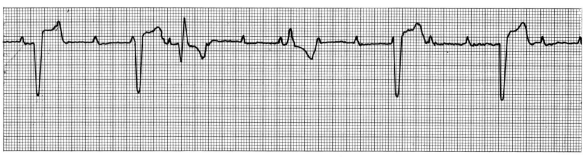

(c) Third-degree or complete heart block

impulse transmission. The PR interval is greater than 0.20 second, and each P wave is followed by a QRS complex. Second-degree AV block (Figure 11-17(b)) is present when one or more sinus impulses are followed by atrial depolarization, but failure in the conduction system results in nonventricular depolarization. There exists at least one nonconducted P wave. Second-degree block may also exist in a fixed ratio of originating impulses and impulses conducted. For example, in a two-to-one block, one impulse out of two is conducted. Third-degree AV block (Figure 11-17(c)) is depicted by a disjunction between atrial impulses and ventricular depolarization. There is no relationship between atrial depolarization and ventricular depolarization. Ventricular rates may range between 40 and 70 per minute.

Ventricular Arrhythmias

A common ventricular arrhythmia is the premature ventricular contraction (PVC), also known as a ventricular premature contraction, ventricular extrasystole, or ventricular ectopic beat (Figure 11-18(a)). The normal QRS complex follows a P wave, is of greater width, and frequently is followed by a compensatory pause. PVC's are the result of impulses originating in the ventricles; thus the pacemaker for this premature beat is located in the ventricles, as opposed to the atria (sinus rhythm) or AV node (nodal rhythm). Ventricular tachycardia (Figure 11-18(b)) is present when the ventricles initiate impulses at a rate above that which is normally generated from the ventricles, and when atrial impulses are not

FIGURE 11-18
Electrocardiographic tracings of ventricular arrhythmias: (a) premature ventricular contraction; (b) ventricular tachycardia; (c) ventricular fibrillation.

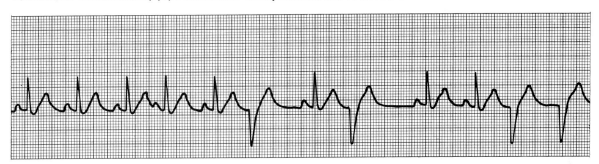

(a) Premature ventricular contraction

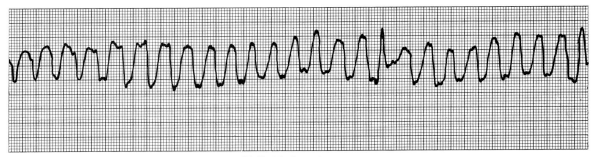

(b) Ventricular tachycardia

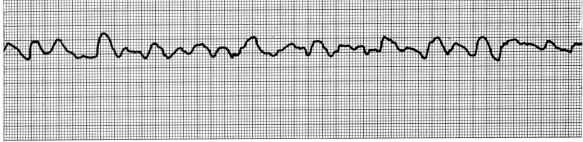

(c) Ventricular fibrillation

conducted through the AV node. The normal ventricular rate is between 20 and 40 beats per minute. When the ventricular rate is between 60 and 100, it is termed slow ventricular tachycardia. If the rate is greater than 100, it is termed fast ventricular tachycardia or paroxysmal ventricular tachycardia.

Ventricular fibrillation (Figure 11-18(c)) exists when no distinct QRS complex is seen on the tracing. This indicates that the cardiac muscles are functioning ineffectively and cardiac output is absent. Coarse waves, which demonstrate ven-tricular fibrillation, are indicative of recent onset; fine waves are indicative of fibrillation in late stages. Unless corrected, ventricular fibrillation is a lethal condition.

Other ventricular arrhythmias that indicate pathology are bundle branch blocks. These blocks can be of right or left origin and affect the QRS complex. They are demonstrated best in lead tracings other than lead II.

For greater depth in ECG interpretation, the nurse is advised to consult references primarily oriented to this topic.

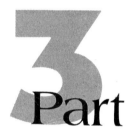

Part 3

STUDY GUIDE QUESTIONS

In the following client situations, identify and describe the subjective and objective data to be collected, the specific tools and procedures to be utilized in the collection of those data, and the rationale for the nursing assessment.

1. Mr. Dale Peterson, a 56-year-old male, is hospitalized for a possible MI one week ago. You are preparing to administer his daily dose of digoxin.

2. Mrs. Martha Taylor is a 70-year-old active widow who lives in a senior-citizen high-rise complex. She comes to you in the high-rise clinic for her annual "heart check-up" and physical exam.

3. Baby girl Hargrove is a 1-hour old infant. During your cursory exam, you note the presence of a heart murmur.

SAMPLE FORMAT TO BE USED IN RESPONDING TO THE STUDY GUIDE QUESTIONS

SUBJECTIVE DATA TO BE COLLECTED	OBJECTIVE DATA TO BE COLLECTED	SPECIFIC TOOLS AND PROCEDURES TO BE UTILIZED	RATIONALE FOR NURSING ASSESSMENT

BIBLIOGRAPHY

BASIC SYSTEMS, INC. "Correcting Common Errors in Blood Pressure Measurement," *American Journal of Nursing,* October 1965, 65, No. 10, pp. 134–164.

BASTA, LOFTY, L., PETRONIO T. LERONA, and LEWIS E. JANUARY, "Physical and Radiologic Examination of the Lung in the Evaluation of Cardiac Disease," *American Heart Journal,* August 1975, pp. 255–264.

BERGMAN, STUART A., and C. GUNNAR BLOMQUIST, "Amplitude of the First Heart Sound at Rest and During Exercise in Normal Subjects and in Patients with Coronary Heart Disease," *American Heart Journal,* December 1975, pp. 714–720.

DURASAY, F., "Heart Volume and Its Relationship to Body Weight in Trained Sportsmen," *Journal of Sports Medicine, Physical Fitness,* September 1974, pp. 178–182.

EVANS, WILLIAM F., *Anatomy and Physiology* (2nd ed), pp. 246–297. Englewood Cliffs, N.J.: Prentice-Hall, Inc., 1976.

FOWLER, NOBEL, O., *Examination of the Heart, Part Two: Inspection and Palpation of Venous and Arterial Pulses.* New York: American Heart Association, 1973.

FRANK, MARTIN J., and SERGIO V. ALVAREZ-MENA, *Cardiovascular Physical Diagnosis.* Chicago: Year Book Medical Publishers, Inc., 1973.

HOCHSTEIN, ELLIOT, and ALBERT L. RUBIN, *Physical Diagnosis,* pp. 128–275. New York: McGraw-Hill Book Company, 1964.

HOLLINSHEAD, W. HENRY, *Textbook of Anatomy* (2nd ed.), pp. 71–94, 525–559. New York: Harper & Row, Inc., 1967.

HURST, J. WILLIS, ed., *The Heart* (3rd ed.), New York: McGraw-Hill Book Company, 1974.

————, and ROBERT C. SCHLANT, *Examination of the Heart, Part Three: Inspection and Palpation of the Anterior Chest.* New York: American Heart Association, 1973.

IBRAHIM, M. MOSHEM, ROBERT C. TARAZI, and HARRIET P. DUSTAN, "Orthostatic Hypotension: Mechanisms and Management," *American Heart Journal,* October 1975, pp. 513–520.

JUDGE, RICHARD D., and GEORGE D. ZUIDEMA, ed., *Physical Diagnosis: A Physiologic Approach to the Clinical Examination* (2nd ed.), pp. 165–225. Boston: Little, Brown and Company, 1968.

KIRKENDALL, WALTER M., and others, *Recommendations for Human Blood Pressure Determination by Sphygmomanometers.* New York: American Heart Association, 1967.

LEHMAN, SISTER JANET, "Auscultation of Heart Sounds," *American Journal of Nursing,* July 1972, pp. 1242–1246.

LEONARD, JAMES J., and FRANK W. KROETZ, *Examination of the Heart, Part Four: Auscultation.* New York: American Heart Association, 1973.

LEVINE, SAMUEL A., and W. PROCTOR HARVEY, *Clinical Auscultation of the Heart* (2nd ed.). Philadelphia: W. B. Saunders Company, 1959.

LITTMANN, DAVID, *Examination of the Heart, Part Five: The Electrocardiogram.* New York: American Heart Association, 1973.

PEREZ, G. L., and others, "Incidence of Murmurs in the Aging Heart," *Journal of American Geriatrics Society,* January 1976, pp. 29–31.

PRIOR, JOHN A., and JACK S. SILBERSTEIN, *Physical Diagnosis* (4th ed.), pp. 223–282. St. Louis, Mo.: The C. V. Mosby Company, 1973.

RAVIN, ABE, *The Clinical Significance of the Sounds of Korotkoff.* West Point, Pa.: Merck, Sharp, and Dohme, June 1973.

SCHLANT, ROBERT, and J. WILLIS HURST, "Assessment of Cardiac Function at the Bedside," *Geriatrics,* June 1975, pp. 49–53.

SEGAL, BERNARD, WILLIAM LINKOFF, and JOHN H. MAYER, eds., *The Theory and Practice of Auscultation.* Philadelphia: F. A. David Company, 1964.

SILVERMAN, MARK E., *Examination of the Heart, Part One: Data Collection: The Clinical History.* New York: American Heart Association, 1973.

TURNER, RICHARD W. D., *Auscultation of the Heart* (3rd ed.). Edinburgh and London: E. and S. Livingston, Ltd., 1968.

12

The Breast

OBJECTIVES

REVIEW OF STRUCTURE AND FUNCTION

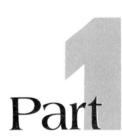

The mammary glands or breasts lie anterior to the pectoralis major muscle and extend transversely across the chest wall from the sternum to the mid-axillary line. The portion of the breast tissue extending to the mid-axillary line is called the tail of Spence. Vertically, the breasts are located between the second and sixth or seventh ribs. Fibrous bands of tissue, termed Cooper's ligaments, travel through the tissue and attach to the fascia of the muscle of the chest wall (Figure 12-1).

The breasts are composed of fatty, connective, and glandular tissue, with a high concentration of glandular tissue in the upper outer quadrant. Each breast has about 15 to 20 lobes, which are subdivided into numerous smaller lobules. The lobules contain milk-producing acini cells, and are served by a network of collecting ducts that unite to form a single exiting duct emerging at the nipple. Prior to emerging on the surface of the nipple, lactiferous sinuses are formed by the ducts. These sinuses, also called ampullae, serve as small milk reservoirs (Figure 12-2). Each breast also contains numerous lymph nodes that form a lymphatic drainage system (Figure 12-3).

In the neonate, breast tissue is nodular in size and can give an indication of gestational age, with 2 mm indicating 36 weeks or less, 4 mm indicating 37 to 38 weeks, and 7 mm indicating 39 weeks or more. The size of the breast in the adult varies, depending upon genetic factors, presence and degree of obesity, and the level of the hormone progesterone. Generally, the breasts are symmetrical in size, but it is common to have one breast slightly larger than the other. Extremely large breasts may be abnormal, and especially so if enlargement is unilateral. Any discomfort experienced from large breasts should also be considered abnormal, except during pregnancy and lactation. A slight fullness, often associated with tenderness, is not uncommon during menses.

The general shape of the breast is conical as it protrudes convexly from the thoracic wall. Large breasts may maintain a conical shape. Breasts that sag or hang are described as pendulous. Whatever the position of the breast, the structures should be bilaterally symmetrical. Asymmetrical shape may develop with underlying masses or inflammatory responses. Asymmetry

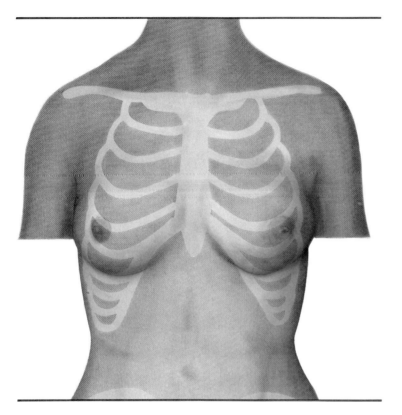

FIGURE 12-1
Anatomical location of the breast.

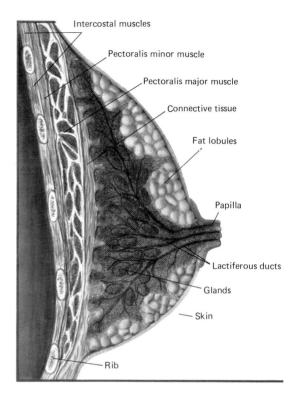

FIGURE 12-2
Structure of the breast.

FIGURE 12-3
Lymphatic drainage system of the breast.

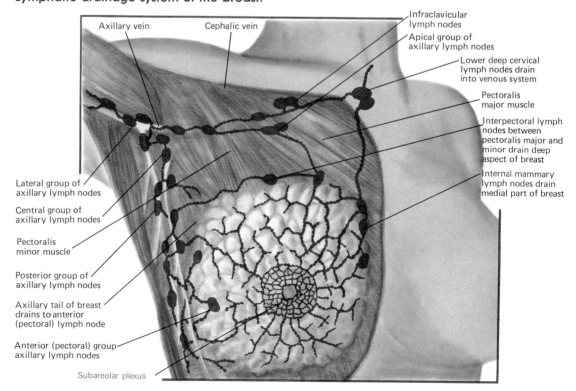

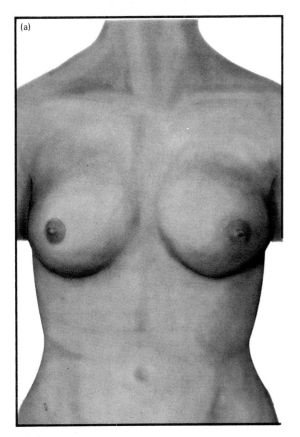 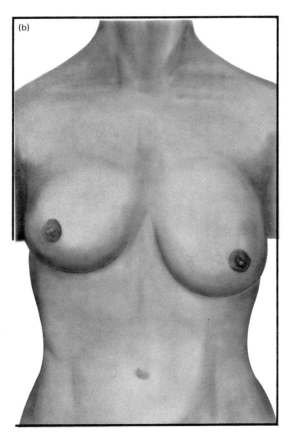

FIGURE 12-4

Contour of the breast: (a) symmetrical; (b) asymmetrical.

may present as retraction of the skin, puckering, or dimpling (Figure 12-4).

The color of the breast varies with the degree of integumentary pigmentation. Linear blue coloration that is bilateral may be the result of underlying vascular structures. If bluish coloration is unilateral and localized, it is generally considered a deviation from normal. Striae that are red are of a recent origin; pale, whitish-colored striae have been present for at least 6 months. Reddened or erythematous areas should be considered a deviation from the normal. The skin of the breast is normally smooth in appearance. Blockage of the lymph-node drainage system causes the skin to become edematous, protruding up and around the pores, giving an orange-peel effect (Figure 12-5).

The areola is normally located centrally on the breast and varies in size from 1 to 2½ cm in diameter. The degree of areolar pigmentation varies widely, ranging from a dark brown to an ex-

FIGURE 12-5

Orange-peel effect of the breast.

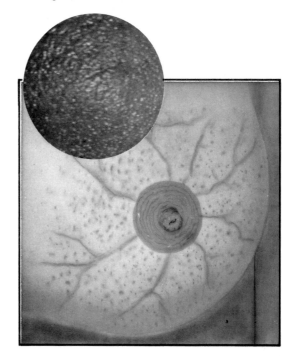

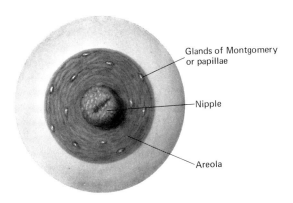

FIGURE 12-6
Areola and associated structures.

Glands of Montgomery or papillae

Nipple

Areola

tremely light pigmentation with the margins minimally demarcated from the surrounding skin. The surface of the areola is smooth and contains sebaceous glands, which appear as projections and are termed papillae, areolar glands, or glands of Montgomery (Figure 12-6). These glands produce a fatty substance, the purpose of which is thought to be for nipple lubrication during lactation. The papillae are most fre-

FIGURE 12-7
Nipple:
(a) protruding; (b) inverted.

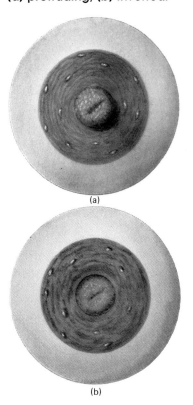

(a)

(b)

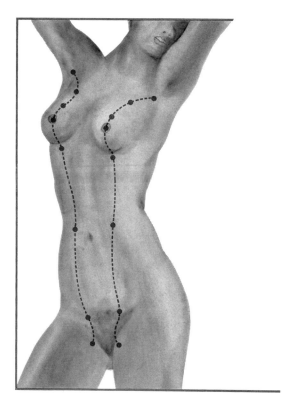

FIGURE 12-8
Milk lines and the location of supernumerary nipples.

quently asymmetrical with variations in presenting patterns. Retraction or bulging of the areola is abnormal and is frequently associated with underlying masses. The areola frequently has hair follicles around its periphery.

The nipple, composed of erectile tissue, is central within the areola and contains milk duct openings. It is generally circular in shape, and may be flush with the surrounding surface, may protrude or protrude with stimulation, or may be inverted (Figure 12-7). Shapes other than circular may be abnormal. Nipples generally possess a fine texture and are intact. Individuals may have supernumerary nipples, which are generally accompanied by a small areola. Supernumerary nipples are generally located in the "milk lines" (Figure 12-8).

Lesions of the nipple are abnormal. Normally, there is no discharge from the nipple unless lactation or pregnancy exist. Thick yellowish discharge can indicate an inflammation of a terminal duct; bloody discharge can be indicative of neoplastic disease.

HEALTH ASSESSMENT OF THE BREAST

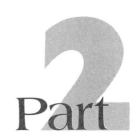

Inspection and palpation are the two methods used in examining the breast tissue. Inspection of the breast is accomplished with the anterior thoracic wall exposed, thus allowing bilateral comparison to be made while the individual is in the sitting and supine positions.

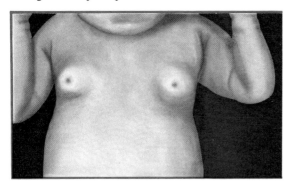

FIGURE 12-9 (above)
Swollen breast tissue of the newborn.

INSPECTION

Observe the position, shape, and contour of the breast and nipple, recognizing that many normal variations exist in the size and shape of the breast. In the newborn, breast tissue may be swollen, and the secretion of "witch's milk," a whitish discharge, may be observed (Figure 12-9). Involutional changes of the neonate's breast tissue occur in 2 to 3 weeks after stimulation from maternal hormones ceases. At puberty, growth of periductal tissue, enlargement of lobules, and deposition of fat causes breast growth. The areola and nipple become more pigmented at this time also. At the completion of puberty, the breasts are generally firm, conical in shape, and some superficial veins may be seen (Figure 12-10).

FIGURE 12-10 (below)
Development of the female breast.

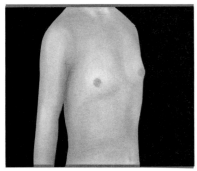

STAGE 1. The breasts are preadolescent. There is elevation of the papilla only.

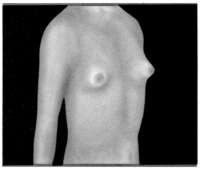

STAGE 2. Breast bud stage. A small mound is formed by the elevation of the breast and papilla. The areolar diameter enlarges.

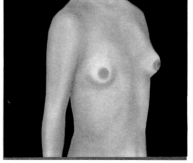

STAGE 3. There is further enlargement of the breast and areola with no separation of their contour.

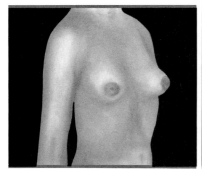

STAGE 4. There is a projection of the areola and papilla to form a secondary mound above the level of the breast.

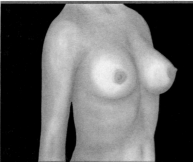

STAGE 5. The breasts are those of a mature female as the areola has recessed to the general contour of the breast.

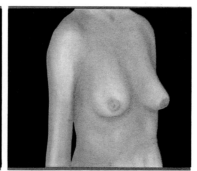

STAGE 6. The breast tissue becomes atropic following menopause.

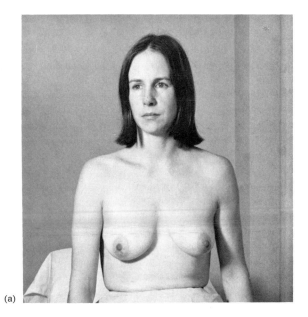
(a)

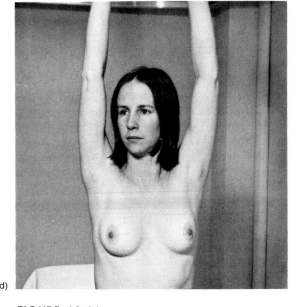
(d)

FIGURE 12-11
Positions assumed by the client during breast examination: (a) sitting upright, arms at the sides; (b) sitting, leaning forward; (c) sitting with hands on hips; (d) sitting with arms over the head.

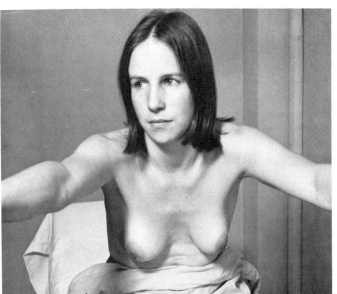
(b)

(c)

The breasts are inspected for symmetry, smoothness, areas of retraction, and orange-peel effect. These variables are assessed while the client assumes the following positions (see Figure 12-11(a), (b), (c) and (d)):

1. Sitting in a straight upright position with arms at the sides.
2. Sitting, leaning forward with arms extended.
3. Sitting with hands on hips, applying pressure in an isometric manner.
4. Sitting with arms raised over the head.

PALPATION

Palpation of the breast is performed with the palmar surfaces of the fingers, using a rotating motion. Pressure of the palpating fingers is first light, and then gradually increased to allow for both superficial and deep tissue examination. The client is seated, the arms are supported at the shoulder height, and the tail of Spence and lymph areas of the axillary region are palpated (Figure 12-12).

190

Following axillary palpation, the client is assisted to a supine position and a folded towel or small pillow is placed under the shoulder of the side on which breast palpation is to occur (Figure 12-13). The towel serves to flatten breast tissue against the thoracic wall, making irregularities more palpable. Tenderness during palpation is unusual in the normal individual, unless palpation of the breast tissue is performed during puberty, during engorgement of the breasts just prior to menses, or during pregnancy and lactation. Some irregularities, nodularities, or glandular sensations are palpable in the normal breast. After lactation or menopause, multiple nodular sensations are common. Tenderness upon palpation in states other than those previously identified may indicate underlying inflammation. Tumors rarely produce pain until later in their development. Benign masses are movable in the tissue, and present a firm, elastic, or fluctuant sensation. These masses do not adhere to the skin or underlying chest wall, and the edges are usually easily located and well defined.

Probable neoplastic changes are most frequently recognized first by the client when lumps or masses and/or nipple discharge are observed in the home setting. A cancerous mass frequently presents itself as a solitary, unilateral, hard, painless, nontender, immobile lump that is irregular in shape and has poor delineation of the margins. The most common site for neoplastic changes to occur is in the upper outer quadrant of each breast.

Palpation, using a circular motion with the palmar surface of the fingers, is carried out systematically to ensure that all areas of the breast are examined. The breast may be divided into quadrants (Figure 12-14). Each quadrant is palpated from the periphery to the center. If the breasts are large and pendulous, supporting the breast with one hand while the other is palpating the tissue of a designated quadrant will help to ensure that all areas of the breast are examined.

The areola is palpated next, using the same gentle rotating motion with slight compression to determine the tissue consistency. Finally, the nipple is gently squeezed between the thumb and index finger to elicit any discharge (Figure 12-15). The areola may also be gently squeezed to determine the possible presence of exudate in the terminal collecting ducts that are located under it.

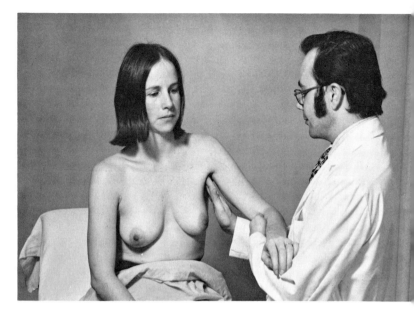

FIGURE 12-12
Palpation of the axillary lymph nodes.

FIGURE 12-13

Palpation of breast tissues with the client supine and shoulder elevated.

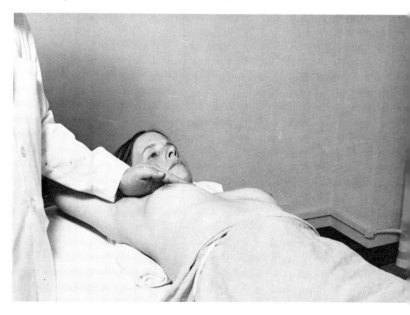

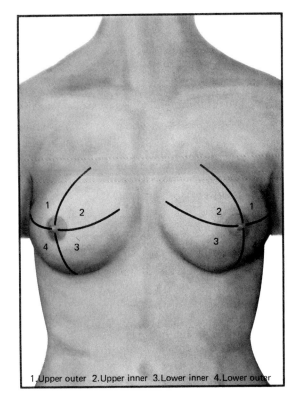

1.Upper outer 2.Upper inner 3.Lower inner 4.Lower outer

FIGURE 12-14 (above)
Quadrant division of the breast.

FIGURE 12-15 (right)
Gentle compression of the areola
and nipple.

The nipple, areola, and rudimentary breast tissue of the male is frequently not examined. The incidence of health-related problems in the male breast is low. Nevertheless, the region should be palpated for tenderness and nodularity, with special attention given to the nipple and areolar area where deviations from normal are generally located. Axillary lymph-node palpation is also completed with the male as with the female.

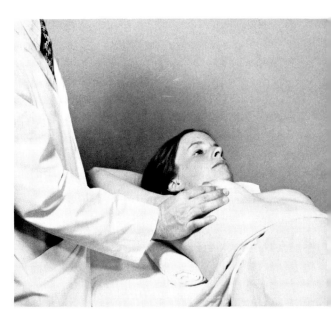

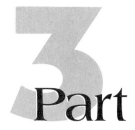

Part

STUDY GUIDE QUESTIONS

In the following client situation, identify and describe the subjective and objective data to be collected, the specific tools and procedures to be utilized in the collection of those data, and the rationale for the nursing assessment.

1. Tessy Carlson, a 26-year-old single female who has a strong familial history of breast cancer (mother, four maternal aunts, and one sister), requests information concerning the structure and function of the breast and a thorough method of performing a self-breast exam.

SAMPLE FORMAT TO BE USED IN RESPONDING TO THE STUDY GUIDE QUESTIONS

BIBLIOGRAPHY

BETHUNE, GORDON W., "Office Evaluation of Breast Problems," *Primary Care,* pp. 263–275. Philadelphia: W. B. Saunders Company, 1976.

BUCHAN, N. G., "Breast Exam in Obese Patients," *Lancet,* January 1976, p. 48.

BURNSIDE, JOHN W., *Adams Physical Diagnosis* (15th ed.), pp. 89–93. Baltimore, Md.: The Williams & Wilkins Company, 1974.

DEGOWIN, ELMER L., and RICHARD L. DEGOWIN, *Bedside Diagnostic Examination* (3rd ed.), pp. 248–259. New York: Macmillan Publishing Company, Inc., 1976.

JUDGE, RICHARD D., and GEORGE D. ZUIDEMA, *Physical Diagnosis: A Physiologic Approach to the Clinical Examination* (3rd ed.), pp. 301–311. Boston: Little, Brown and Company, 1968.

PAWSON, I. G., and N. L. PETRAKES, "Comparisons of Breast Pigment Among Women of Different Racial Groups," *Human Biology,* December 1975, pp. 441–450.

PRIOR, JOHN A., and JACK S. SILBERSTEIN, *Physical Diagnosis* (4th ed.), pp. 209–222. St. Louis, Mo.: The C. V. Mosby Company, 1973.

REGENIE, SANDRA, LYNETTE RUSSELL, and ALICE KIRKMAN, "The Self-Instructional Package: An Educational Resource—Breast Disease," *Journal of Nurse-Midwifery,* Vol XX, No. 4, Winter 1975, pp. 8–15.

STRAX, PHILEP, "Control of Breast Cancer Through Mass Screening," *Journal of American Medical Association,* April 1976, pp. 1600–1602.

13

The Abdomen

OBJECTIVES

1. Describe the anatomical location of the major abdominal organs.
2. Describe the general function of the identified major abdominal organs.
3. Systematically assess and describe:
   a. Abdominal contour
   b. Abdominal integument
   c. Abdominal movement
   d. Auscultated abdominal sounds
   e. Density of the abdomen and location of the major organs through percussion
   f. Palpated superficial and muscular structures
   g. Liver, spleen, and kidneys
   h. Pulsations of the abdominal aorta

REVIEW OF STRUCTURE
AND FUNCTION

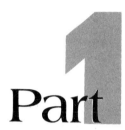

The abdomen can be divided into four anatomical quadrants; the upper right, lower right, upper left, and lower left. The vertical midline that divides the right and left sides of the abdomen must also be included as an important anatomical division. Several of the major organs located in each quadrant of the abdomen are illustrated in Figure 13-1.

The abdomen may also be divided into nine regions. Figure 13-2 illustrates major organ content in each region.

Figures 13-3 through 13-13 inclusive illustrate the anatomical positions of the major abdominal organs within the abdominal cavity. The captions for each of these eleven figures present a discussion in summary form of some of the functions of the abdominal organs. Included are discussions of the liver, the gallbladder, the pancreas, the stomach, the small intestine (including the duodenum, the jejunum, and the ileum), the large intestine (including the cecum, the ascending colon, the transverse colon, the descending colon, the sigmoid colon, and the rectum), the spleen, the ovary, the kidney, the urinary bladder, and the uterus.

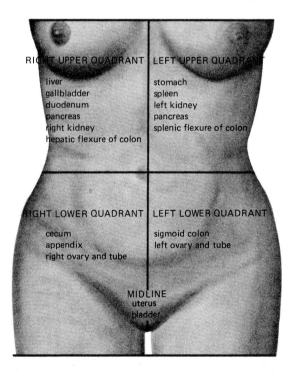

FIGURE 13-1

Abdominal quadrants and major structures located in each quadrant.

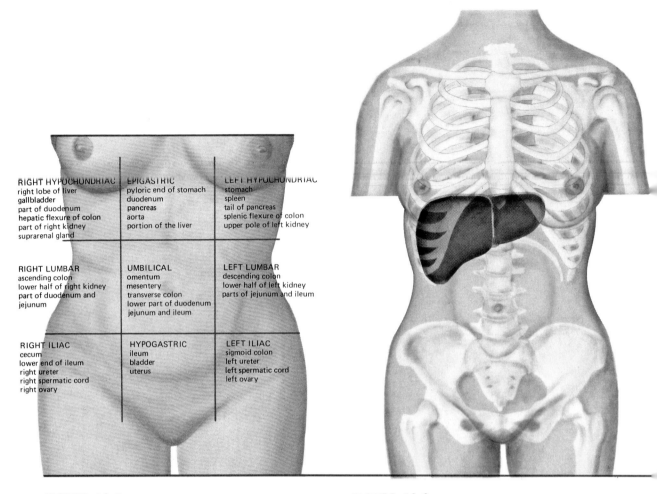

RIGHT HYPOCHONDRIAC
right lobe of liver
gallbladder
part of duodenum
hepatic flexure of colon
part of right kidney
suprarenal gland

EPIGASTRIC
pyloric end of stomach
duodenum
pancreas
aorta
portion of the liver

LEFT HYPOCHONDRIAC
stomach
spleen
tail of pancreas
splenic flexure of colon
upper pole of left kidney

RIGHT LUMBAR
ascending colon
lower half of right kidney
part of duodenum and
jejunum

UMBILICAL
omentum
mesentery
transverse colon
lower part of duodenum
jejunum and ileum

LEFT LUMBAR
descending colon
lower half of left kidney
parts of jejunum and ileum

RIGHT ILIAC
cecum
lower end of ileum
right ureter
right spermatic cord
right ovary

HYPOGASTRIC
ileum
bladder
uterus

LEFT ILIAC
sigmoid colon
left ureter
left spermatic cord
left ovary

FIGURE 13-2

Division of the abdomen into nine regions, with the major organ content in each region.

FIGURE 13-3

Anatomical location of the **liver.** The liver: (1) receives blood that has circulated through vessels of the digestive tract; (2) engages in phagocytosis and detoxification of bacteria and some foreign materials; (3) produces erythrocytes in the embryo; (4) is involved in the hematopoietic process and synthesis of the necessary products for clotting; (5) produces bile, which is necessary for digestion of fatty materials; (6) stores glycogen; (7) stores fat-soluble vitamins A, D, E, and K, and water-soluble vitamin B_{12}; (8) is involved in the metabolism of carbohydrates, fats, and proteins; (9) conjugates products of metabolism and chemical breakdowns for excretion; and (10) synthesizes essential body enzymes.

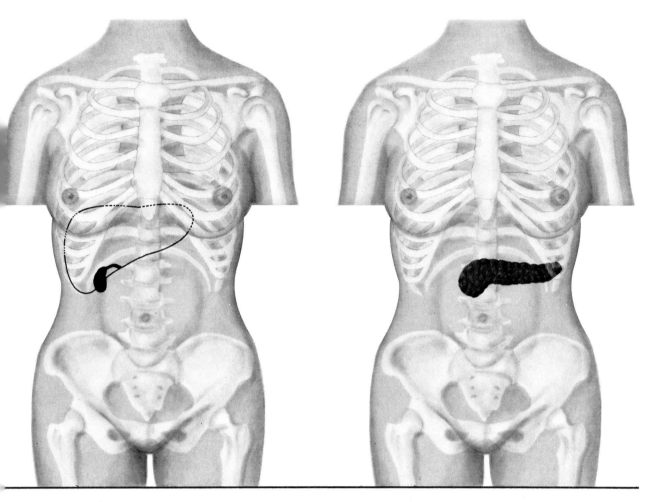

FIGURE 13-4
Anatomical location of the **gallbladder.**
The gallbladder stores bile and emulsifying
substances.

FIGURE 13-5
Anatomical location of the **pancreas.** The
pancreas (1) produces digestive enzymes;
and (2) produces and secretes the hormones
insulin and glucagon.

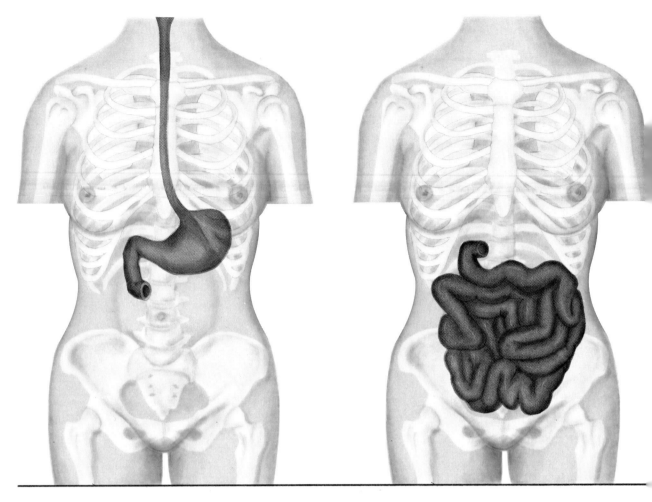

FIGURE 13-6

Anatomical location of the **stomach.** The stomach (1) receives ingested substances; (2) secretes juices, hydrochloric acid, and digestive enzymes necessary for initial catabolism of ingested substances; (3) stores ingested substances and controls emptying rate of contents into duodenum; and (4) engages in minimal absorption of ingested substances.

FIGURE 13-7

Anatomical location of the **small intestine** (small bowel), consisting of the duodenum, the jejunum, and the ileum, in that order. The duodenum (1) receives the churned food or chyme from the stomach; (2) possesses a highly alkaline environment, with a pH greater than 7.0; and (3) receives secretions of bile from the bile ducts and pancreatic enzymes for digestion. The small intestine as a whole (1) absorbs nutrients from ingested substances; and (2) propels ingested substances through itself using peristaltic waves, pushing the substances forward and rotating them for maximum exposure to intestinal secretions and the absorption structures lining the intestinal wall. The ileocecal valve permits entry of the contents of the small intestine into the large intestine.

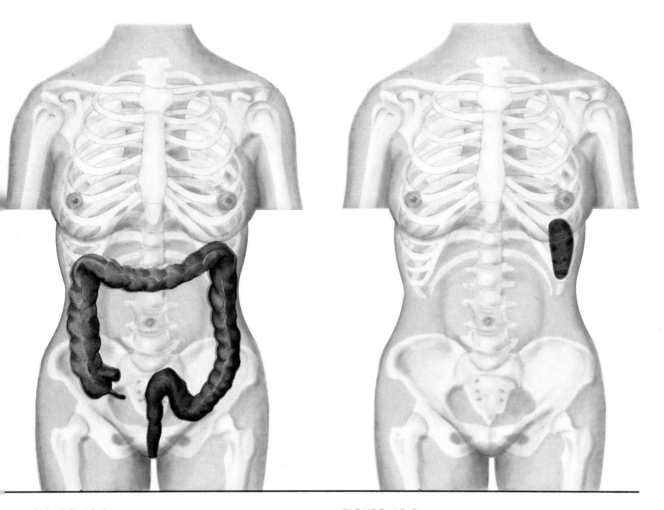

FIGURE 13-8

Anatomical location of the **large intestine** (large bowel), consisting of the cecum, the ascending colon, the transverse colon, the descending colon, the sigmoid colon, and the *rectum,* in that order. The appendix is attached to the cecum near the ileocecal junction and has no identified function. The large colon absorbs a high percentage of the fluid remaining in the bulk content of the intestine. At the proximal end of the large colon, vitamin K is synthesized by some of the resident bacteria. The sigmoid colon and the rectum serve as storage areas for the feces.

FIGURE 13-9

Anatomical location of the **spleen.** The spleen (1) destroys old red blood cells; (2) influences production and release of blood cells from bone marrow; (3) produces antibodies; and (4) stores and filters blood.

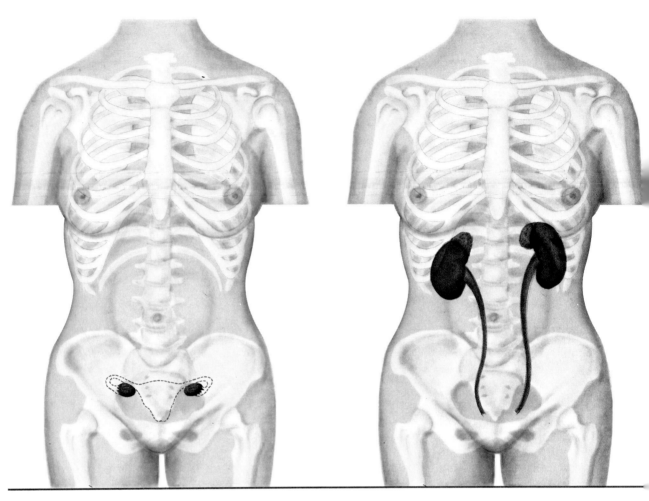

FIGURE 13-10

Anatomical location of the **ovaries.** The ovaries are the female reproductive organs. They (1) store, mature, and expel ova; and (2) produce feminizing hormones.

FIGURE 13-11

Anatomical location of the **kidneys.** The kidneys (1) serve as channels through which blood serum is filtered; (2) collect body waste products in preparation for excretion; (3) prevent excess fluid loss through reabsorption of water; (4) are involved in controlling blood pH and electrolyte balance; and (5) excrete fluid into the bladder through the ureters. In the adult, approximate excretion is 1500 ml/day, depending on age; children excrete 400 to 500 ml/day.

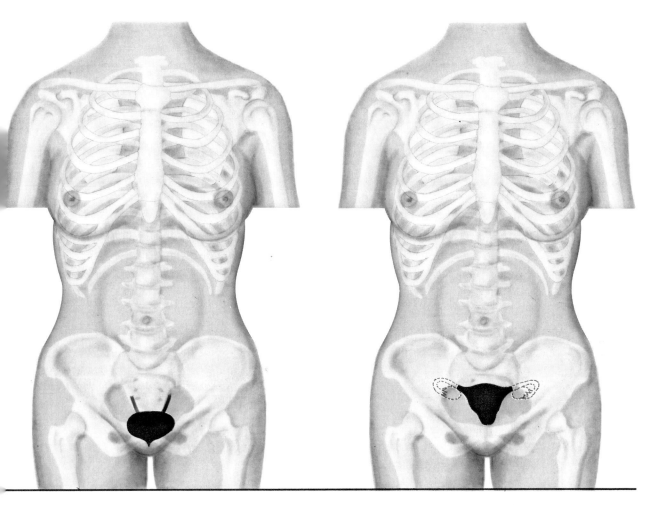

FIGURE 13-12
Anatomical location of the **urinary bladder.** The urinary bladder (1) stores urine until excretion (also known as micturition or voiding) occurs; and (2) expels urine from the body through the urethra. Normally, the adult is capable of storing 300 to 350 ml of urine prior to the occurrence of tension stimulation for voluntary micturition.

FIGURE 13-13
Anatomical location of the **uterus.** The uterus (1) functions as a passageway for sperm going to the fallopian tubes; (2) serves as a reservoir and provides nutrients for the developing fetus; and (3) expels the developed fetus following a normal gestation of ten lunar months. The internal wall of the uterus, or endometrium, is influenced by the cyclical secretion of female sex hormones and serves as the site for the implantation of a fertilized ovum.

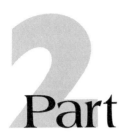

HEALTH ASSESSMENT OF THE ABDOMEN

Part 2

Evaluation of the abdomen employs the skills of inspection, auscultation, percussion, and palpation, in that sequence. The following provisions are facilitating to obtain accurate data in assessing the abdomen:

1. Adequate lighting
2. Warm environment
3. Warmed stethoscope
4. Warm hands
5. Short fingernails
6. Use of a systematic process including inspection, auscultation, percussion, and palpation

The abdomen is generally examined with the client in a supine position. The client's knees should be slightly flexed, as this maneuver relaxes the abdominal musculature. The subject's arms should be at his or her side or folded across the chest. In the male, the chest and abdomen are exposed down to the pubis, whereas in the female, the breasts are covered and exposure is from the lower thoracic wall down to the pubis. In the neonate, all body areas are kept covered except the abdomen to ensure temperature maintenance.

INSPECTION

When beginning the assessment of the abdomen, note the position assumed by the client. Normally, the client is able to recline in what appears to be a comfortable position. If pain is present, the client may assume a position to relieve it. One example is flexion of the right leg. This is frequently observed in splinting when appendicitis is present. Physical movements may coincide with cramping sensations in the abdomen. Constant motion may also indicate physiological or psychological discomfort.

The abdomen should be viewed as if it were divided into the four quadrants, and a vertical midline section. Initially, inspect the skin of the abdomen, observing its color (pink, jaundice, bronze), pigmentation lines such as the linea nigra, hair pattern, and the presence or absence of petechiae, spider angiomas, and excoriations.

The three abdominal contours commonly observed in the adult are as follows:

1. Flat, in which the abdomen is even from the chest to the pubis.
2. Scaphoid, in which the abdomen is concave when observing from the costal margins to the pubis. A scaphoid abdomen is typical of the very thin or emaciated individual.

3. Rounded, in which the abdomen presents a mounded appearance. The degree of rounding is dependent upon the degree of obesity. The highest point of a rounded abdomen is observed at the umbilicus while the client is in a supine position. When sitting or standing its farthest protruding point is located between the umbilicus and the symphysis pubis.

Infants through the toddler stage generally present a cylindrical, slightly protruding, or rounded abdomen. Children in this age range who present a scaphoid abdomen need further evaluation. Other deviations from normal, in both children and adults, are the indrawn and distended abdomen. The indrawn abdomen is under high muscular tension and is more pronounced when seen in adolescents and adulthood, owing to the developmental characteristics of the abdominal musculature. It generally indicates the presence of a pathological process occurring in the abdomen or back. The distended abdomen may be due to a gas- or fluid-filled bowel or a fluid-filled abdominal cavity. Frequently, if distention occurs as a result of small

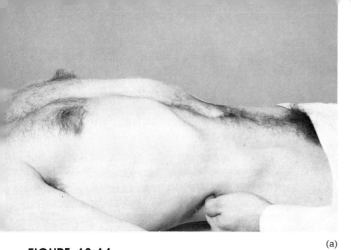

(a)

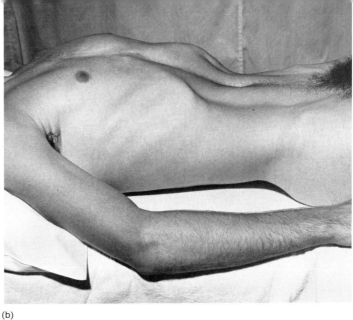

(b)

FIGURE 13-14
Abdominal contours: (a) flat; (b) scaphoid;
(c) rounded; (d) indrawn; (e) distended;
(f) cylindrical rounded abdomen of a toddler.

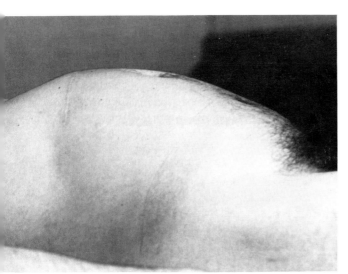

(c)

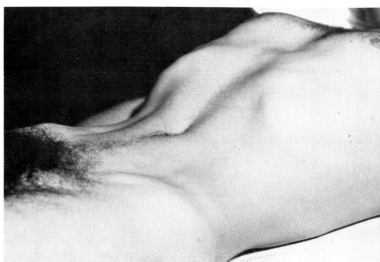

(d)

(e)

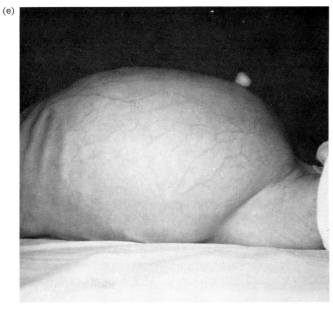

(f)

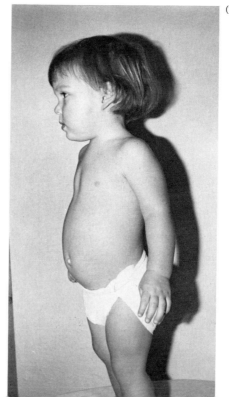

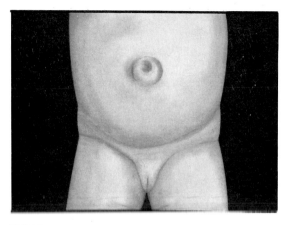

FIGURE 13-15
Umbilical hernia
(frontal view of umbilical protrusion).

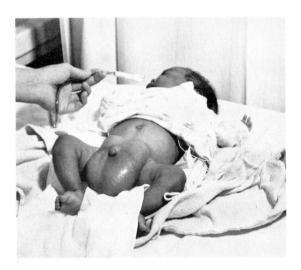

FIGURE 13-16
Direct bilateral hernias in a neonate.

FIGURE 13-17
Incisional hernias.

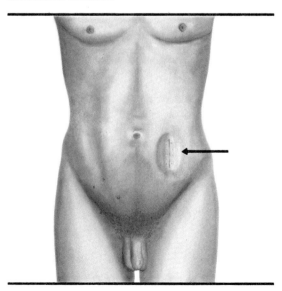

bowel dilation, the distention of the abdomen appears asymmetrical, whereas dilation of the large bowel will often yield a more symmetrical distention. Intense, prolonged distention of the abdomen may result in the abdominal skin appearing very tense, smooth, and shiny. If distention is created by a large volume of intra-abdominal fluid, the flanks may bulge when the client is supine, whereas the lower abdomen protrudes when the client is erect or sitting. Figure 13-14(a) through (f) illustrates the various contours.

Herniation or a disruption of the abdominal wall that allows protrusion of the abdominal contents may also present an asymmetrical appearance of the abdomen. Umbilical hernias (Figure 13-15) are the result of weak muscle structure and/or the failure of its closure at the site of the umbilicus. Umbilical hernias in the adult may follow pregnancy. The color of the herniated umbilicus becomes bluish in color when bowel infarction has occurred. Generally, the umbilicus in infants, toddlers, and young children should appear even with the skin surface. As growth continues, the umbilicus may assume a depressed appearance. The degree of inversion is also affected by the presence and degree of obesity. Direct inguinal hernias (Figure 13-16) may present bulging in the inguinal area of the abdominal wall and are more characteristic in the male than the female. Inguinal hernias, described as indirect, may enter the scrotal sac of the male. The assessment of scrotal hernias will be discussed in Chapter 14. Bulging may also be seen along an incisional scar line. This is called an **incisional hernia** (Figure 13-17). Increase in intra-abdominal pressure by the infant crying, or the adult performing the Valsalva maneuver "or bearing down," may yield a protrusion that otherwise would not be seen. Standing in the erect position or assumption of a knee to chest position may also help to produce an observable protruding sac.

Striae, or stretch marks (Figure 13-18), may also be observed on the skin of the abdomen. Striae that have developed recently have a reddish or bluish hue; those of long-standing duration take on a silvery white color. Striae are caused by excessive stretching of the skin, resulting in rupture of the elastic fibers. Predisposing factors to striae formation are obesity and pregnancy.

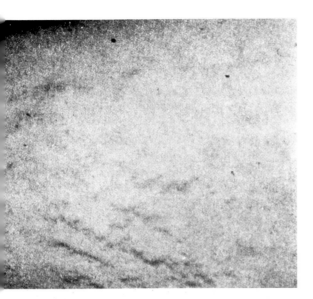

FIGURE 13-18
Striae or stretch marks on the
abdomen of a primigravida at term.

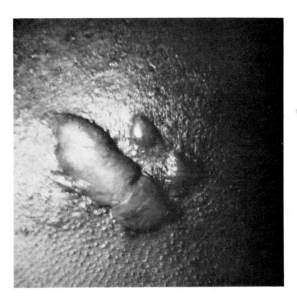

FIGURE 13-19
Keloidal tissue.

The presence of scars indicates surgical or other traumatic wounds. A recent scar is red and gradually turns into a pinkish color. At approximately 6 months, the scar tissue is the color of the skin, but gradually becomes more pale. If the wound healed by first intention, the scar line is thin; healing by second intention produces a wider scar. Traumatic scar tissue is frequently jagged, and scars from drainage sites are often puckered. Some individuals develop keloidal tissue or hypertrophied scar tissue (Figure 13-19).

Normally, in the adult, the abdominal veins are minimally visible, unless the subcutaneous tissue is thin, as in the infant and young child. In children, the abdominal veins are more readily visible but not prominent. In the elderly, loss of subcutaneous tissue makes the veins appear more prominent if the abdomen is thin. During pregnancy, dependent upon genetic factors, presence or absence of obesity, and the trimester, abdominal veins may become more visible. Abdominal veins above the umbilicus flow in an upward direction; blood flow in the veins below the umbilicus is in a downward direction.

The trauma line or belt line of the abdomen should be inspected carefully for color change, moles, or lesions. Some lesions may either be caused or irritated by friction. At times, the belt line has increased pigmentation compared to the surrounding skin. This is the result of tight constrictive clothing, such as a belt, that has been applying continuous pressure.

The abdomen is also inspected for involuntary abdominal movement. Normal peristaltic waves can be seen during inspection as undulations under the skin of children or thin adults with a less-developed abdominal musculature. In the normal adult with a well-developed abdominal wall, peristaltic waves are not revealed unless they are of increased intensity. When visible, these waves appear near the left upper quadrant

FIGURE 13-20
Direct percussion of the abdomen
to stimulate peristaltic waves.

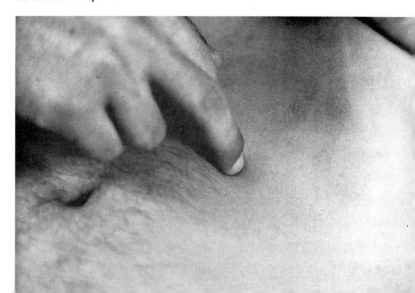

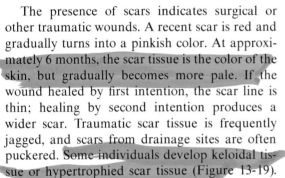

and generally move in a downward direction to the right. If the examiner is unsure that peristaltic waves were seen, tapping the abdomen with the index finger (Figure 13-20) may be sufficient stimulation to initiate bowel contraction and subsequent visible undulations. Pulsations of the abdominal aorta may also normally be seen in thin clients. These pulsations are especially notable in the epigastrium.

Respiratory movements are also observed. Generally, males, more often than females, are abdominal breathers. Increased movement of the abdominal wall during respiration may indicate intrathoracic disease; a decrease in the amount of abdominal movement may indicate intra-abdominal pathology.

AUSCULTATION

Next proceed to auscultation of the abdomen. This skill must be carried out prior to palpation and percussion, as bowel sounds may be increased or decreased due to the disturbing manipulation. Increased bowel sounds may, in turn, hide any vascular sound present. An unwarmed hand or stethoscope will cause the abdominal muscles to contract, and these contractions may

FIGURE 13-21
Abdominal auscultatory sites.

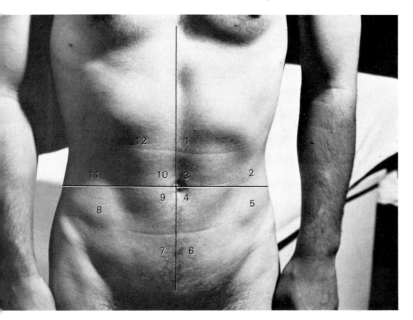

be heard during auscultation. Auscultate all quadrants of the abdomen in a clockwise fashion. Change the auscultatory site 2 or 3 in. with each move, as illustrated in Figure 13-21. Each time that the location of the stethoscope is changed, remove it from the abdomen, and then replace it. Dragging the stethoscope across the abdomen is irritating to the client and frequently causes involuntary muscle spasms.

Peristaltic sounds are high-pitched, gurgling noises that occur five or more times a minute, and are best transmitted using the diaphragm headpiece of the stethoscope. Two abnormal types of bowel sounds are the following:

1. Absence of or extremely weak and infrequent sounds. This type of sound or absence of sound could indicate bowel immotility, which is characteristic of peritonitis or paralytic ileus. The absence of bowel sounds cannot be determined unless auscultation is performed for 3 to 5 minutes.
2. Frequent, loud, rushing, high-pitched sounds may indicate a mechanical obstruction or hypermotility of the bowel.

It is important to identify the temporal relationship between the client's last meal and auscultation of the abdomen in order to determine the significance of unusual sounds. Shortly after or long after eating, bowel sounds may be increased, and are loudest when a meal is long overdue. This is a normal phenomenon. Bowel sounds may seem continuous when auscultating over the region of the ileocecal valve as a result of its permitting entry of small bowel contents into the colon. This event may occur 4 to 7 hours after a meal. The thickness of the abdominal wall, relative to both muscles and obesity, affects the relative ease and close proximity at which the sounds are heard.

The abdominal cavity should be auscultated for other abnormal sounds, such as bruits and peritoneal friction rubs. Bruits are peripheral murmurs that are characteristic of aortic aneurysms and other pathological conditions. Peritoneal friction rubs sound like two pieces of leather rubbing or grating together. Sometimes the rub is palpable by laying the palmar surface of the hand lightly over the area. Peritoneal friction rubs can indicate peritoneal inflammation. Rarely are venous hums heard in the abdomen.

PERCUSSION

Percussion follows auscultation of the abdomen. Using the mediated method (Figure 13-22), percuss the abdomen to determine density of the area and to map out underlying structures. Awareness of expected organ location is essential in interpreting the results of this procedure. Normally, sounds produced upon percussion range from tympany to dullness; flatness is an abnormal sound. Percussion over the stomach, epigastric area, or upper midline section normally yields a tympanic sound. Normally, the spleen is difficult to identify through percussion owing to the presence of gastric tympany. Tympanic sounds may also interfere with identification of splenic boundaries. Any dullness extending above the ninth intercostal space in the left mid-axillary line should raise suspicions of either an enlarged spleen, lower lung consolidation, or left liver lobe enlargement, and indicates need for further evaluation. A full bladder, a pregnant uterus that has risen above the pelvic brim, and the liver will also yield a dull sound.

If a dull sound is obtained upon percussion and the presence or absence of fluid needs to be determined, the examiner can percuss for a fluid wave. To do so, have the client or a co-worker place an arm longitudinally along the midline of the subject's abdomen. This prevents fat waves from traveling across the abdomen and being interpreted as fluid waves. Place the fingertips of the receiving right hand in the subject's lumbar area. With the left hand, quickly thrust your approximated fingers into the opposite lumbar region. If fluid is present, the receiving hand will feel the wave. Percussion for a fluid wave is illustrated in Figure 13-23.

The determination of free-floating intra-abdominal fluid or encapsulated fluid within the bowel is accomplished through percussion. With the client supine, percuss the abdomen to determine where the level of dullness resides. Then have the client assume a lateral position, and percuss the abdomen for the level of dullness. Turning the client in different positions determines the mobility of the fluid. Fluid within the abdominal cavity should be mobile, and therefore it should shift in the direction of gravity pull. Excess fluid within the bowel does not significantly shift in the direction of gravity pull when the client's position is changed. Figure 13-24

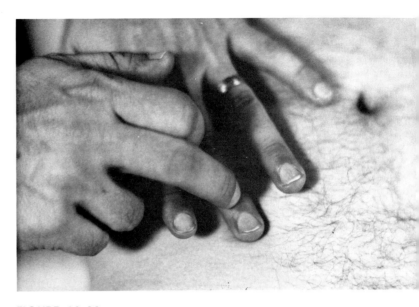

FIGURE 13-22
Mediated percussion of the abdomen.

FIGURE 13-23
Percussion for an abdominal fluid wave. The examiner quickly and gently thrusts approximated fingers into the lateral abdominal wall while the opposite fingers are placed in the opposite lateral abdominal wall.

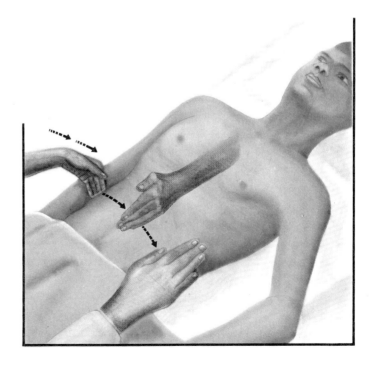

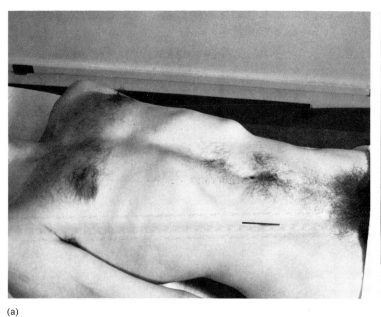 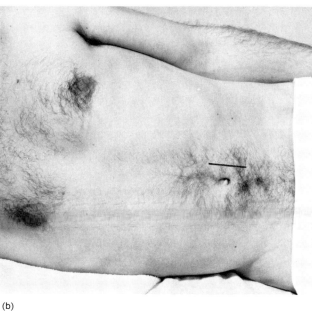

(a)   (b)

FIGURE 13-24
Position change of the client to differentiate free abdominal fluid from
encapsulated abdominal fluid: (a) supine; (b) lateral.

FIGURE 13-25
Percussion of liver borders:
(a) beginning in the mid-clavicular
mid-chest region;
(b) beginning in the lower abdomen
moving toward the chest.

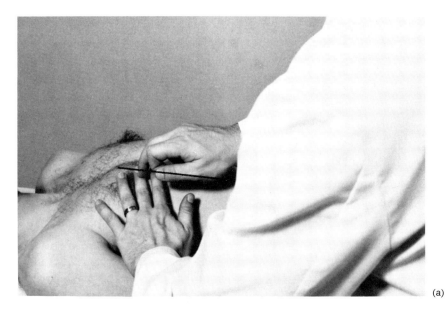

(a)

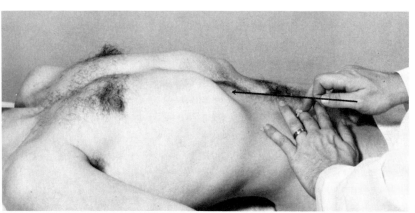

(b)

illustrates gravitational changes of free and encapsulated abdominal fluid.

Finally, percuss the outline of the liver. Begin in the mid-clavicular line at the mid-sternal level and proceed in a downward direction. When the upper edge of the liver is encountered, a dull sound will be produced. It is generally located between the fifth and seventh intercostal spaces. Continue percussing downward, until the lower liver margin is located. The upper and lower boundries should not be more than 10 cm apart. Percussion of the liver border gives the examiner an indication of liver location when initiating palpation of that organ. Figure 13-25 illustrates percussion of the liver borders.

PALPATION

Begin palpation by employing the light technique. The right hand, with the palmar surface down and fingers closely approximated, is placed on the abdomen to a depth of approximately 1 cm, or the depth of the subcutaneous tissue, and is moved in a circular motion (Figure 13-26). Palpate one quadrant thoroughly before proceeding to the next. If the client is ticklish, have him or her place his or her hand on top of or underneath yours. This tends to lessen the amount of ticklishness and subsequent muscle tenseness. Light palpation of the abdomen is utilized to determine the characteristics of the skin and subcutaneous tissue, as well as to elicit any tenderness of these superficial structures. If the client has indicated the presence of any tender areas, palpate these last.

Guarding of the abdomen may be voluntary or involuntary. Involuntary guarding persists in both the inspiratory and expiratory phases of respiration and results in a tensed abdominal musculature. Voluntary guarding is paramount during inspiration, whereas expiration results in a lessening of muscle tension. Guarding affects the examiner's ability to assess the superficial as well as the deep structures of the abdomen. Light palpation of the inguinal area frequently yields the presence of small lymph nodes, 0.5 to 1 cm in diameter. These nodes are termed shotty, and are most frequently present after biological maturity and throughout adulthood. Figure 13-27 illustrates the location of inguinal nodes. Normally, light palpation yields the characteristics of smoothness and mobility of surface structures.

Deep palpation can be performed using the bimanual method. The right hand is placed palmar surface down on the abdomen. Its purpose is sensory or tactile only. The fingers of the left hand press upon the interphalangeal joints of the right hand. The left hand applies pressure and creates the motion for the underlying hand. The depth of deep palpation should be 4 or 5 cm, or a suitable distance beyond the subcutaneous tissue.

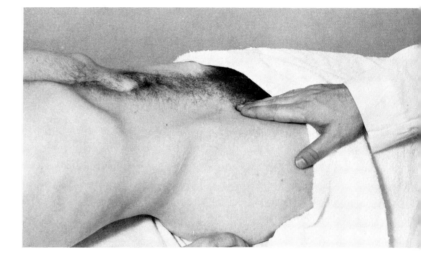

FIGURE 13-26
Light palpation of the abdomen.

FIGURE 13-27
Anatomical location of the inguinal lymph nodes.

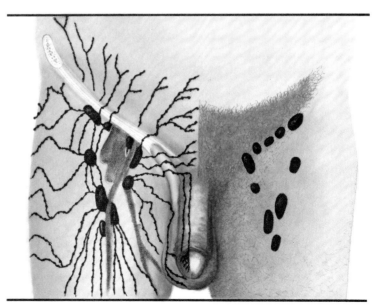

All quadrants of the abdomen are palpated at this depth to assess the underlying contents and structure. In deep palpation of the liver, spleen, and kidneys, let the descent of the diaphragm with deep inspiration through the mouth bring the organ to you.

Another method of deep palpation for the liver, spleen, and kidneys is accomplished by placing the left hand on the posterior flank, between the twelfth rib and the iliac crest to support and direct the structures anteriorly. Place the right hand on the anterior abdomen, using it to apply pressure and discriminate tactile sensations.

FIGURE 13-28

Two methods of palpating the liver: (a) one hand on the anterior abdomen with the opposite hand placed posteriorly; (b) both hands placed on the anterior abdomen.

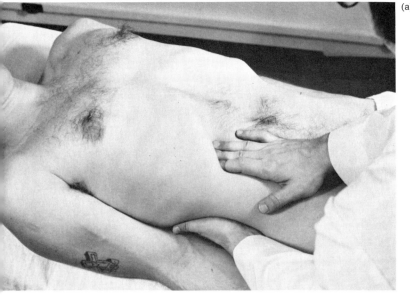

(a)

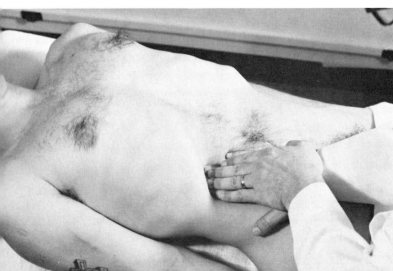

(b)

The liver is palpated in the right upper quadrant by placing the right hand parallel to the rectus muscle, just beneath the most inferior angle of the right costal margin, or approximately 2.5 cm below the level of the percussed lower liver border. Request the client to inspire deeply, letting the abdominal hand ride with the protruding abdominal wall. During expiration, exert a slow and gentle downward and forward pressure with the abdominal hand. In the adult a depth of 4 to 5 cm should be reached. During expiration, the abdominal wall is relaxed and facilitates deep palpation. Once the appropriate depth is reached, the hand is maintained in place without motion, and the client is requested to inspire deeply. Inspiration then aids the descent of the liver. The abdominal hand must resist the abdominal musculature minimally in order to palpate the liver, but it also must rise with the abdominal wall or great discomfort may result. The liver edge feels firm, with a sharp ridge of regular and relatively straight contour. It is generally located at or above the right costal margin in the adult, whereas in the infant it can be 2 cm below the right costal margin, and requires light palpation of 1 to 2 cm depth using only fingertips. Figure 13-28(a) and (b) illustrates the two methods of liver palpation.

Although the spleen is normally not palpable in either the adult or child, the splenic area is palpated. Palpation for the spleen (Figure 13-29) is accomplished on the left side, lateral to the mid-clavicular line, by the same method used for palpating the liver. Splenic enlargements have been graded as slight (1 to 4 cm below costal margin), moderate (4 to 8 cm below costal margin), and great (8 cm or more below the costal margin). The use of such words as slight, moderate, or great add little value to the data, whereas the use of centimeters creates a more explicit data base. When palpating the spleen, gentleness is an absolute, as this organ may be ruptured.

Palpation of the kidney (Figure 13-30) is performed by pressing directly upward beneath the costal margin at the mid-clavicular line while the client takes a deep breath. As the diaphragm is displaced downward, the inferior margin of the kidney is likewise depressed and may be felt. This is especially true of the right kidney as it is anatomically located lower than the left. Normally the kidneys are not palpable in the adult unless the individual is thin, and then only the lower pole is palpable. In elderly persons who are thin

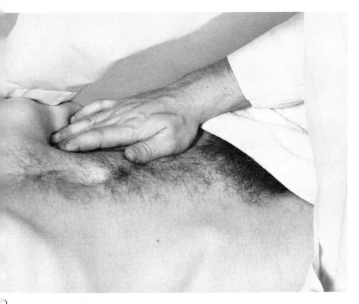

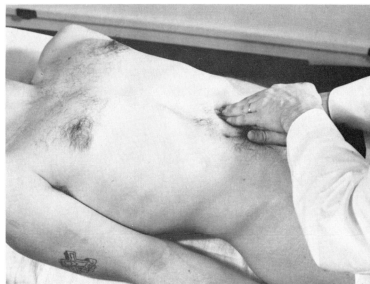

(b)

FIGURE 13-29
Two methods of palpation of the spleen:
(a) one hand on the anterior abdomen with
the opposite hand placed posteriorly;
(b) both hands placed on the anterior
abdomen.

and have relaxed abdominal musculature, the inferior portion of the kidney may be palpable. The kidneys are generally palpable in the neonate and the cooperative infant or thin child. If excessive pressure is applied when the kidney is palpated, a sickening discomfort can result.

Large masses, as well as a gravid uterus or distended bladder, may also be palpable in the abdominal region. Large masses may be found in any quadrant when deep palpation is performed. Minimal manipulation of the mass should be done, although it is essential to determine its size and characteristics. In the infant, 3 ounces of urine or 90 cc are required to distend the bladder above the pelvic brim; in the adult, 6 ounces or 180 cc is generally needed. Palpation of the bladder is accomplished bimanually by placing the palmar surfaces of the fingers between 2.5 and 5 cm above the pubic area (Figure 13-31), and gently pressing downward, curving the fingers back toward the hand. If the bladder is distended with urine, the fingers may need to be placed higher on the abdomen to determine the location of its most superior portion. A description of its location in centimeters from the umbilicus or pubic area is recorded. Guided practice and validation by an expert are required for a safe and interpretable assessment to occur using deep palpation.

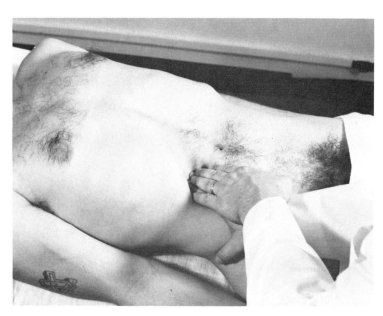

FIGURE 13-30
Bimanual palpation of the kidney.

FIGURE 13-31
Palpation of the urinary bladder.

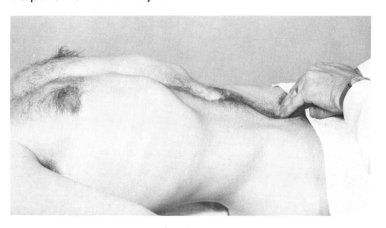

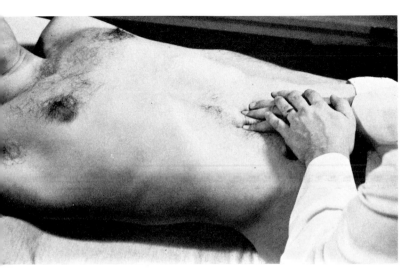

The abdominal portion of the descending aorta is palpated to determine the rate, rhythm, and quality of its pulsations. The examiner's findings are then compared to the palpable femoral pulses. Assessment of a pulsation of large diameter in the area of the aorta is accomplished through palpation. The index and second finger are placed, one on each side of the pulsating area (Figure 13-32). The divergence of the fingers during palpation may yield some information as to the possible existence of an aortic aneurysm.

Upon completing the assessment of the abdomen, the client's comfort should be acknowledged by covering the previously exposed abdomen. This is especially important in the neonate for whom conservation of body heat is essential.

FIGURE 13-32
Palpation of the abdominal aorta.

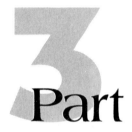
Part

STUDY GUIDE QUESTIONS

In the following client situations, identify and describe the subjective and objective data to be collected, the specific tools and procedures to be utilized in the collection of those data, and the rationale for the nursing assessment.

1. Mr. Anderson, a single 68-year-old male who is paraplegic and confined to his home, tells you during your weekly home visit that his abdomen feels full and he has not had a bowel movement for 4 days.

2. Mary Johnson, a 3-year-old female of slight build, is being examined by you for admission to preschool. Initially, while observing the abdomen, you question the presence of visible peristaltic waves.

3. Mrs. Ada Jensen, a 49-year-old female, is hospitalized for abdominal pain that coincides with cramping sensations. Her physician is particularly concerned about the possibility of abdominal obstruction.

4. Ralph Watson, a 22-year-old obese male, is now 8 hours post-op from an emergency appendectomy. One of your responsibilities is to determine when he is ready for his first clear liquids.

5. Colleen O'Malley is a 6-month-old infant whose mother has complained about her "protruding belly button." She returns to the well-baby clinic again with the same complaint.

6. Mr. Mark Schneider, a 57-year-old male, is admitted to the in-patient chemical dependency ward of your hospital with the diagnosis of alcoholism. You are concerned about his apparently acute abdominal distention.

SAMPLE FORMAT TO BE USED IN RESPONDING TO THE STUDY GUIDE QUESTIONS

OBJECTIVE DATA (what you observed)	SUBJECTIVE DATA (client's report)	TECHNIQUES AND PROCEDURES you utilized	RATIONALE FOR nursing assessment

BIBLIOGRAPHY

ALEXANDER, MARY M., and MARIE S. BROWN, *Pediatric Physical Diagnosis for Nurses,* pp. 149–163. New York: McGraw-Hill Book Company, 1974.

———, "Physical Examination, Part 13: Examining the Abdomen," *Nursing 76,* January 1976, pp. 65–70.

BURNSIDE, JOHN, *Adam's Physical Diagnosis* (15th ed.), pp. 160–172. Baltimore, Md.: The Williams & Wilkins Company, 1974.

COPE, SIR ZACHARY, *The Early Diagnosis of the Acute Abdomen.* New York: Oxford University Press, 1972.

DEGOWIN, ELMER L., and RICHARD L. DEGOWIN, *Bedside Diagnostic Examination* (3rd ed.), pp. 460–569. New York: Macmillan Publishing Company, Inc., 1976.

DENNIS, HUGH, JAMES DOWLING, and ROBERT F. RYAN, *Abdominal Hernias.* New York: Appleton-Century-Crofts, 1975.

HOLLINSHEAD, W. HENRY, *Textbook of Anatomy* (2nd ed.), pp. 561–678. New York: Harper & Row, Inc., 1967.

PRIOR, JOHN A., and JACK S. SILBERSTEIN, *Physical Diagnosis* (4th ed.), pp. 283–302. St. Louis, Mo.: The C. V. Mosby Company, 1973.

14

The Male Genitalia

REVIEW OF STRUCTURE AND FUNCTION

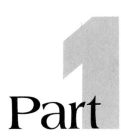

Two basic components of the genitourinary system are the urinary structures, which consist of the kidneys, ureters, bladder, and urethra, and the genital organs, which are composed of the penis, urethra, and scrotum with its contents (Figure 14-1(a)). The genital organs of the male are concerned with excretion, sexuality, and reproduction.

The penis is composed of cavernous tissue, which is structured in three longitudinal columns. The two lateral columns are called the corpora cavernosa. The medial column, which contains the urethra and forms the glans penis, is termed the corpus spongiosum. Figure 14-1(b) and (c) illustrates the structural columns of the penis. The proximal portion of the penis or junction between the penis and pubis is called the root. The neck of the penis refers to that area between the glans of the corpus spongiosum and the body of the penis.

Sexual stimuli, whether from psychological or physiological origin, can result in engorgement of the cavernous tissue with blood. Engorgement is the result of parasympathetic impulses that cause vasodilation and venous constriction to occur, thereby regulating blood flow into and out of the penis. This firming distention of the penis is called an erection. At the distal end of the penis is the glans through which the urethra forms its external opening, the urinary or urethral meatus. Normally, the meatus is located in the midline of the tip of the glans. However, congenital misplacements of the meatus can occur.

The urethra serves two purposes: (1) an exiting passageway for fluid waste products from the body in the form of urine, and (2) the exiting passageway for semen. The pathway that the urethra assumes from the bladder to the urethral meatus is characteristically S shaped. The urethra can be divided into four anatomical segments, the prostatic urethra, membranous urethra, bulbous urethra, and the penile or pendulous urethra. The prostatic segment of the urethra is circumscribed by the prostate gland and contains the orifices of the ejaculatory ducts. The Cowper's glands lie on each side of the membranous urethra as it progresses through the urogenital diaphragm. The bulbous urethra extends through the bulb of the corpus spongiosum and is followed by the penile or pendulous urethra, the longest section of the urethra. The penile urethra contains numerous tubular glands called glands

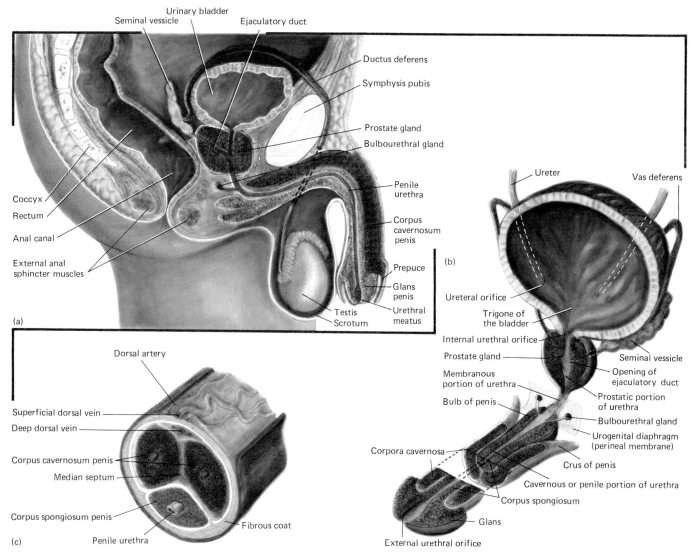

FIGURE 14-1

Male reproductive organs: (a) sagittal section of the pelvis;
(b) the three sections of the urethra; (c) cross section of the penis.

of Littré. These glands are of greatest concentration in the anterior surface of the urethra. The glands of Littré empty into recesses called the lacunae of Morgagni. Following acute infections of the urethra, these glands frequently develop chronic infectious states.

The skin of the penile shaft is composed of a single layer of tissue. It is loose and possesses mobility as far as the glans. The skin covering the glans, called the prepuce or foreskin, folds back upon itself. Its outer surface resembles the skin on the shaft, whereas the inner surface possesses more of a mucosal characteristic. The prepuce or

foreskin is retractable and is attached to the ventral side of the penis at the base of the glans by the frenulum. Surgical removal of the prepuce is known as circumcision and is frequently done when a male infant is approximately 2 to 3 days of age. Figure 14-2 illustrates a comparison of a circumcised and uncircumcised penis.

The scrotum, located behind the penis, is a saclike structure composed of smooth muscle. Upon contraction of the scrotal musculature, the scrotum is drawn toward the body; during relaxation of the musculature, the scrotum falls away from the body and assumes its normal pendulous position. The purpose of this muscular activity is to maintain the testes at an optimum temperature range for the production and viability of spermatozoa. The midline of the scrotum is a cordlike ridge called the raphe. Embryonically, this is formed by the junction of three muscle groups, which, with maturation of the fetus, develops into the septum; the scrotal septum divides the internal scrotal structure into two components, one for each testicle. The testes originate in the abdomen and then descend into the scrotum. Each testis is encapsulated by a fibrous sheath and is internally segmented by fibrous septa. Each segment or lobule contains convoluted or seminiferous tubules. The lining of these tubules is composed of a germinal epithelium that is specialized for spermatogenesis. The convoluted tubules within the lobules gradually converge, forming the efferent ductules, which lead into the epididymis. Newly formed sperm are transported to the epididymis, where, after approximately 18 hours, they become motile. Leydig cells, located between the matrix of the convoluted tubules, are responsible for the production of the androgenic hormone, testosterone.

The epididymis is a single convoluted duct and is continuous with the ductus deferens or vas deferens. Spermatozoa are transported into the lower abdominal cavity through the ductus deferens. The nerves, lymphatic and blood vessels, and the ductus deferens follow a similar pathway, and the composite of these structures forms the spermatic cord. The ductus deferens separates from the spermatic cord in the abdomen and enters the prostate gland posteriorly, where the seminal vesicles, ejaculatory duct, and bulbourethral glands are located. The seminal vesicles are equated to diverticula or appendages and are located laterally at the superior portion or base of the prostate. The seminal vesicles are involved in the production and secretion of seminal fluid.

The prostate gland, encapsulated in connective tissue, is located at the base of the bladder surrounding the urethra, and is separated from the rectum by a thin layer of tissue. It is composed of muscular and glandular tissue. The prostate is frequently referred to by lobes. The right and left lobe (consider the urethra as a midpoint reference) comprise the major portion of the gland. Between the right and left lobe is a medial sulcus or groove. The middle lobe, composed of glandular tissue, lies between the ejaculatory duct and the urethra. The posterior lobe is used as a reference when palpation of the gland occurs. The posterior lobe is subdivided into the base (uppermost portion) and the apex (the lowermost portion).

Puberty usually ensues during the approximate age range of 12 to 16 for the male. In this maturational process, the endocrine system plays an important role in the development of the genitalia and the secondary sex characteristics.

FIGURE 14-2
Penis: (a) external appearance of the circumcised penis; (b) external appearance of the uncircumcised penis.

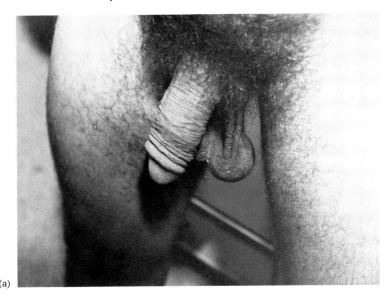

(a)

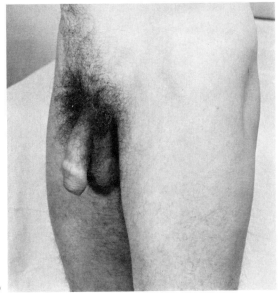

(b)

The prepubertal phase is heralded by development of hair on the scrotum similar to that of the abdomen. As puberty ensues, sparse, downy, straight hair grows at the base of the penis. At the same time, the testes and scrotum enlarge, the scrotal skin reddens, and proceeds through texture changes. As maturation progresses, the pubic hair takes on darker pigmentation and spreads over the entire pubic region; concurrent with this, facial hair begins to grow. It is during this time that the prostate gland enlarges, preparing itself for sexual activity.

At the completion of puberty, the skin of the penis and scrotum has a dark pigmentation, and the pubic hair is dense and curly, forming a diamond shape from the umbilicus to the anus. There is no hair on the penile shaft. The characteristic end products of sexual development remain throughout adult life until approximately the age of 50, when some atrophy of the external genitalia occurs gradually, and the pubic hair may thin out. These changes are due to decreasing amounts of androgenic hormone production (Figure 14-3(a) and (b)).

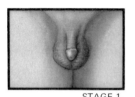 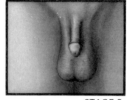 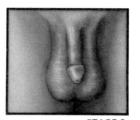 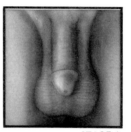 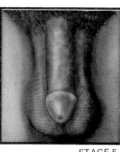

STAGE 1.

STAGE 2.

STAGE 3.

STAGE 4.

STAGE 5.

(a)

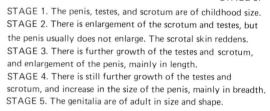

STAGE 1. The penis, testes, and scrotum are of childhood size.
STAGE 2. There is enlargement of the scrotum and testes, but the penis usually does not enlarge. The scrotal skin reddens.
STAGE 3. There is further growth of the testes and scrotum, and enlargement of the penis, mainly in length.
STAGE 4. There is still further growth of the testes and scrotum, and increase in the size of the penis, mainly in breadth.
STAGE 5. The genitalia are of adult in size and shape.

FIGURE 14-3

Developmental changes in the male pubic-hair pattern and genitalia:
(a) stages of genitalia development;
(b) stages of pubic hair development.

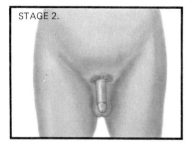 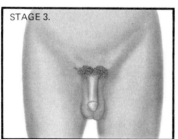 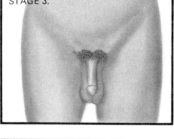

STAGE 2.

STAGE 3.

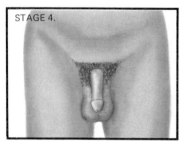 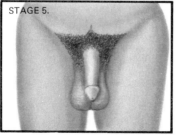

STAGE 4.

STAGE 5.

STAGE 1. (Not illustrated). There is no pubic hair.
STAGE 2. Initial growth, primarily at the base of the penis, of sparse, long, slightly pigmented, downy, straight, or slightly curled hair.
STAGE 3. Pubic hair is sparse, spreading over junction of the pubic region. Hair has greater pigmentation and is more curled.
STAGE 4. Pubic hair is long, thick, coarse and curled and covers as smaller area than in the adult.
STAGE 5. Pubic hair is adult in type and covers the pubic area forming an inverted triangle.

(b)

HEALTH ASSESSMENT OF THE MALE GENITALIA

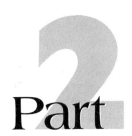

Part 2

To ensure a systematic process when collecting objective data, the tools of inspection and palpation are used for assessment of the male genitalia.

INSPECTION AND PALPATION

If appropriate to the chronological age, observe the color, density, and pattern of the pubic hair. Perineal hair growth prior to 10 years of age may indicate pathology of endocrine origin. Determine the developmental level of the genitals. The size of the penis shaft varies, as does the size and pendulousness of the scrotum. The left side of the scrotum hangs somewhat lower than the right. Observe the skin for color and presence of moles and lesions. If lesions are observed, wear rubber gloves to prevent spread of possible infectious agents. Lesions that are encrusted can be scraped with a tongue blade, and a sample of exudate obtained with a sterile applicator for culture and sensitivity. To ensure good observation, observe the dorsal, lateral, and ventral surfaces of the penis and scrotum.

In the uncircumcised male, inspection of the glans requires retraction of the foreskin. Nor-

mally, in the child and adult it retracts easily when grasping the penis behind the glans with the thumb and index finger and moving these fingers in the direction of the penile root. In some adults, the prepuce does not cover the glans entirely. Nevertheless, it is retracted to enable inspection of the entire structure. When the prepuce is retracted, it must be replaced once inspection is completed.

At birth, the glans penis is covered entirely by the prepuce. This structure is not retractable in the neonate, and frequently is nonretractable until 4 to 6 months of age. The patency of the urinary meatus is determined by the first voiding of the infant. The first voiding generally occurs within 12 hours of life and should, at the maximum, occur within the first 24 hours.

A condition in which the prepuce is so tight that it cannot be retracted is called **phimosis.** Phimosis (Figure 14-4) is generally due to strictures of the prepuce in the older male and adhesions in the newborn and young child. If the prepuce is tight and becomes entrapped behind the glans, the condition is called paraphimosis (Figure 14-5). A short frenulum, either due to congenital malformation or trauma such as a

FIGURE 14-4
Phimosis, a constricting foreskin covering the glans penis.

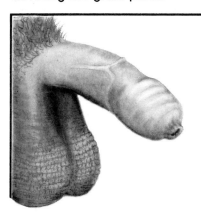

FIGURE 14-5
Paraphimosis, a constricting foreskin located behind the glans penis.

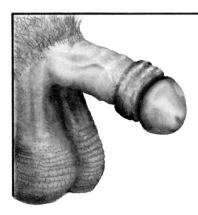

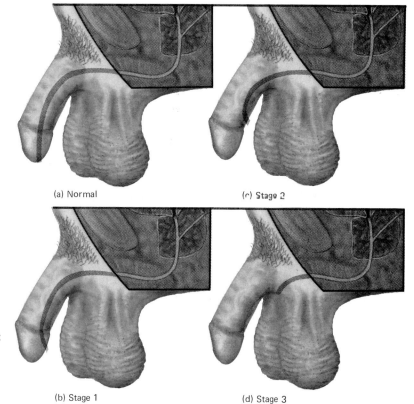

FIGURE 14-6

Normal urethral pathway compared to the three most common stages of hypospadias:
(a) normal urethral pathway;
(b) stage one;
(c) stage two;
(d) stage three.

(a) Normal

(c) Stage 2

(b) Stage 1

(d) Stage 3

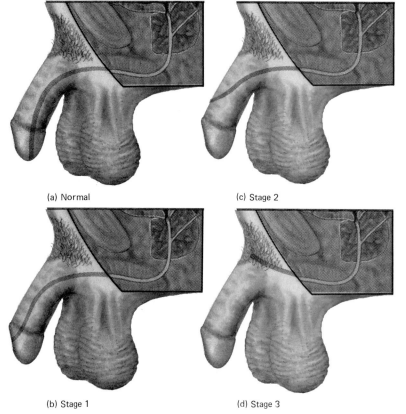

FIGURE 14-7

Normal urethral pathway compared to the three most common stages of epispadias:
(a) normal urethral pathway;
(b) stage one;
(c) stage two;
(d) stage three.

(a) Normal

(c) Stage 2

(b) Stage 1

(d) Stage 3

laceration, may cause retraction of the foreskin or a downward curvature of the glans, dependent upon the frenulum length.

The size and shape of the glans penis is evaluated for appropriateness relative to age. The structure of the glans is broad and smooth without protrusions or induration. Its greatest diameter is at the corona. A very conically shaped glans can indicate a tight or constricting prepuce that inhibited the development of breadth. In the adult Caucasian male, the glans is pink in color. In races with greater pigmentation, the glans is proportionately more pigmented. In the newly circumcised neonate, the glans frequently appears reddened, which may be due to forced dehiscence of the prepuce from the glans, as well as any other trauma received.

Observe the corona, retroglandular sulcus, and frenulum for the presence of lesions and type of hygiene. The sebaceous glands at the coronal sulcus appear as tiny projections and secrete a cheesy white substance called **smegma.** Collection of this material is due to inadequate hygiene and can lead to a foul odor. Smegma deposits predispose the client to bacterial colonization and subsequent inflammation.

Balanitis, an inflammation of the glans, may be due to various causes, such as ammoniacal diaper rash or inadequate hygiene. The degree of redness and edema is dependent upon the severity of the inflammation.

The meatus should be located at the tip of the glans. Congenital misplacements of the meatus are (1) hypospadias, in which the meatus is below the midline tip on the ventral surface, and (2) epispadias, in which the meatus is located above the tip on the dorsal surface of the penis. Figure 14-6 illustrates the three most common stages of hypospadias and compares them to the normal placement of the meatus; Figure 14-7 illustrates the three most common stages of epispadias and compares them to the normal anatomical placement.

With the thumbs of both hands, spread the lips of the meatus to determine if any strictures, lesions, or exudates are present. Figure 14-8 illustrates palpation of the glans to determine urethral patency.

Palpate the penis from the bulb to the urethral meatus, noting consistency and the presence or absence of indurations. Palpation of the penile shaft and glans is accomplished by using the index finger and thumb of both hands. This en-

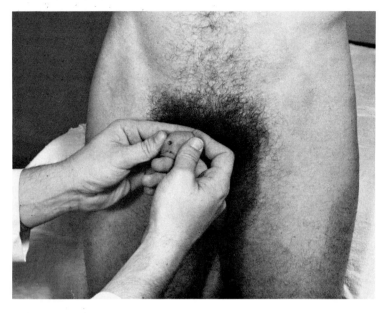

FIGURE 14-8
Inspection of the urethral meatus to determine patency.

ables all surfaces to be palpated at once (Figure 14-9). The normal penis is soft, but not flabby until old age, and contains no indurations. Fibrotic thickening, indurations (caverns), or protrusions are indicative of underlying disease processes such as abscess in the cavernous tissue or urethral diverticula. Palpable small nodules or shotlike bodies in the midline of the ventral surface of the penile body may be due to occluded periurethral glands. Bimanual palpation of the penile shaft also allows the examiner to strip the urethra and determine presence or absence of discharge. Normally, there is no discharge.

FIGURE 14-9
Palpation of the penile shaft.

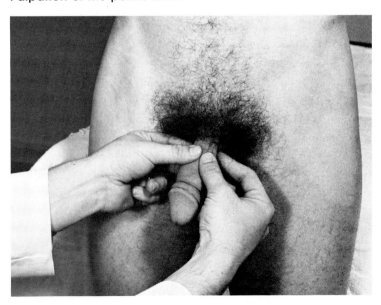

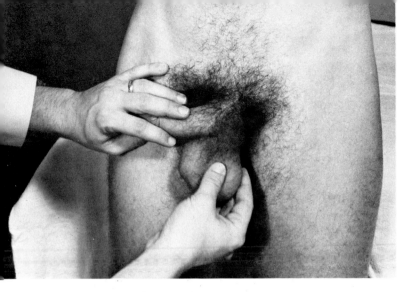

FIGURE 14-10
Palpation of the testes.

Next, assess the scrotum. In the premature neonate, the scrotum is frequently smooth, without rugation and closely approximated to the perineum. In the full-term infant and adult the scrotum is rugated. Spread the rugae between the fingers to facilitate inspection of the skin more closely. Sebaceous cysts appear as small yellowish raised nodules on the scrotal skin and are the result of sebaceous gland blockage. Prominent, dilated, tortuous veins within the scrotal skin are varicosities. Frequently, these veins are of little significance unless creating pain, although they may be related to an underlying metastatic cellular proliferation. An edematous scrotum may appear smooth, shiny, taut, and almost translucent.

FIGURE 14-11
Bilateral inguinal occlusion,
enabling palpation of the testes
in the newborn and young child.

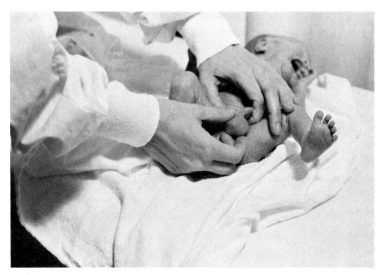

Following inspection of the scrotum, palpate each testicle bilaterally for location, size, shape, symmetry, consistency, mobility, and tenderness (Figure 14-10). In the adult the testis should feel smooth, firm, and rubbery, but not hard or soft. From middle age on, the testes begin to shrink in size and become softer in consistency. Palpable nodules should not be squeezed. Clients in whom nodules are assessed need to be referred to a specialist. Each testicle should be mobile within its fascial cleft and should be tender under pressure. In the full-term male infant, the testes are normally in the scrotum, while in the premature neonate, they are frequently found in the inguinal canal. In the neonate, evaluation of the testes is generally related to their presence and location, relative to the scrotal sac or inguinal canal. Frequently, touching the scrotum stimulates a retracting response, and the testes ascend into the inguinal canal, making confirmation of presence more difficult. To prevent this occurrence, the examiner can occlude the inguinal canal simultaneously by placing gentle pressure bilaterally at the opening of each canal with the thumb and one finger of one hand, thus leaving the other hand free to palpate the testes (Figure 14-11).

The tunica vaginalis lies anteriorly and laterally on the testicle. This is the region of fluid collection in hydroceles. Congenital hydroceles, common in the neonate, frequently resolve without intervention. They may occur in association with a hernia (Figure 14-12). Acquired hydroceles are of several origins and occur in various age groups, most frequently after the age of 40. Palpation of a hydrocele that envelops the testicle yields a soft fluctuating sac or a smooth, firm, or tense sac depending upon the amount of encapsulated fluid. The presence of a hydrocele may change the configuration of the scrotum.

On the upper pole of the testis lies the globus major or head of the epididymis. The body of the epididymis is on the posterior surface of the testis. Normally, the epididymis, when palpated between the index finger and thumb, is a soft, flaccid structure that feels like an appendage to the firm, rubbery testicle (Figure 14-13). The epididymis becomes continuous with the vas deferens, which eventuates into the spermatic cord. Bilaterally, place the index finger posteriorly and the thumb anteriorly to the scrotal sac. Locate the spermatic cord near the root of the scrotum and, with gentle compression, roll it between the thumb and finger following it downward toward

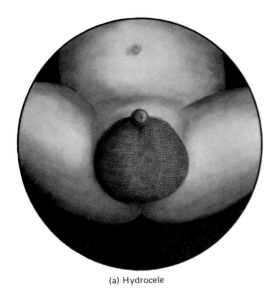

(a) Hydrocele

FIGURE 14-12
Hydrocele:
(a) scrotal appearance with
bilateral hydrocele in an infant;
(b) normal scrotum;
(c) simple hydrocele;
(d) hydrocele with a hernia
within the scrotal compartment.

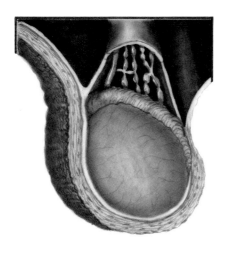

(b) Normal scrotum

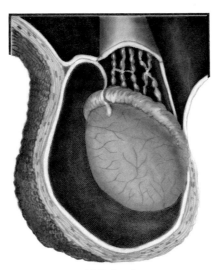

(c) Hydrocele

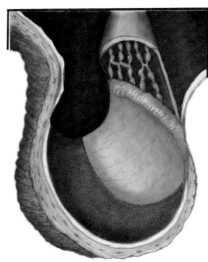

(d) Hydrocele with hernia

FIGURE 14-13
Palpation of the epididymis.

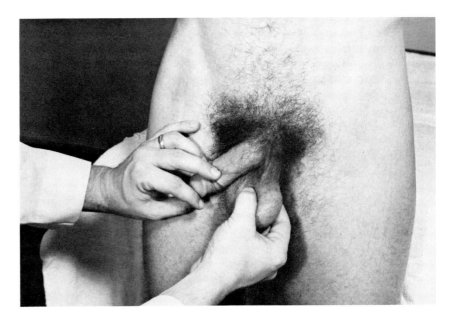

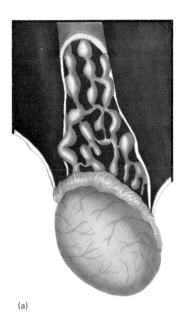
(a)

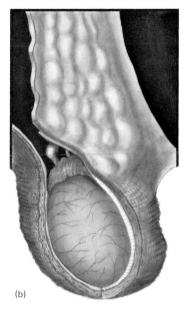
(b)

FIGURE 14-14
Varicocele: (a) normal scrotum;
(b) varicocele within the scrotal compartment.

the testicle. Another method is to locate the cord immediately proximal to the testis and follow it distally to the root of the scrotum. Normally, the spermatic cord feels "cordlike," rounded, smooth, and firm with resilience. A soft fluctuating, spindlelike mass along the cord may be indicative of a hydrocele of the cord. Varicoceles, varices, or varicose veins are most frequently palpated on the left spermatic cord and yield a hard, nodular elongated form, which may be likened to noodles or characteristically described as a bag of worms (Figure 14-14). Varicose veins are palpable when the client is in a standing position. In a supine position the veins decompress and are no longer palpable.

If a bulge is evident in the scrotum, grasp the root of the scrotum to determine how high the mass extends. If the fingers can be approximated above the mass, an indirect hernia is not likely, and probably the mass is of scrotal origin. Figure 14-15(a) illustrates finger approximation at the root of the scrotum; Figure 14-15(b) illustrates a scrotal mass that does not allow the examiner's fingers to approximate.

FIGURE 14-15
Approximation of palpating fingers to assess the origin of a scrotal mass:
(a) expected approximation of the fingers;
(b) fingers not approximated at root of scrotum due to the presence of a mass descending into the scrotum.

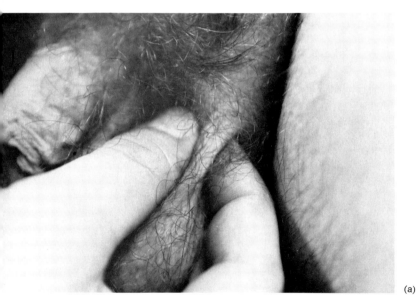
(a)

(b)
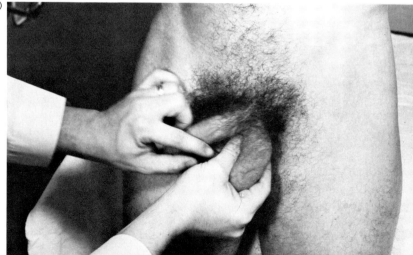

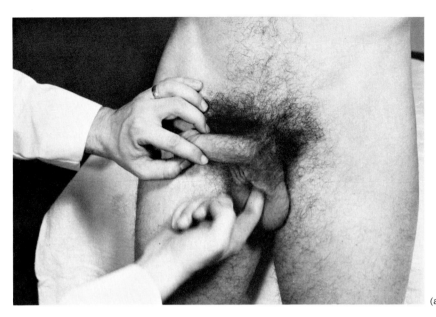

(a)

FIGURE 14-16
Assessment of inguinal ring integrity:
(a) invagination of the scrotal skin with index
finger to enable palpation of inguinal ring;
(b) palpation of the inguinal ring.

(b)

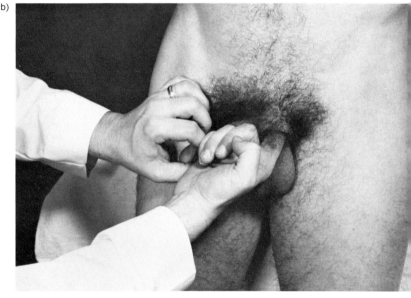

If one testicle feels larger than the other, nodular, hard, or of fluid consistency, the scrotal sac can be transilluminated. To accomplish transillumination, shine a light on the posterior surface of the scrotum behind the mass, with the scrotal skin stretched tautly. Fluid will transilluminate, whereas bowel loops will appear opaque. A darkened room is needed for this procedure.

To evaluate the inguinal ring (Figure 14-16(a) and (b)), unilaterally invaginate the lower part of the scrotum with the index finger and follow the spermatic cord upward until contact is made with the pubic bone. Be very careful not to pinch the skin or spermatic cord as a sickening pain may develop. Locate the slitlike ring $\frac{1}{2}$ in. above and lateral to the pubic tubercle. Normally, a protruding mass is not felt (Figure 14-17). Request the client to cough or bear down. Note any pulsation or sliding sensations against the finger. Normally, a slight pulsation may be felt against the finger. If a sliding sensation is felt, a hernia is likely and a judgment as to its size is made.

FIGURE 14-17
Normal scrotum (a), and scrotum
showing inguinal hernia (b).

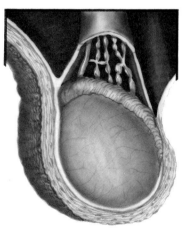

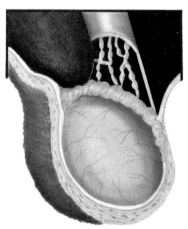

(a) Normal scrotum   (b) Inguinal hernia

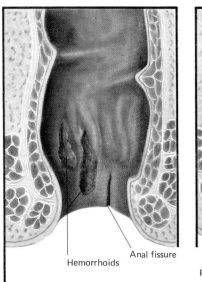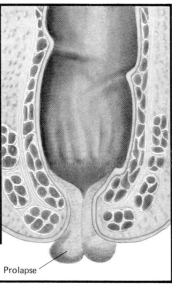

Hemorrhoids   Anal fissure

Prolapse

FIGURE 14-18
Abnormalities of the anus and rectum.

RECTAL EXAMINATION

The rectal examination enables assessment of the prostate as well as completion of the abdominal examination. The purpose of the rectal examination is to determine the skin condition around the rectal area, to determine the presence or absence of hemorrhoids, and to determine the size, shape, and consistency of the prostate gland, a part of the genital organs. Place the client in a knee-to-chest position, lithotomy position, or left lateral recumbent position, or have him stand with hips flexed and bent over a table for support. In the healthy young adult, these structures are generally assessed with the client standing flexed at the hips; in the elderly, the recumbent left lateral position is frequently used. In children, examination of the anus and rectum is accomplished with the child supine and frog legged.

FIGURE 14-19
Positioning of the client for palpation of the anus, rectum, and prostate gland:
(a) semiflexed bending over examination table; (b) left lateral recumbent position.

(a)   (b)

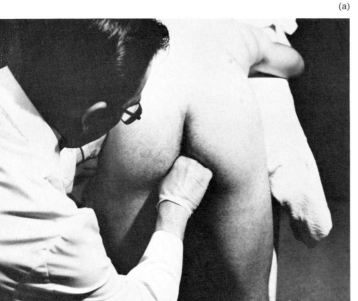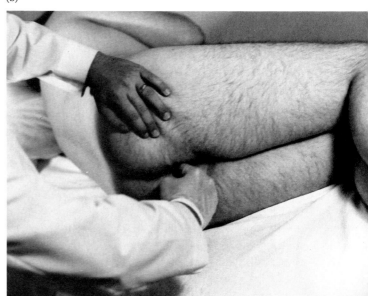

Inspection and Palpation

First, inspect the skin around the anus for signs of inflammation, excoriation, and external hemorrhoids. Normally, the anus appears drawn or puckered and of reddish-brown coloration. In children, it appears more reddish in color. Hemorrhoids are dark red, full, or tenselike protrusions composed of distended veins. Healed hemorrhoids or hemorrhoidal tags are small, loose skin structures. Ask the client to bear down and observe for internal hemorrhoids, polyps, or prolapsed rectal mucosa that may be exposed (Figure 14-18). Prolapsed rectal mucosa may appear velvety in consistency (surface characteristic) and reddish in color. Digital palpation is done with a well-lubricated gloved finger. Ask the client to bear down, pressing the index finger against the anal tissue for a brief period of time and then gently inserting your finger (Figure 14-19). Bearing down reduces sphincter tension, thus making entrance into the anus easier and more comfortable for the client. Evaluate the tonus of the external sphincter muscle. Normally, it is tight. A loose sphincter may indicate underlying disease processes. Insertion of the finger approximately $1\frac{1}{4}$ in. places it in the anal canal. Palpate the anal canal for polyps and other masses. The rectum is 5 in. in length and its walls should also be evaluated for masses.

The prostate gland rests along the anterior wall of the rectum and projects into the rectal lumen approximately 1 cm. Define the upper limits, generally the widest portion of the gland, the lateral margins, medial sulcus, and the lower margins; the apex is normally the narrowest section of the prostate gland. In the adult, the normal prostate is approximately 4 cm in diameter, and is characteristically described as the shape of a chestnut. The seminal vesicles extend upward and laterally along the upper margin of the prostate. The seminal vesicles cannot be felt unless inflamed. Generally, consistency of the prostate is smooth and rubbery and normally nontender. The prostate examination may produce an uncomfortable sensation, a sensation frequently associated with the need to void.

Palpation of a painful prostate results in reflex closure of the anal sphincter and a tensing of the buttocks. The prostate can feel hot, boggy in consistency, raised, with margins blending into

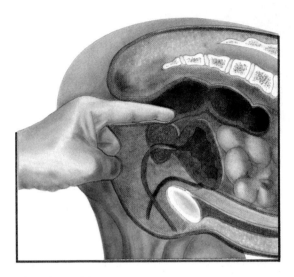

FIGURE 14-20

Sagittal section illustrating the position of the examiner's finger inserted into the rectum to assess the prostate gland.

the surrounding tissue. These signs may mean the presence of an inflammatory process with resultant congestion. A hard nodule, which may or may not be raised, and is well demarcated may be indicative of neoplastic changes.

Protrusion of the prostate gland into the rectal lumen more than 1 cm is abnormal, and is considered a state of hypertrophy. Frequently, centimeters of protrusion are recorded in a grading system. A grade I represents 1 to 2 cm of projection; a grade II represents 2 to 3 cm. Grade III is 3 to 4 cm, and grade IV is 4-cm protrusion into the rectal lumen. Prostate irregularities in size, shape, and consistency should be referred for medical evaluation. Figure 14-20 illustrates finger positioning to achieve evaluation of the prostate gland.

The rectal examination is indicated on a routine basis from puberty and thereafter. In the neonate, rectal examinations are never routine. Inspection of the anal opening and evaluation of anal sphincter control and patency of the anus are sufficient. One method through which anal patency can be determined is by gentle insertion of a lubricated thermometer, a maximum of 1 cm. Anal patency is usually confirmed by the appearance of the first stool, which generally occurs within the first 24 hours of life.

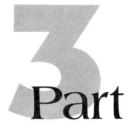

Part 3

STUDY GUIDE QUESTIONS

In the following client situations, identify and describe the subjective and objective data to be collected, the specific tools and procedures to be utilized in the collection of those data, and the rationale for the nursing assessment.

1. Two-week-old Johnny is brought to clinic by his mother for a 2-week check. His mother is concerned about the uneven size of his scrotum.
2. Jimmy Norr, a 3-year-old male, is brought to clinic by his mother, who recently discovered that he was not circumcised and requests an evaluation to determine if circumcision is necessary.
3. Craig Hannon, a 27-year-old male, states he has noted a fullness of his scrotum on the right side, which subsides when lying down.
4. George Rudolph, a 66-year-old male, comes to the annual neighborhood cancer-screening clinic. You are to assess the genitourinary system.

SAMPLE FORMAT TO BE USED IN RESPONDING TO THE STUDY GUIDE QUESTIONS

SUBJECTIVE DATA TO BE COLLECTED	OBJECTIVE DATA TO BE COLLECTED	SPECIFIC TOOLS AND PROCEDURES TO BE UTILIZED	RATIONALE FOR NURSING ASSESSMENT

BIBLIOGRAPHY

ALEXANDER, MARY M., AND MARIE S. BROWN, *Pediatric Physical Diagnosis for Nurses,* pp. 166–185. New York: McGraw-Hill Book Company, 1974.

CAMPBELL, MEREDITH F., *Principles of Urology.* Philadelphia: W. B. Saunders Company, 1957.

Children Are Different, pp. 127–130. Columbus, Ohio: Ross Laboratories, 1970.

DEGOWIN, ELMER L., and RICHARD L. DEGOWIN, *Bedside Diagnostic Examination* (3rd ed.), pp. 571–603. New York: Macmillan Publishing Company, Inc., 1976.

HOLLINSHEAD, W. HENRY, *Textbook of Anatomy* (2nd ed.), pp. 124–129, 728–751. New York: Harper & Row, Inc., 1967.

JUDGE, RICHARD D., and GEORGE D. ZUIDEMA, eds., *Physical Diagnosis: A Physiologic Approach to the Clinical Examination.* Boston: Little, Brown and Company, 1963.

KAPLAN, HELEN S., *The New Sex Therapy,* pp. 1–61. New York: Brunner/Mazel Publishers, 1974.

KATCHADOURIAN, HERANT A., and DONALD T. LUNDE, *Fundamentals of Human Sexuality* (2nd ed.), pp. 21–143. New York: Holt, Rinehart and Winston, Inc., 1975.

PRIOR, JOHN A., and JACK S. SILBERSTEIN, *Physical Diagnosis* (4th ed.), pp. 306–312. St. Louis, Mo.: The C. V. Mosby Company, 1973.

SMITH, DONALD R., *General Urology.* Los Altos, Calif.: Lange Medical Publications, 1972.

TURNER, RODERICK D., ed., *Office Urology.* New York: McGraw-Hill Book Company, Inc., 1963.

The Female Genitalia

15

OBJECTIVES

1. Identify the structures of the female genitalia.
2. Describe the functions of the structures of the female genitalia.
3. Describe the characteristics of the female genitalia throughout the life cycle.
4. Systematically assess and describe:
   a. Pubic hair pattern
   b. Integument of the genitalia and perineal region
   c. External genitalia
   d. Paraurethral and greater vestibular glands
   e. Vaginal walls and cervix through the use of inspection and instrumentation
   f. Vaginal muscle tone
   g. Characteristics of cervix through the use of palpation
   h. Characteristics and position of the uterus and adnexa
   i. Anus, sphincter tone, and rectal walls
   j. Posterior cul-de-sac

REVIEW OF STRUCTURE AND FUNCTION

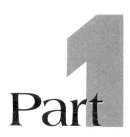

Part **1**

The female urinary system is composed of the kidney, ureters, bladder, and urethra. In contrast to the male, many of the genital structures are housed within the pelvic cavity, with only a few of those structures being external (Figure 15-1).

FIGURE 15-1

Sagittal section of the female pelvis.

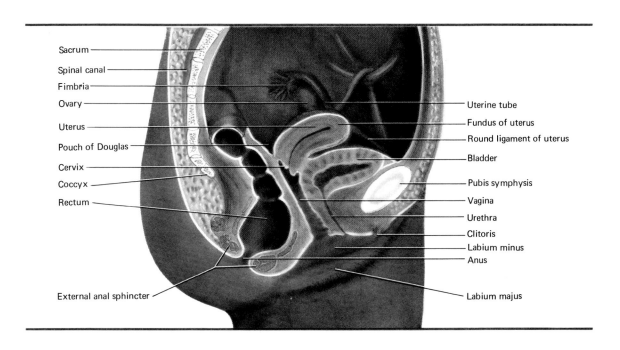

Sacrum

Spinal canal

Fimbria

Ovary

Uterus

Pouch of Douglas

Cervix

Coccyx

Rectum

External anal sphincter

Uterine tube

Fundus of uterus

Round ligament of uterus

Bladder

Pubis symphysis

Vagina

Urethra

Clitoris

Labium minus

Anus

Labium majus

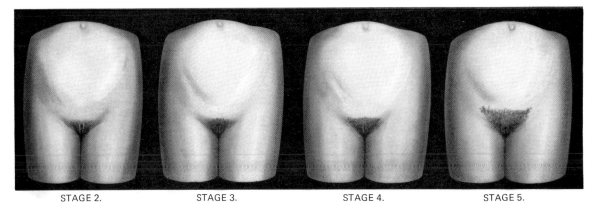

| STAGE 2. | STAGE 3. | STAGE 4. | STAGE 5. |

STAGE 1. (Not illustrated) There is no pubic hair.
STAGE 2. There is sparse growth of long, slightly pigmented, downy hair, straight or only slightly curled, primarily along the labia.
STAGE 3. The hair is considerably darker, coarser, and more curled. The hair spreads sparsely over the junction of the pubes
STAGE 4. The hair, now adult in type, covers a smaller area than in the adult.
STAGE 5. The hair is adult in quantity and type.

FIGURE 15-2
Stages of pubic hair development in the female.

EXTERNAL GENITALIA

Collectively, the external female genitals are called the vulva. The mons pubis overlies the pubic symphysis and is composed of fatty tissue. The area covered by pubic hair is called the escutcheon. Generally, the hair pattern of a mature female forms an inverted triangle, with the upper edge of the mons pubis and the point or tip extending posteriorly, covering the outer surfaces of the labia majora. Variations of this pattern exist, such as a diamond shape that has an anterior point progressing toward the umbilicus and a posterior point progressing toward the anus. The pubic hair may also include a portion of the inner thigh. Generally, the hair pattern is formed between the ages of 11 and 12. The hair is curly, coarse, and generally dense, until the postmenopausal state, when thinning and softening of texture occurs (Figure 15-2).

The labia majora consist of skin folds that form liplike structures and are most prominent near the anterior point of origin, the pubis. Their pigmentation is generally greater than that of the surrounding tissue. The labia contain both sebaceous glands and sweat glands. Posteriorly, the

labia majora lose their prominence and merge with the tissue above the anus, the perineum. In the premature newborn, the labia majora appear small, resulting in protrusion and exposure of the labia minora. In the term infant, the labia majora approximate each other and appear edematous. The labia majora remain infantile until puberty, when feminizing hormones stimulate deposition of fat, resulting in enlargement and prominence. The pudendal cleft, or space between the labial lips, is most often visible only when the lips are parted, and presents an inner surface that is smooth and hairless. Close approximation of the labial lips generally continues until after a vaginal delivery. In postmenopausal females, the labia majora atrophy, and lose their prominence and smooth skin appearance to a retiring and wrinkled appearance.

The labia minora present as two folds of pinkish, wrinkled, hairless skin located between the labia majora. Posteriorly, the labia minora merge with the labia majora. Anteriorly, they are joined, forming the prepuce, a sheath surrounding the clitoris. Immediately inferior to the clitoris are two folds of skin that form the frenulum of the clitoris. The anterior–posterior extension of the labia minora forms the vestibule, an area in which the clitoris, external urethral orifice, hymen, vaginal orifice, and paraurethral and greater vestibular glands are contained.

The surfaces of the labia minora are closely approximated, which can lead to labial agglutination during childhood. After vaginal delivery, with the separation of the majora, the labia minora appear slightly prominent. With menopause, and the marked decrease in estrogenic stimuli, the labia minora become atrophic.

In the neonate, the clitoris appears hypertrophic and may protrude through the labia minora, whereas in the premature it characteristically protrudes through the labia majora (Figure 15-3). Involution of the hypertrophic clitoris occurs by the end of the neonatal period. In the child and adult, the clitoris remains decreased in prominence. In the adult, it is approximately 2 cm in length and 1 cm in width. Following menopause, the clitoris decreases in size owing to diminished levels of feminizing hormones. The clitoris is composed of cavernous erectile tissue, which is highly vascular and contains numerous nerve endings. Anatomical divisions of the clitoris are the glans, body, and the crura. The clitoris becomes engorged with blood during sexual excitement, resulting in an erection of the tissue. The numerous nerve endings are the source of its great sensitivity.

The urethra in the female, in contrast to the male, acts as a conveying passageway for urine only and is not involved with reproductive functions. It is generally found in the midline between the frenulum of the clitoris and the vaginal orifice. The urethral meatus is circular or slitlike, and generally blends into the surrounding tissue color. The paraurethral glands are located approximately at the 4 and 8 o'clock positions. These glands are located proximal to the internal meatal lips or, most frequently, proximal to the external meatal lips. The paraurethral glands are also called the urethral glands or Skene's glands. Figure 15-4 illustrates the location of the labia minora, clitoris, urethra, and paraurethral glands.

The introitus, vaginal orifice or vaginal opening, is located between the labia minora and occupies a major portion of the posterior vestibule. The hymen, a thin, highly vascularized membrane, separates the vaginal orifice from the vestibule. It may be described in several ways. A complete or imperforated hymen occludes the entire vaginal orifice. In complete occlusion, menstrual flow is impeded and may cause a forward bulge. A hymen that does not completely occlude the vaginal orifice is termed incomplete or partial. In the newborn, a hymenal tag may be seen in addition to the hymen. This extra tag of tissue involutes by the end of the neonatal period. The hymen may be torn at any time during the life cycle and does not necessarily indicate sexual activity. Once the hymen is perforated, the edges retract and hymenal tags form along the periphery of the vaginal orifice. Increased fragmenta-

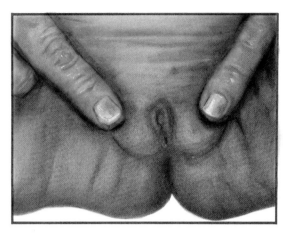

FIGURE 15-3
Clitoral protrusion in the premature.

FIGURE 15-4
Anatomical location of the external female organs of reproduction.

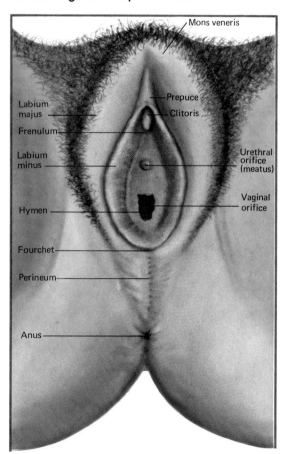

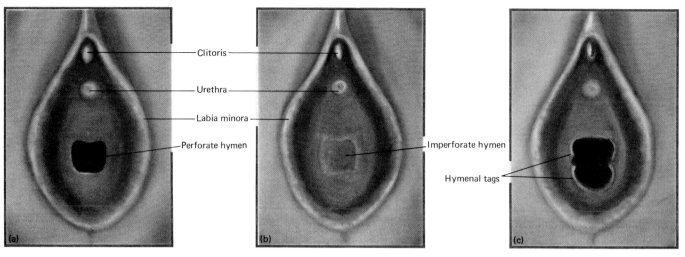

FIGURE 15-5

Hymen: (a) perforate; (b) imperforate; (c) hymenal tags.

tion of these tags with reduction in size occurs following a vaginal delivery (Figure 15-5).

At birth the walls of the vaginal orifice are closely approximated. With the onset of sexual activity and especially following a vaginal delivery, the orifice is open. A widely open vaginal orifice is described as gaping. Bartholin's glands or the greater vestibular glands are located in approximately the 4 and 8 o'clock positions and are immediately adjacent to the vaginal opening. The maximum size of these glands is 5 mm (Figure 15-6).

FIGURE 15-6

Anatomical location of the greater vestibular glands and paraurethral glands.

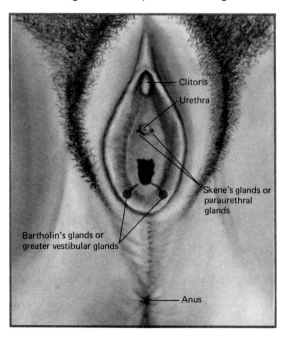

INTERNAL SEXUAL ORGANS

The vagina is a distensible, tubular, muscular sheath that is directed downward and forward. The vaginal walls are pink in color and are rugated in the adult female. Atrophy occurs after menopause and immediately postpartum, resulting in a pale pink mucosa with a smooth surface. In the postpartum breast-feeding mother, the vaginal mucosa may show a bright red hue, with few rugations. The surfaces of the vaginal walls are generally moist owing to a secretion of clear colorless or slightly whitish substance.

The vaginal walls should be firm, without bulging. After vaginal delivery, various degrees of change in the muscle tone occur, and slight bulging may result. Generally, the degree of muscle relaxation is minimal.

It is through the tubular structures of the vagina that sexual intercourse occurs, menstrual discharge is excreted, and fetal passage occurs. Normally, urine does not pass through the vagina, but is excreted from the urethra located superior to the vaginal opening.

The uterus is slightly pear shaped until after pregnancy, when a more defined pear shape results (Figure 15-7). The uterus consists of three basic structures—the fundus or superior rounded portion, the body, or main portion, and the cervix, which has a necklike appearance and projects into the vagina (Figure 15-8).

Uterine tissue consists of three layers. The peritoneum, or serosa, is the outermost layer, and the myometrium is the middle, thick, muscular layer of interlaced fibers that yields strength and elasticity to the uterus. It is the contraction of the myometrium that pushes the fetus into the external world and "ligates" the interepithelial vessels to prevent hemorrhage after delivery. The endometrium is the innermost tissue layer of the uterus. It is highly vascular and serves as the site for implantation of the fertilized ovum. The thickness of this layer varies with the monthly reproductive cycle, as estrogen and progesterone reach their peak blood levels. Sloughing of the endometrial lining results in menstrual flow, and begins between the ages of 10 and 14. This is called **menarche.** If menarche has not ocurred by the age of 17, and all other primary and secondary sexual characteristics are present, menarche is termed delayed.

The size of the uterus varies. In the prepubescent female, it is approximately 2.5 to 3 cm in length; between the ages of 11 and 12 it begins to increase in size, and following puberty it varies from 5.5 to 8 cm in length and 3.5 to 4 cm in width. During pregnancy the uterus hypertrophies after which it remains slightly larger. The surface characteristics of the uterus are smooth and firm owing to the muscular structures.

The cervix of the uterus appears to protrude into the vaginal vault. In the mature nongravid female, cervical projection into the vaginal vault is approximately 1 to 2 cm; in the gravid female its projection ranges from 2 to a maximum of 3 cm. During menopause the cervical tissue begins to atrophy, and in the postmenopausal female it becomes flush with the vaginal wall. The cervix is smooth, pink, rounded, glistening, and 2.5 to 3.5 cm in diameter.

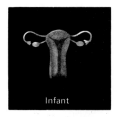
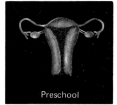
Infant
Preschool

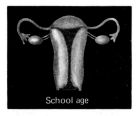
School age

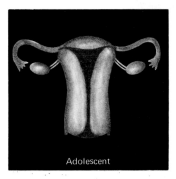
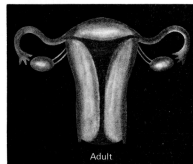
Adolescent
Adult

FIGURE 15-7
Shape of the uterus at various ages.

FIGURE 15-8
Uterus and associated structures:
(a) fundus, body, and cervix, with
fallopian tubes and ovaries
(b) ovarian and uterine ligaments
and blood vessels.

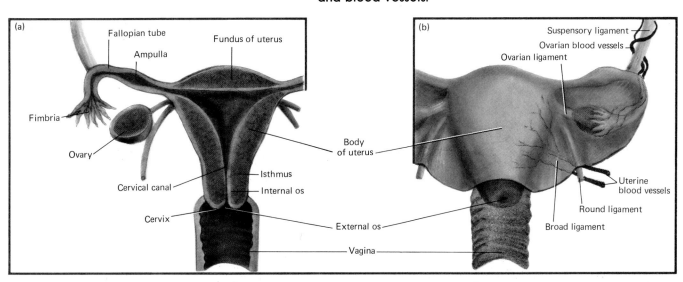

(a) Fallopian tube, Ampulla, Fundus of uterus, Fimbria, Ovary, Cervical canal, Cervix, Isthmus, Internal os, Body of uterus, External os, Vagina

(b) Suspensory ligament, Ovarian blood vessels, Ovarian ligament, Body of uterus, Uterine blood vessels, Round ligament, Broad ligament

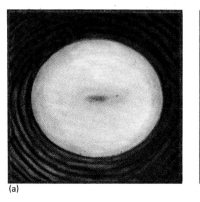
(a)

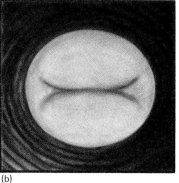
(b)

FIGURE 15-9
Cervical os: (a) circular os of a nulliparous female; (b) stellate os of a parous female.

The cervical os or opening is located centrally on the cervix. In the nulliparous female, it appears closed and round in shape. In contrast, the parous state presents a slit or transverse and partially inverted posterior lip, a stellate appearance, resulting in a slight structural asymmetry (Figure 15-9). The squamocolumnar junction appears more velvety, yet smooth, and red in color compared to the surrounding pink. This junctional area may be located outside of the cervical os and on the cervix, in which case it is described as on the ectocervix, or it may be located within the cervical os and its location described as endocervical. The squamocolumnar junction is generally round and symmetrical in appearance (Figure 15-10).

The ovaries lie in a vertical position, flank the uterus bilaterally, and are held in place by the ovarian ligaments. They are surrounded by the ovarian capsule. The ovaries vary in size, relative to the individual's maturational stage. The ovary may reach 6 cm in size near ovulation, after which the size decreases to 3 to 4 cm in diameter.

FIGURE 15-10
Squamocolumnar junction of the cervix.

Squamous epithelium   Squamocolumnar junction   Columnar epithelium

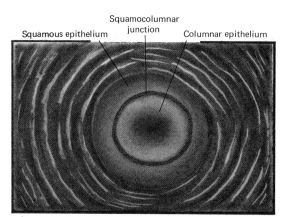

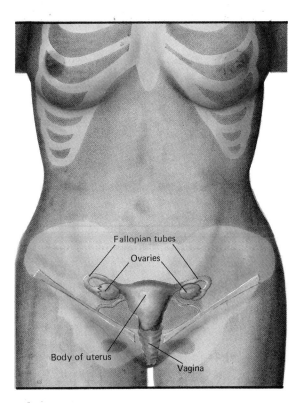

Fallopian tubes

Ovaries

Body of uterus

Vagina

FIGURE 15-11
Location of the ovaries and fallopian tubes.

The peripheral portion of the ovary is composed of follicles that contain the ova; the central portion contains a rich vascular supply. At birth there are approximately 400,000 immature ova in the female.

The ovaries are oval or almond in shape, firm in consistency, and smooth prior to the beginning of ovulation. After sexual maturity, with rupture of the follicles and ovulation, the ovarian surfaces begin to scar, resulting in a roughened nodular surface.

The fallopian tubes are hollow structures, approximately 10 cm long, that serve as a passageway for the ova to enter the uterus. The ovarian end of these tubes is called the **infundibulum.** The fallopian tubes are funnel shaped, with projections called **fimbriae.** These projections are closely approximated to the ovary. Distal to the ovary, the uterine tube enters the lateral margin of the uterus slightly inferior to the fundus. Ova, unlike sperm, do not possess mobility and depend upon the sweeping motion of the cilia that line the uterine tube to propel them to the uterus. The fallopian tube is generally the site where fertilization of the ovum by the sperm cell occurs. Figure 15-11 illustrates the anatomical location and structures of the fallopian tubes.

HEALTH ASSESSMENT OF THE FEMALE GENITALIA

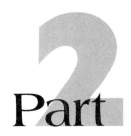

In children, only inspection and external palpation are indicated for the collection of objective data; when working with young adults, adults, and the elderly, internal (vaginal) palpation and special equipment are employed. In children the legs are placed in a frog-leg position; with adults, an examination table with stirrups is generally used. This position is termed lithotomy (Figure 15-12). The frog-leg position may also be utilized with the adult client supine in bed, and the buttocks down toward the end of the bed.

INSPECTION AND PALPATION

The examiner begins the systematic process by inspection of the escutcheon. Until puberty, hair growth presents an abnormal physiological function; at puberty it is an indicator of normal hormonal functions. Second, the skin of the pubis, vulva, and perineal region is inspected, noting the skin color and the presence or absence of lesions. In infants and toddlers who are not toilet trained, diaper rash is a commonly found lesion. Intertrigo, a mild type of diaper rash, presents chafing of the skin and pinkish-erythematous areas. Ammonia lesions are papulovesicular and may present ulcerated, bleeding, and indurated areas. The surrounding skin of the ammonia lesion is pinkish in color. Monilial infections in the diaper-wearing child present bright red lesions, which are scaly, papulovesicular, and have well-defined borders.

Following inspection of the hair pattern and skin characteristics, the examiner informs the client by touching the leg and through verbalization that the internal structures will be inspected next. Internal examination requires skillful instrumentation and is therefore seldom employed by the beginning-level practitioner. A gooseneck lamp is an essential piece of equipment, as it enhances inspection of external structures and enables visualization of the vaginal vault and cervix.

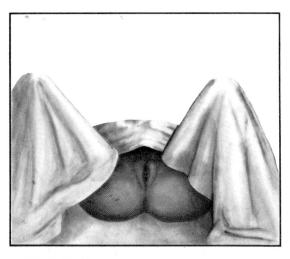

FIGURE 15-12
Lithotomy position used for pelvic assessment.

FIGURE 15-13
Finger separation of the labia minora to enable inspection.

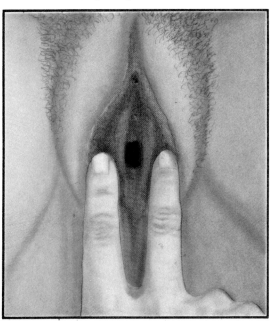

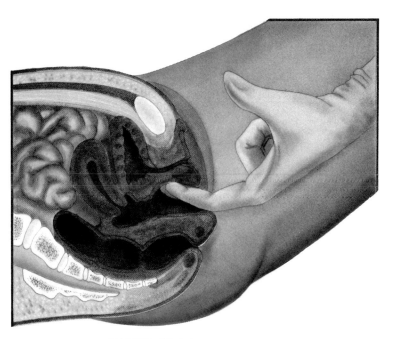

FIGURE 15-14
Palpation of the urethra.

FIGURE 15-15
Palpation of the greater
vestibular glands.

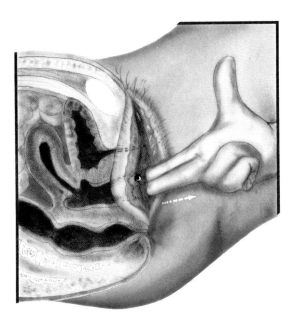

The labia majora are separated by using the thumbs of both hands or the thumbs and index finger or the second and third digits of a single hand (Figure 15-13). With the lips of the labia majora separated, the labia minora, clitoris, urethral meatus, paraurethral glands, hymen, vaginal orifice, and Bartholin's glands are inspected (Figure 15-14).

Labial agglutination or adhesion of the labia minora lips may be seen in infants and toddlers. The labia minora may be only partially separable, which would allow visualization of the introitus. If the area of adhesion of the surfaces is extensive, voiding may be difficult for the child. These children may also have a predisposition to urinary tract infections, as a urine reservoir may be present, yielding a bacterial medium.

In the neonate, the labia majora are soft and somewhat resilient to palpation; in the reproductively mature female, the labia majora are firmer in consistency. The presence of hypertrophic, indurated, soft or hard tissue is abnormal. Between the folds of the labia majora and the labia minora, smegma, a cheese-like substance can collect and become odiferous.

The prepuce covering the clitoris should be easily retractable by palpation, and the size of the clitoris can then be estimated. The urethra, located between the clitoral frenulum and vaginal opening, is assessed for its structural design and color. Erythema and pouting of the meatal lips may indicate a deviation from normal. The paraurethral glands are rarely visible. Palpation of the urethra (Figure 15-14) is accomplished by placing the finger on the anterior surface of the vaginal vault and gently applying pressure while bringing the finger forward toward the vaginal orifice. Upon palpation, the urethra feels like a soft tubular structure. Discharge from the urethra noted upon inspection or with compression is abnormal. The hymen is described as complete or imperforate, incomplete or partial, torn or with fragmented tags. The vaginal opening or orifice is described as closed, open, or gaping. The presence or absence of discharge is recorded.

The area of the greater vestibular glands is also observed. Normally, these glands are not visible. Compression or stripping of the glandular area is achieved by placing one finger inside the vaginal vault and compressing the area while bringing the finger toward the vaginal opening (Figure 15-15). Discharge, erythema, and prominence of glandular ducts are abnormal.

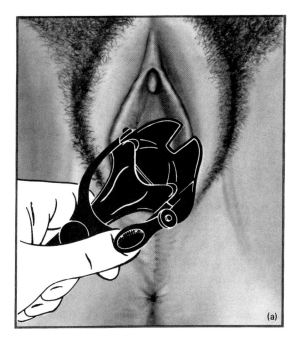 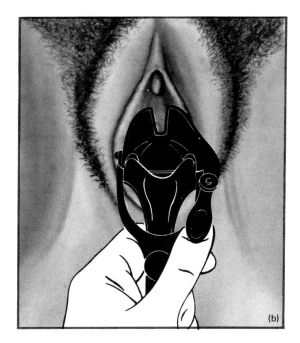

FIGURE 15-16
Insertion of the vaginal speculum: (a) initial insertion at an oblique angle,
approximately 45 degrees; (b) completing speculum insertion on a
horizontal plane.

INSTRUMENTATION

To inspect the internal vaginal walls and cervix, a water-lubricated, warm speculum is used. Speculum sizes are small, medium, and large. Frequently small- or medium-sized speculums are used in adolescent females and in postmenopausal females; the medium-to-large speculums are frequently utilized in the young adult and adult age groups. It is inserted into the introitus at an oblique plane and gently rotated to a horizontal plane as insertion continues in a forward and downward angle (Figure 15-16). The blades are opened at the completion of the insertion, exposing the posterior vaginal wall and the cervix. If the open blades do not expose the cervix, the speculum may be anterior to the cervix, in which case the presenting vaginal tissue appears rugated. If the blades are posterior to the cervix, the vaginal tissue appears smooth. If the cervix has not been exposed, the blades are relaxed and the speculum is withdrawn half the distance of the vaginal vault and reinserted at a different plane. Figure 15-17(a), (b), and (c) illustrates, respectively, the speculum blades anterior to the cervix, posterior to the cervix, and correctly positioned, revealing the cervix.

The cervix is inspected for its color and diameter. The cervical color is pink and glistening during the reproductive phases of life and pale after menopause. It ranges in diameter from 2.5 to 3.5 cm. The smaller diameter is frequently associated with nulliparity; the larger diameter is more characteristic of parity. It is also inspected for characteristic texture, shape, and symmetry. The cervical os is inspected for location, color, texture, and symmetry. Deviations from normal may indicate the presence of pathology.

After the cervix is inspected, specimens for cytological studies are obtained. The cervical os, in particular the squamocolumnar junction, is scraped with a spatula to obtain cell-laden secretions (Figure 15-18(a) and (b)). This specimen is then prepared by the method recommended by the agency laboratory. If the cervix bleeds slightly as a result of the scraping, it is described as friable, unless the client is pregnant and has an ectopia or eversion of the columnar epithelium. A second specimen is taken from the cervical pool, an area immediately below the cervix, using a second spatula or the opposite end of the first one. This specimen is prepared the same as the first one for laboratory evaluation.

As the speculum is withdrawn, the blades are gradually released and rotated to allow for inspection of the lateral, anterior, and posterior vaginal walls, noting color, muscle tone, and moisture or secretions.

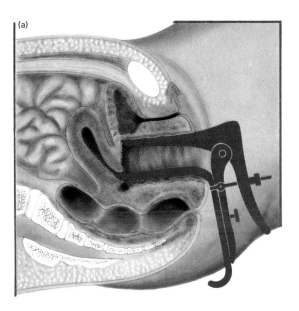

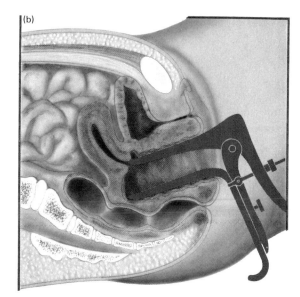

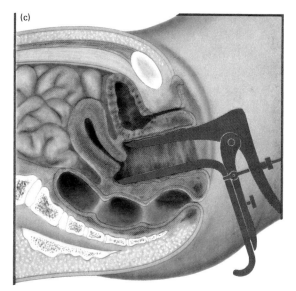

FIGURE 15-17

Sagittal sections showing possible
positions of the speculum:
(a) anterior to the cervix;
(b) posterior to the cervix;
(c) revealing the cervix.

FIGURE 15-18

Obtaining a cytologic specimen using
a cervical spatula:
(a) insertion of speculum with spatula;
(b) rotation of spatula.

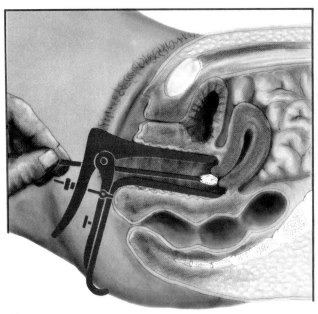

(a)

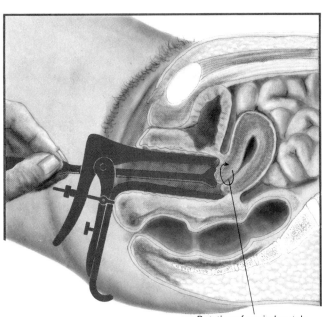

Rotation of cervical spatula

(b)

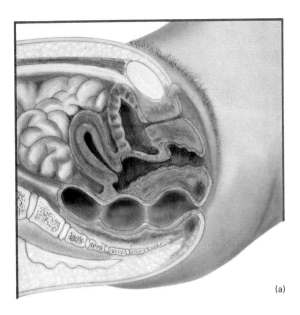

(a)

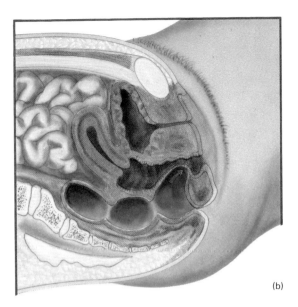

(b)

FIGURE 15-19

Abnormalities of the vaginal wall:
(a) cystocele, a deviation in the
anterior vaginal wall;
(b) rectocele, a deviation in the
posterior vaginal wall.

Characteristics other than the normal firm muscle tone of the vaginal wall may be abnormal. The anterior wall presenting a forward or a forward and downward bulging might indicate the presence of a cystocele; an upward or an upward and forward bulging (Figure 15-19(a) and (b)) of the posterior vaginal wall may be indicative of a rectocele. Deviations from the characteristic pinkish color, firm muscle tone, clear colorless moisture, and absence of secretions may be abnormal.

PALPATION

At the completion of inspection of the vaginal vault, a bimanual assessment of the cervix, uterus, and adnexa is initiated. Generally, a vaginal orifice that appears open will admit two fingers. The vaginal floor is palpated to determine muscular tone both with the individual relaxed, and with her bearing down. Next, the cervix is palpated with the palmar surface of the inserted fingers to determine surface characteristics, consistency, and mobility. Nodules palpable on the surface of the cervix may be a Nabothian cyst. Gentle pushing on the cervix determines its mobility. Movement of the cervix also creates movement of the uterus and associated adnexa. If the cervix is pushed to the right, the uterus moves to the left. Tenderness or pain resulting from uterine and adnexal movement may indicate the existence of an inflammatory process (Figure 15-20).

FIGURE 15-20

Palpation of cervical characteristics
and uterine mobility.

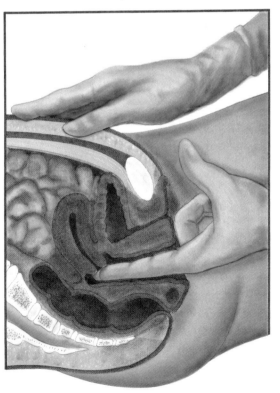

241

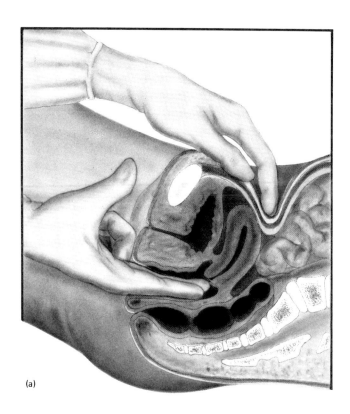

(a)

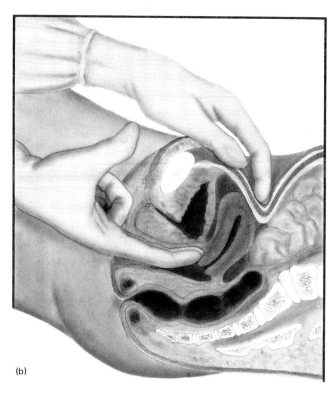

(b)

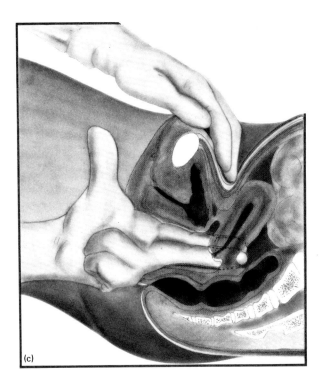

(c)

FIGURE 15-21

Bimanual palpation of the uterus:
(a) capturing the uterus;
(b) vaginal fingers palpating the anterior uterus and abdominal fingers palpating the posterior uterine wall;
(c) vaginal fingers palpating the posterior uterine wall and the abdominal fingers palpating the anterior uterine wall.

After cervical palpation is completed, the free hand is placed on the abdomen approximately half the distance from the pubis to umbilicus in midline. Downward and forward pressure is utilized, drawing the hand toward the pubis. If the uterus is palpable, this maneuver allows it to be captured and palpated by the abdominal hand. Keep the abdominal hand still and bring the structures up to the abdominal hand for examination. Moving the abdominal hand, especially using the fingers in a digging manner, is painful and does not contribute any more information.

The inserted fingers, when placed on top of or anterior to the cervix, can be gently moved forward, allowing for palpation of the anterior uterine wall. Placement of the vaginal fingers below or posterior to the cervix, using the same gentle forward movement, enables the examiner to palpate the posterior wall of the uterus. Manipulation of the uterus with the inserted fingers brings the uterus to the abdominal hand for palpation (Figure 15-21(a), (b) and (c)). When palpated, the uterus feels firm and smooth. A nodular or irregular surface is described as such.

The adnexa are palpated next. Frequently, the ovaries are not palpable and rarely, either, are the fallopian tubes palpable. The nearer the individual is to ovulation with resulting ovarian distention, the easier it may be to palpate the ovaries. If palpated, the ovary should feel oval in shape, firm, smooth or slightly nodular, and movable (Figure 15-22). Excessive pressure applied to the ovary during palpation can cause intense pain and should be avoided.

The rectovaginal exam follows the abdominal vaginal exam. Muscle tone and several structures are assessed by this procedure. They are anal sphincter tone, rectal mucosa, rectovaginal septum, posterior cul-de-sac, the posterior and lateral portions of the pelvis, the cervix, and the posterior uterine wall. While the client bears down, the middle finger is gently inserted into the rectum after a slight pressure has been applied to the anal area. The index finger is placed into the vagina. Palpation through the rectal wall is done with the palmar surface of the finger. The rectal wall should feel smooth without projections, and the rectovaginal septum, resilient. It is through the rectovaginal septum that the posterior cul-de-sac, or pouch of Douglas, is palpated (Figure 15-23). This area is normally nontender to the pressure of palpation, but tenderness may develop with inflammatory processes. Dependent upon the position of the uterus within the pelvic area, the cervix may be palpable immediately anterior to the cul-de-sac, while the body of the uterus may be palpable posterior to the cul-de-sac. Assessment of the right uterosacral ligament is accomplished through palpation with the palmar surface of the fingers, beginning at the 12 o'clock position and proceeding in a semicircular counterclockwise manner to the 6 o'clock position; the left uterosacral ligament is assessed in a similar manner going clockwise from the 12 o'clock to 6 o'clock positions.

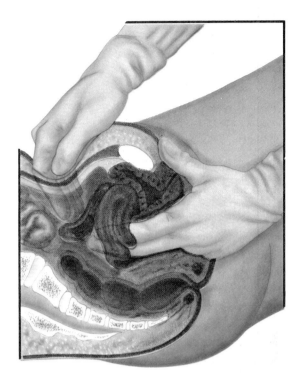

FIGURE 15-22
Bimanual palpation of the adnexa.

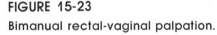

FIGURE 15-23
Bimanual rectal-vaginal palpation.

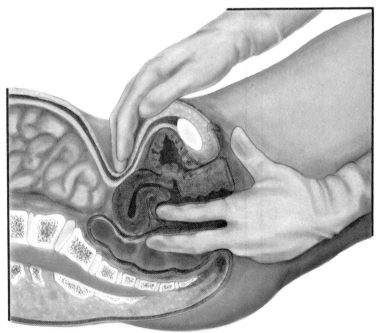

TABLE 15-1
Pelvic Examination Findings with a Client in the Lithotomy Position

CLASSIFICATION OF UTERINE POSITION	POSITION OF CERVIX ON INSPECTION AND PALPATION	PORTIONS OF THE UTERUS PALPABLE WITH THE ABDOMINAL HAND IN BIMANUAL PALPATION	PORTIONS OF THE UTERUS PALPABLE WITH FINGERS IN THE VAGINA	PALPABLE STRUCTURE IN THE POSTERIOR	
ANTEVERTED	Directed posteriorly	Superior 1/4 of the posterior uterine body fundus. Superior 1/4 to 1/2 of the anterior uterine body	With vaginal fingers anterior to cervix 1/2 to 3/4 of anterior uterine wall. With vaginal fingers posterior to cervix up to 1/2 of posterior uterine wall	Posterior cervical wall. Cul-de-sac	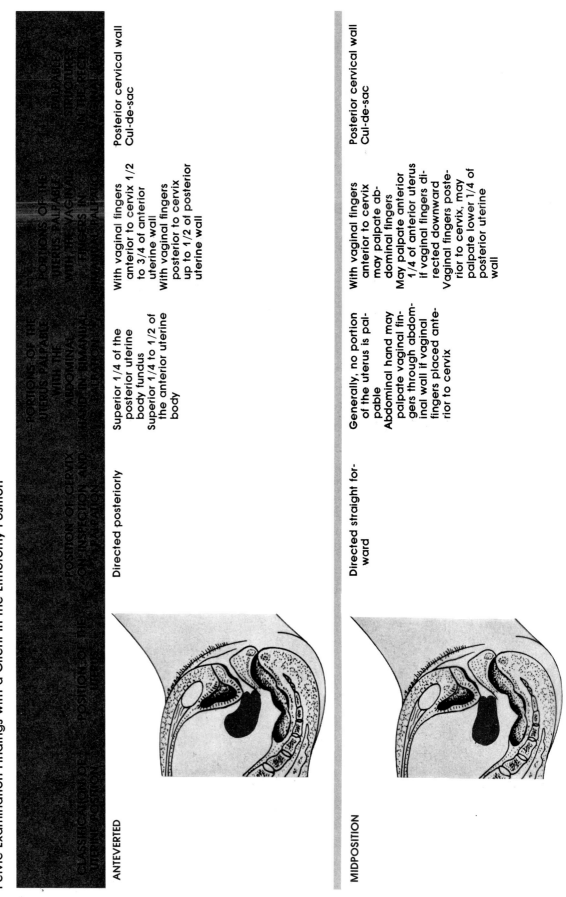
MIDPOSITION	Directed straight forward	Generally, no portion of the uterus is palpable. Abdominal hand may palpate vaginal fingers through abdominal wall if vaginal fingers placed anterior to cervix	With vaginal fingers anterior to cervix may palpate abdominal fingers. May palpate anterior 1/4 of anterior uterus if vaginal fingers directed downward. Vaginal fingers posterior to cervix, may palpate lower 1/4 of posterior uterine wall	Posterior cervical wall. Cul-de-sac	

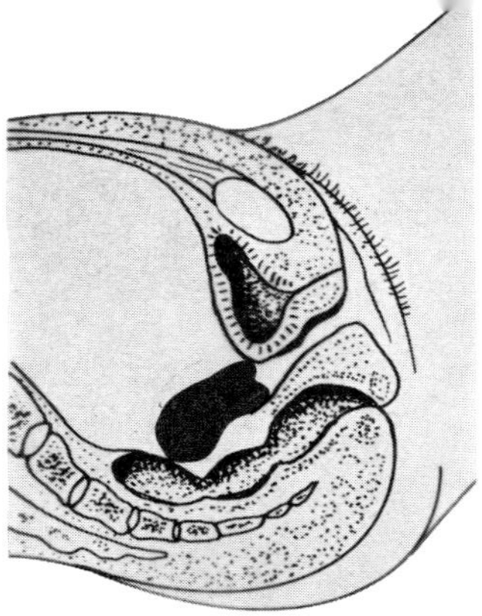

Cul-de-sac
1/4 of anterior uterine wall
Fundus
1/4 of posterior uterine wall

rior to cervix may palpate cervix and small amount of anterior uterine wall
With vaginal fingers posterior to cervix, 1/2 of posterior uterine wall palpable

pable with the abdominal hand
May palpate vaginal fingers which are anterior to the cervix

ANTEFLEXED

Small amount of the posterior cervical wall
Cul-de-sac

Vaginal fingers palpate a mass like structure anterior to the cervix
Unable to palpate anterior uterine wall
Vaginal fingers posterior to cervix, may palpate abdominal fingers if abdominal musculature thin and degree of uterine flexion maximal
1/4 to 1/2 of posterior uterine wall palpable

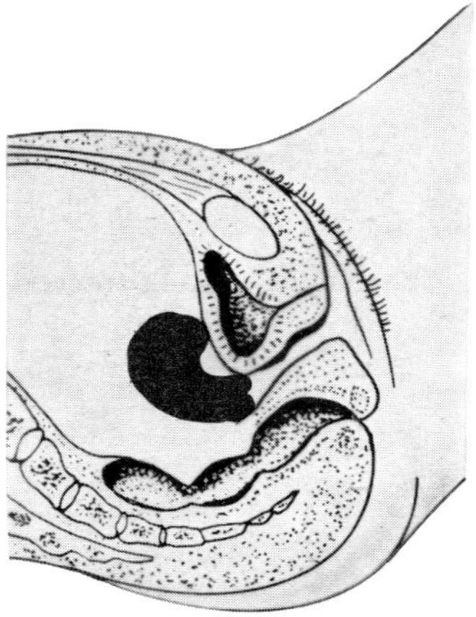

Directed posteriorly

Up to 1/2 of posterior uterine wall is palpable
Fundus may not be palpable if anteflexion extreme

RETROFLEXED

May or may not be able to palpate posterior cervical wall
May palpate up to 1/2 of anterior uterine wall
Cul-de-sac may be obliterated

With vaginal fingers anterior to cervix, a maximum of 1/4 of anterior uterine surface may be palpable
With vaginal fingers posterior to cervix, may palpate a mass-like structure. Posterior uterine wall not palpable

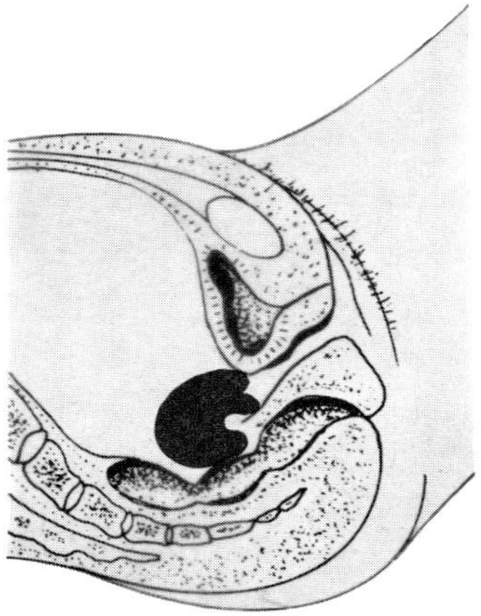

Directed anteriorly

Abdominal hand and vaginal fingers anterior to cervix may meet and be palpable
A maximum of 1/4 of the anterior uterine wall may be palpable

On occasion the uterosacral ligament can be located in the cul-de-sac. This is determined by the patient's sudden discomfort when the examiner is palpating close to the cervix posteriorly. Endometriosis of the uterosacral ligament enlarges the structure and causes pain. Clients with a history of severe cramps and heavy bleeding with menses should be suspected of having this condition. The examiner must be cautious not to confuse this pain with the pain caused by manipulating the cervix in a client who has an ectopic pregnancy associated with bleeding in the peritoneal cavity.

Dependent upon the position of the uterus, various structures are palpable or not palpable through the abdomen, vagina, and rectum. Table 15-1 presents various positions of the uterus and the associated findings upon palpation.

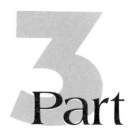

Part 3

STUDY GUIDE QUESTIONS

In the following client situations, identify and describe the subjective and objective data to be collected, the specific tools and procedures to be utilized in the collection of those data, and the rationale for the nursing assessment.

1. In your bimonthly visit to the home of Brian and Anita Saunders, Mrs. Saunders asks you to look at her 6-month-old daughter Jennifer's diaper rash.
2. Dorothy Mason is an 18-year-old college coed who comes to you at the student health service for her first pelvic exam and pap smear.
3. Gertrude Little is a 68-year-old female who complains of urine incontinence when she coughs, sneezes, or laughs.
4. Mary Olson, a 30-year-old married female, comes to you at the clinic with a complaint of vaginal discharge.

SAMPLE FORMAT TO BE USED IN RESPONDING TO THE STUDY GUIDE QUESTIONS

SUBJECTIVE DATA TO BE COLLECTED	OBJECTIVE DATA TO BE COLLECTED	SPECIFIC TOOLS AND PROCEDURES TO BE UTILIZED	RATIONALE FOR NURSING ASSESSMENT

BIBLIOGRAPHY

BROWN, MARIE S., and MARY M. ALEXANDER, "Physical Examination, Part Fifteen: Female Genitalia," *Nursing 76,* March 1976, pp. 39–41.

Children Are Different, pp. 79–85. Columbus, Ohio: Ross Laboratories, 1970.

DEGOWIN, ELMER L., and RICHARD L. DEGOWIN, *Bedside Diagnostic Examination* (3rd ed.), pp. 603–623. New York: Macmillan Publishing Co., Inc., 1976.

GREEN, THOMAS H., *Gynecology.* Boston: Little, Brown and Company, 1965.

HOLLINSHEAD, W. HENRY, *Textbook of Anatomy* (2nd ed.), pp. 124–129, 728–751. New York: Harper & Row, Inc., 1967.

JUDGE, RICHARD D., and GEORGE D. ZUIDEMA, *Physical Diagnosis: A Physiologic Approach to the Clinical Examination* (3rd ed.), pp. 313–327. Boston: Little, Brown and Company, 1968.

KATCHADOURIAN, HERANT A., and DONALD T. LUNDE, *Fundamentals of Human Sexuality* (2nd ed.), pp. 21–143. New York: Holt, Rinehart and Winston, Inc., 1975.

PRIOR, JOHN A., and JACK S. SILBERSTEIN, *Physical Diagnosis* (4th ed.), pp. 312–330. St. Louis, Mo.: The C. V. Mosby Company, 1973.

PRITCHARD, JACK A., and PAUL C. MACDONALD, *Williams Obstetrics* (15th ed.). New York: Appleton-Century-Crofts, 1976.

SINGER, ALBERT, "The Uterine Cervix from Adolescence to the Menopause," *British Journal of Obstetrics and Gynecology,* February 1975, pp. 81–99.

ULENE, ARTHUR, *Module, Pelvic Examination, Submodule, Anatomy for Abdominal and Pelvic Examinations.* Raritan, N.J.: Department of Educational Services, Ortho Pharmaceutical Corporation, 1974.

———, *Module, Pelvic Examination, Submodule Pelvic Examination Findings: Description and Classification.* Raritan, N.J.: Department of Educational Services, Ortho Pharmaceutical Corporation, 1973.

16

The Musculoskeletal System

REVIEW OF STRUCTURE AND FUNCTION

Part 1

The musculoskeletal system provides man with structure and protection and, coordinated by the central nervous system, gives man the means for mobility. The muscular component of the system includes muscles, tendons, and ligaments; the skeletal component consists of bones and cartilage.

Bone is a hard form of connective tissue composed largely of inorganic substances such as calcium phosphate and calcium carbonate. Bone stores approximately 99 percent of all the calcium in the body. This rich mineral content gives bone the structural strength to resist compression. Organic substances of bone consist of osteoblasts, osteocytes, osteoclasts, and collagenous connective tissue. Collagenous tissue provides resistance to opposing forces.

Bone is continuously undergoing reabsorption and deposition through the action of osteoclasts and osteoblasts. The activity of the osteoblast is greatest during the longitudinal growth phases of the bone. Molding of the bony contours occurs in response to growth and the pressures resulting from weight bearing and muscle pull.

Two types of bone exist, compact and spongy (Figure 16-1). Compact bone is dense and is

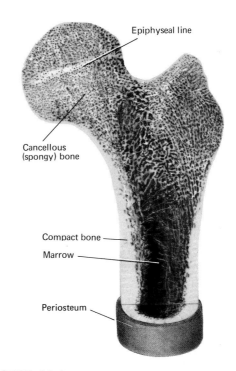

Epiphyseal line

Cancellous (spongy) bone

Compact bone

Marrow

Periosteum

FIGURE 16-1

Portion of a bone showing spongy and compact bone material.

primarily the cortex or outermost bone structure. Within the compact bone is the Haversian system. This system provides pathways for vascular, lymph, and nerve structures to pass through the bone. Spongy bone or cancellous bone appears honeycombed or porous. The spaces within cancellous bone are filled with red marrow. This marrow is involved in hematopoietic functions. The primary bones, which contain red bone marrow, are the sternum, ribs, vertebrae, and pelvic bones. In contrast to red marrow, yellow marrow, composed of fat cells and connective tissue, is found in the hollow shafts of the long bones.

Lining the external and internal surfaces of the bone are connective tissues called the periosteum and endosteum, respectively. The periosteum bonds are strongest in the bone regions where tendon insertions occur.

CARTILAGE

Cartilage is another structure of the skeletal system. It may provide support or a smooth surface upon which movable bony structures articulate. There are three types of cartilage: hyaline, fibrous, and elastic. Hyaline cartilage is the first form of the skeletal structure in the fetus. By the sixth month of fetal development, the ossification process replaces much of this cartilaginous skeletal structure with bone. Hyaline cartilage remains throughout life to cover the articulating surfaces of bones and to form the attachment media between the ribs and the sternum. Hyaline cartilage can also be found in other body areas, such as the nose, trachea, and bronchi.

Fibrous cartilage, the second type, is a denser and less elastic structure than hyaline cartilage. It is found between the vertebrae, and it forms the symphysis pubis. Elastic cartilage, the last of the three types, lends support and resilience to body structures such as the ear and epiglottis.

SKELETAL STRUCTURES

The adult skeletal structure is composed of 206 bones (Figure 16-2); the number of bones in the fetus and newborn is slightly more until ossification of certain bones occurs. By the third month of fetal life, the cartilaginous skeletal structure exists; by the sixth month, bone substance is formed, replacing much of the cartilaginous structure. The skeletal structure is frequently subdivided into the axial and appendicular skeletons.

The axial skeleton is composed of 74 bones, including the skull, vertebral column, ribs, sternum, and hyoid bone. The skull is composed of the 29 cranial and facial bones. Cranial bones consist of one frontal, two parietal, one occipital, two temporal, one sphenoid, one ethmoid, and six auditory ossicles. The facial bones consist of two nasal, two palatine, two maxillary, two zygomatic, two lacrimal, two inferior turbinates, one vomer, and one maxillary bone. In addition, the hyoid bone, a singular bone that does not articulate with other bones, provides support to the tongue.

The vertebral column is composed of 26 vertebrae: seven cervical; twelve thoracic; five lumbar; five sacral; and four coccygeal. By adulthood, the sacral vertebrae are fused, forming the sacrum, and the four coccygeal vertebrae are fused forming the coccyx. The spinal vertebrae vary in size, with the cervical being the smallest and the lumbar the largest. Each vertebra is composed of a disc-shaped anterior body, an arch through which the spinal cord passes, and three processes, two transverse and one directed posteriorly. Each also possesses four articular processes, two superiorly and two inferiorly, which allow for articulation with the corresponding vertebrae. Located between each successive vertebra is an intervertebral disc, which is composed of fibrous cartilage. This structure serves as a shock absorber, deferring compression of the vertebra.

The sternum, a single structure, is another part of the axial skeleton. It consists of the manubrium, gladiolus or body, and the xiphoid process. Articulating with the manubrium on its superior lateral aspects are the clavicles. The sternoclavicular junction is closely followed by the first rib. The second rib attaches approximately at the junction of the manubrium and the body of the sternum. The first seven pairs of ribs articulate directly with the sternum through the costal cartilage structures; the costal cartilage structures of the eighth through tenth ribs are attached to that of the preceding rib. The eleventh and twelfth pairs of ribs do not articulate with the sternum and are called floating ribs. Posteriorly, all the ribs articulate with the thoracic vertebrae.

FIGURE 16-2 (facing page)
Adult skeletal structure in anterior and posterior views.

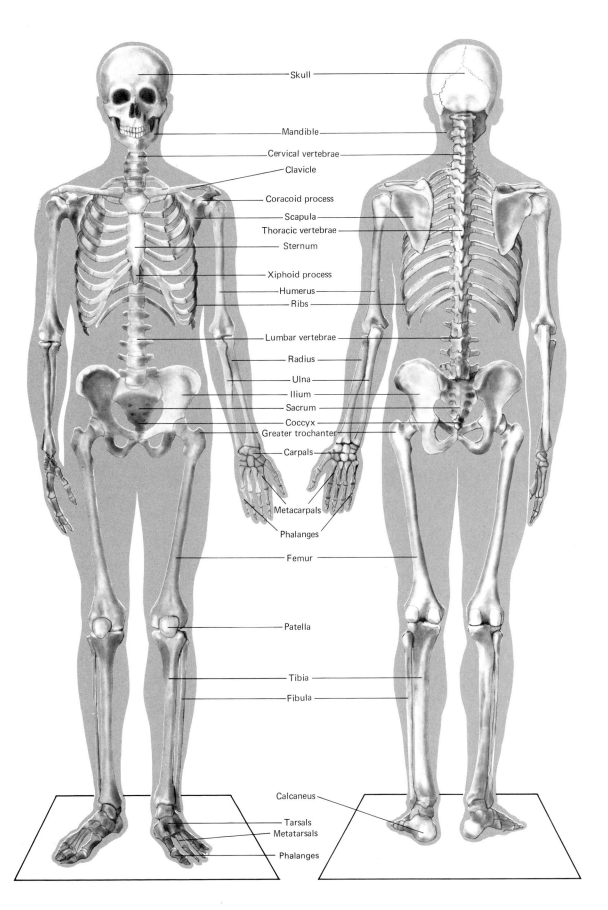

Skull

Mandible

Cervical vertebrae

Clavicle

Coracoid process

Scapula

Thoracic vertebrae

Sternum

Xiphoid process

Humerus

Ribs

Lumbar vertebrae

Radius

Ulna

Ilium

Sacrum

Coccyx

Greater trochanter

Carpals

Metacarpals

Phalanges

Femur

Patella

Tibia

Fibula

Calcaneus

Tarsals

Metatarsals

Phalanges

251

The appendicular skeleton is composed of the bony structures of the upper and lower extremities. In the upper extremities, the bones that exist in pairs are the clavicle, or collar bone, the scapula, humerus, ulna, and radius. There are 16 carpals, 10 metacarpals, and 28 phalanges. The bones of the upper extremities compose the upper portion of the appendicular skeleton. The bones of the lower extremities bilaterally include the ilium, ischium, femur, patella, tibia, and fibula, with 14 tarsals, 10 metatarsals, and 28 phalanges. The pelvis also contains one pubic bone.

Bones comprising the skeletal structure vary in size and shape. The long bones of the appendicular skeleton consist of the radius, ulna, humerus, femur, tibia, and fibula. These bones are divided into segments consisting of the epiphysis, or enlarged ends, and the diaphysis or shaft. Longitudinal bone growth occurs from the epiphyseal portion of the long bones. Short bones, such as the carpals and tarsals, are composed of cancellous bone and a thin layer of compact bone. The scapula and ribs represent flat bones, and are composed of cancellous bone and a thin layer of compact bone. Cancellous bones covered by thin compact bone are called irregular bones because of their irregular shape. The last category of bones is the sesamoid bones, with the largest being the patella.

JOINTS

The joints of the skeletal system are the unions or junctions between two or more bony surfaces. Joints that do not permit movement, such as the sutures of the skull, are classified by the term synarthrosis. At birth, the sutures are movable, permitting molding of the skull during vaginal delivery. As growth occurs, the approximating skull bones articulate through continuous interlacing fibers, thus inhibiting movement at this junction. Amphiarthrosis is another classification of joints. This type of joint is characterized by the formation of an interosseous membrane or ligament, and movement is minimal. The pubic symphysis, radial–ulnar, and sacral–lumbar articulations fall into this category. The third classification of joints is diarthrosis. Joints in this classification provide the greatest range of mobility and are further subdivided according to the shape of the articulating bone surface. The six types of diarthrodial joints are ball and socket, hinge, pivot, condyloid, saddle, and gliding.

MUSCLE COMPOSITION AND ACTION

There are three major types of body muscle: smooth, striated, and cardiac. Smooth muscle responds by contraction to stimuli received from the autonomic nervous system. Cardiac muscle is specific to the heart. It contains an intrinsic property of autorhythmicity; that is, it can initiate its own impulse for contraction.

Striated or skeletal muscle, which is of major importance in this chapter, is composed of cells called **fibers.** Each muscle fiber consists of a variable number of fibrils, also termed **myofibrils.** The myofibril is composed of alternating I bands and A bands. These in turn are composed primarily of protein substances. Within the I bands is a dark line called the **Z membrane.** The section between two Z membranes is the sarcomere, the unit of muscle contraction (Figure 16-3). The myofilaments within each sarcomere slide over each other, thus decreasing its length and resulting in contraction.

Muscle fibers are bound together to form bundles of fasciculi, which are surrounded by connective tissue. Many of these bundles together comprise the muscle mass. Muscles vary in size, shape, anatomical position, attachment, and type of actions performed. These factors are utilized in naming the numerous muscles of the body. Muscles have an origin that is fixed, and an insertion, which provides the mobility of the skeletal structures involved. Generally, the muscle origin is an attachment to bony structure, whereas the insertion is frequently an attachment to another muscle. In the extremities, the muscle origin is proximal, while the insertion is distal. Frequently, muscles are attached indirectly to the underlying skeletal structure by tendons. Tendons are fibrous bands of tissue that are strong and nonelastic. They connect with the periosteum, forming a firm point of attachment, thus enabling skeletal movement.

Movement is rarely carried out by a single muscle, but instead is accomplished by a group of muscles. The agonist, also called the prime mover, is the muscle or muscles that produce the movement. Fixators or synergists are those muscles that assist the agonist in the movement. Antagonists are the muscles that carry out actions opposite to those of the prime mover or agonist. Muscular movement is created by the transmission of impulses from the nerves to the skeletal muscle fibers through the neuromuscular junction. Branches of the terminal myelinated nerve

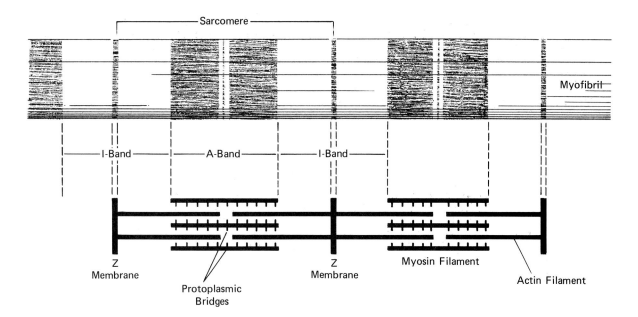

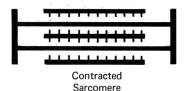

Contracted
Sarcomere

FIGURE 16-3
A sarcomere, the unit of muscle contraction.

fiber form the end plate, which is adherent to the muscle fiber. Muscle contraction is subject to the all or none principle; that is, the impulses must be strong enough to excite the entire muscle unit or contraction does not occur.

Upper Extremities

The major regions of the upper extremities are the shoulder, axilla, arm, elbow, forearm, wrist, hand, and the fingers and thumb. The fingers are frequently called digits and are numbered I through V, with the thumb as the first digit, the index finger as the second digit, the middle finger as the third digit, the ring finger as the fourth digit, and the little finger as the fifth digit. The wrist is also subdivided by the ulnar and radial prominences; the elbow may be divided into the antecubital and cubital regions (Figure 16-4). A competent muscle structure with an intact nerve supply and articulating processes enables the range of motions that can be performed by the joint. These motions may include flexion, extension, rotation, abduction, and adduction.

The upper extremities receive their blood supply through vessels that branch off from the aortic arch. As the subclavian artery enters the axilla, its name changes to the axillary artery, thus corresponding with the body region entered. The axillary artery yields numerous branches and continues into the brachium or arm as the brachial artery. In the elbow or cubital area, the brachial artery branches, forming the radial and ulnar arteries, which extend toward the hand (Figure 16-5). The venous structures closely correspond to the major arteries, each emptying its particular

section of the muscle mass. The major veins of the upper extremities are the brachiocephalic, cephalic, axillary, brachial, median cubital, and basilic (Figure 16-6).

The upper extremities are provided with innervation from the brachial nerve plexus, which is composed of nerves emerging from vertebrae C5 through T1. This nerve plexus descends into the axilla, where five major nerve branches arise from it. These branches are the circumflex or axillary nerve, the musculocutaneous nerve, the ulnar nerve, the median nerve, and the radial nerve (Figure 16-7). The circumflex nerve innervates the deltoid muscle, its overlying integument and the teres minor muscle; the musculocutaneous nerve innervates the biceps, brachialis, coracobrachialis, and provides sensory terminals for the integument in the lateral forearm area. The ulnar nerve innervates the muscles of the forearm and those of the hand. The flexor muscles of the forearm are innervated by the median nerve; the radial nerve innervates the triceps muscle and provides sensory branches to the integument.

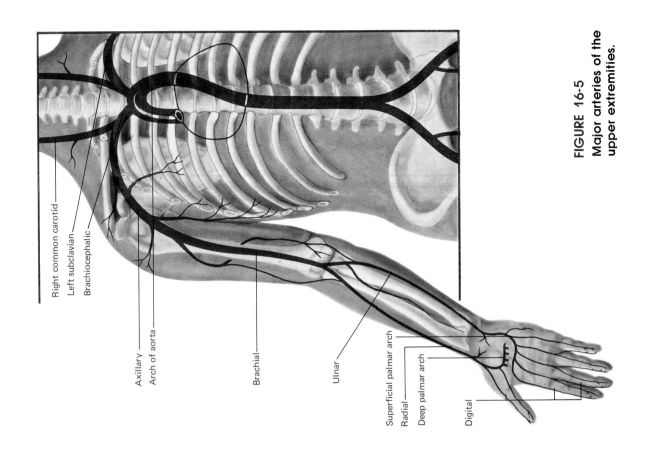

FIGURE 16-5
Major arteries of the upper extremities.

Right common carotid
Left subclavian
Brachiocephalic

Axillary
Arch of aorta

Brachial

Ulnar

Superficial palmar arch
Radial
Deep palmar arch

Digital

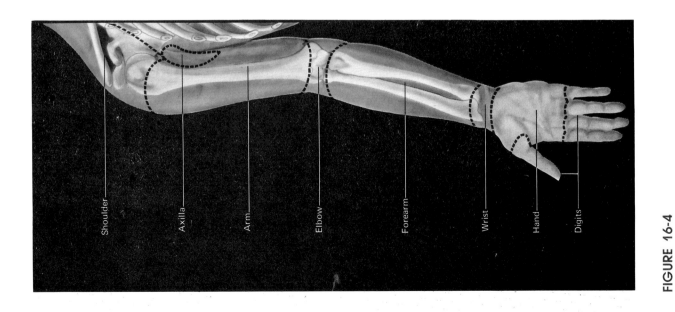

FIGURE 16-4
Major regions of the upper extremities.

Shoulder

Axilla

Arm

Elbow

Forearm

Wrist

Hand

Digits

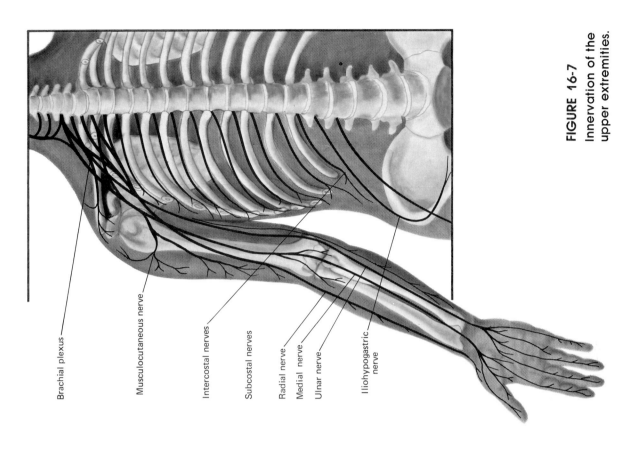

FIGURE 16-7
Innervation of the upper extremities.

Brachial plexus

Musculocutaneous nerve

Intercostal nerves

Subcostal nerves

Radial nerve

Medial nerve

Ulnar nerve

Iliohypogastric nerve

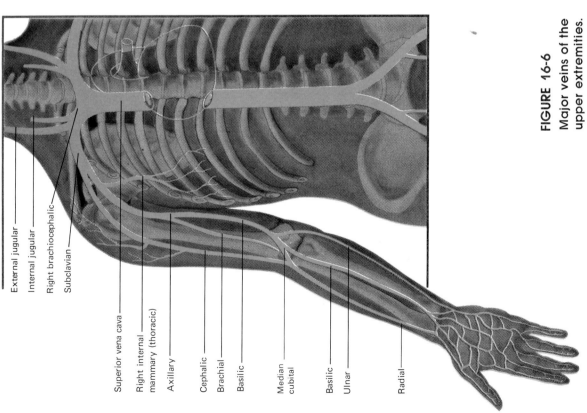

FIGURE 16-6
Major veins of the upper extremities.

External jugular

Internal jugular

Right brachiocephalic

Subclavian

Superior vena cava

Right internal mammary (thoracic)

Axillary

Cephalic

Brachial

Basilic

Median cubital

Basilic

Ulnar

Radial

Back

The muscular structures of the back are numerous. Frequently, fusion between muscle segments occurs, creating a larger muscle mass. Most of the muscular structures of the back have multiple origins and insertions, adding further complexity to the muscular structures.

In general, most of the posterior thoracic muscles are innervated by the dorsal rami of the spinal nerves. The muscles of the back, in combination, produce the movements of flexion, extension, lateral flexion, and rotation of the trunk.

Lower Extremities

Like the upper extremities, the lower extremities can be divided into major regions. These regions are the gluteal region or buttocks, the thigh, the anterior and posterior region of the knee (the popliteal and patellar regions, respectively), the ankle (with its medial and lateral malleoli), and the foot (composed of the heel or calyx, metatarsals, and digits). The toes are numbered one through four, beginning with the great toe. The little toe is termed digitus minimus (Figure 16-8).

FIGURE 16-8
Regions of the lower extremities.

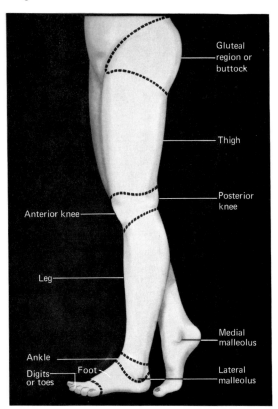

The numerous muscles of the lower extremities, combined with an intact nervous system and articulating processes, enable the range of motions that can be performed by the joints. These motions may include flexion, extension, rotation, abduction, and adduction.

The lower extremities receive their blood supply from the abdominal aorta, which bifurcates slightly below the umbilicus into the right and left iliac arteries. As the iliac artery passes into the femoral area, it is termed the femoral artery. The femoral artery continues until it reaches the poples, and then is termed the popliteal artery. This segment of the vascular system ends in the upper segment of the leg at the point where it divides into the anterior and posterior tibial arteries. The anterior tibial artery supplies the anterior portion of the leg and the dorsum of the foot; the posterior tibial artery supplies the posterior leg and the plantar portion of the foot (Figure 16-9).

Two of the most prominent venous structures of the lower extremities are the greater and lesser saphenous veins. The greater saphenous vein originates in the medial dorsal aspect of the foot and ascends the leg on the medial side. The greater saphenous vein ends in the anterior mid-thigh region and empties into the femoral vein. The lesser saphenous vein originates in the lateral margin of the foot, ascends the leg posteriorly through the calf, and ends in the popliteal area, where it is referred to as the popliteal vein. The lesser and greater saphenous veins communicate with the deep veins of the legs (Figure 16-10).

The lumbar and sacral plexuses provide the basis for muscular innervation from the gluteal region to the foot. The lumbar plexus possesses three major branches, the lateral femoral cutaneous nerve, the femoral nerve, and the genitofemoral nerve. These nerve branches supply the skin on the lateral portion of the thigh, the flexor thigh muscles, and the skin of the anterior thigh, hip, and lower leg. The scrotum and remaining skin of the thigh are innervated by the genitofemoral nerve.

The sciatic nerve originates in the gluteus maximus area from the sacral plexus and descends through the thigh, branching into the tibial and common perineal nerve. Another major nerve arising from the sacral plexus is the pudendal nerve, which supplies muscles of the genitalia, perineal skin, and anal sphincter.

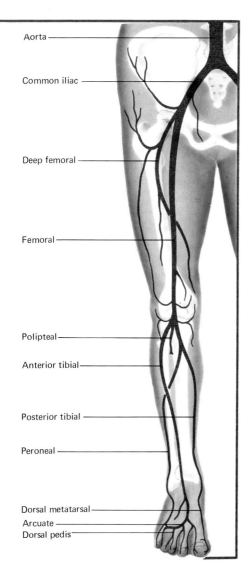

FIGURE 16-9
**Major arteries of the
lower extremities.**

Aorta
Common iliac
Deep femoral
Femoral
Poplteal
Anterior tibial
Posterior tibial
Peroneal
Dorsal metatarsal
Arcuate
Dorsal pedis

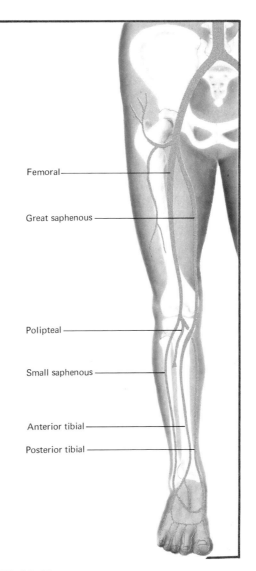

FIGURE 16-10
**Major veins of the
lower extremities.**

Femoral
Great saphenous
Poplteal
Small saphenous
Anterior tibial
Posterior tibial

In summary, innervation of the anterior thigh arises from the lumbar plexus, while the nerves of the posterior thigh and the anterior and posterior lower leg are supplied by the sacral plexus.

MATURATIONAL CHANGES THROUGHOUT THE LIFE SPAN

At birth, the average full-term neonate is approximately 45 to 52.5 cm long. In the first year of life, bony length increases approximately 50 to 75 percent; in the second year of life, the increase averages 12 to 13 cm. From the third year on, length increases by 5 to 6 cm until adolescence.

FIGURE 16-11 (pages 258–265)
Growth curves for females from birth to 36 months ((a) and (b)); growth curves for females from 2 to 18 years of age ((c) and (d)); growth curves for males from birth to 36 months ((e) and (f)); growth curves for males from 2 to 18 years of age ((g) and (h)). Adapted from National Center for Health Statistics: NCHS Growth Charts, 1976. Monthly Vital Statistics Report, Vol. 25, No. 3, Supp. (HRA) 76-1120. Health Resources Administration, Rockville, Maryland, June 1976. Data from the National Center for Health Statistics and from The Fels Research Institute, Yellow Springs, Ohio. Copyright © 1976 by Ross Laboratories. Reproduced with permission.

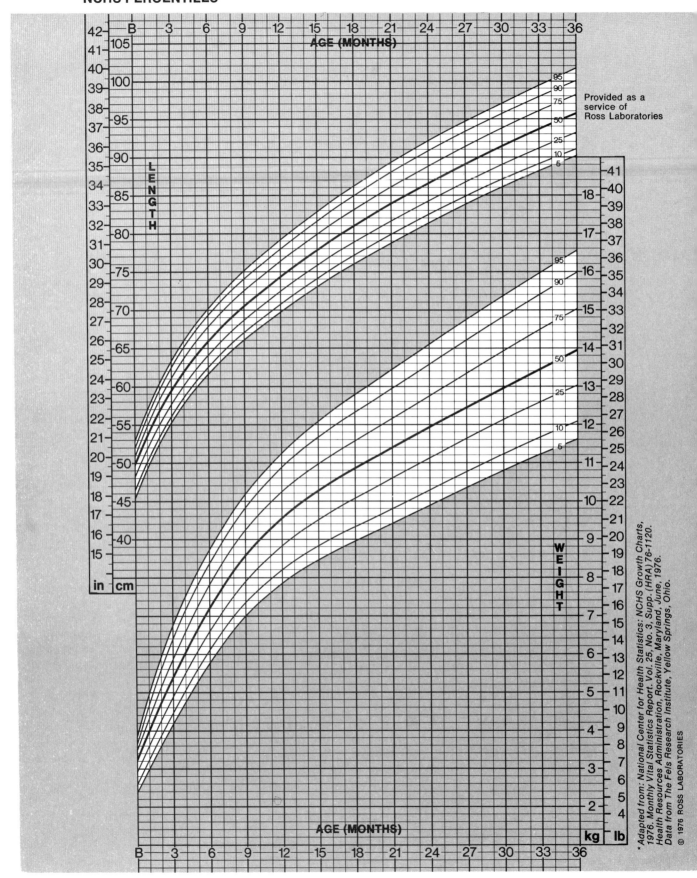

Provided as a
service of
Ross Laboratories

*Adapted from: National Center for Health Statistics: NCHS Growth Charts,
1976. Monthly Vital Statistics Report. Vol. 25, No. 3, Supp. (HRA) 76-1120.
Health Resources Administration, Rockville, Maryland, June, 1976.
Data from The Fels Research Institute, Yellow Springs, Ohio.

© 1976 ROSS LABORATORIES

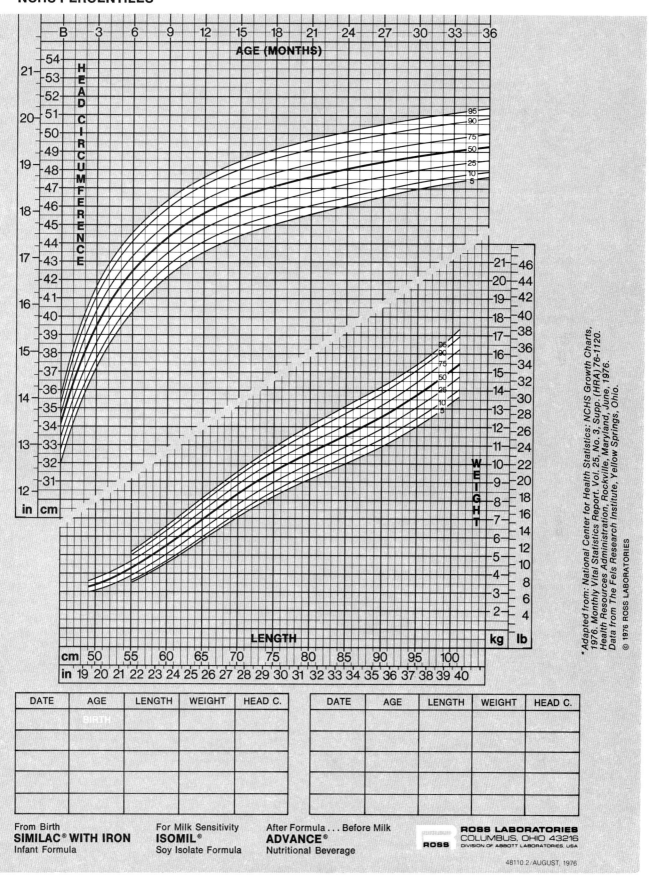

*Adapted from: National Center for Health Statistics: NCHS Growth Charts, 1976. Monthly Vital Statistics Report. Vol. 25, No. 3, Supp. (HRA)76-1120. Health Resources Administration, Rockville, Maryland, June, 1976. Data from The Fels Research Institute, Yellow Springs, Ohio.

© 1976 ROSS LABORATORIES

DATE	AGE	LENGTH	WEIGHT	HEAD C.
	BIRTH			

DATE	AGE	LENGTH	WEIGHT	HEAD C.

From Birth
SIMILAC® WITH IRON
Infant Formula

For Milk Sensitivity
ISOMIL®
Soy Isolate Formula

After Formula . . . Before Milk
ADVANCE®
Nutritional Beverage

ROSS LABORATORIES
COLUMBUS, OHIO 43216
DIVISION OF ABBOTT LABORATORIES, USA

48110.2/AUGUST, 1976

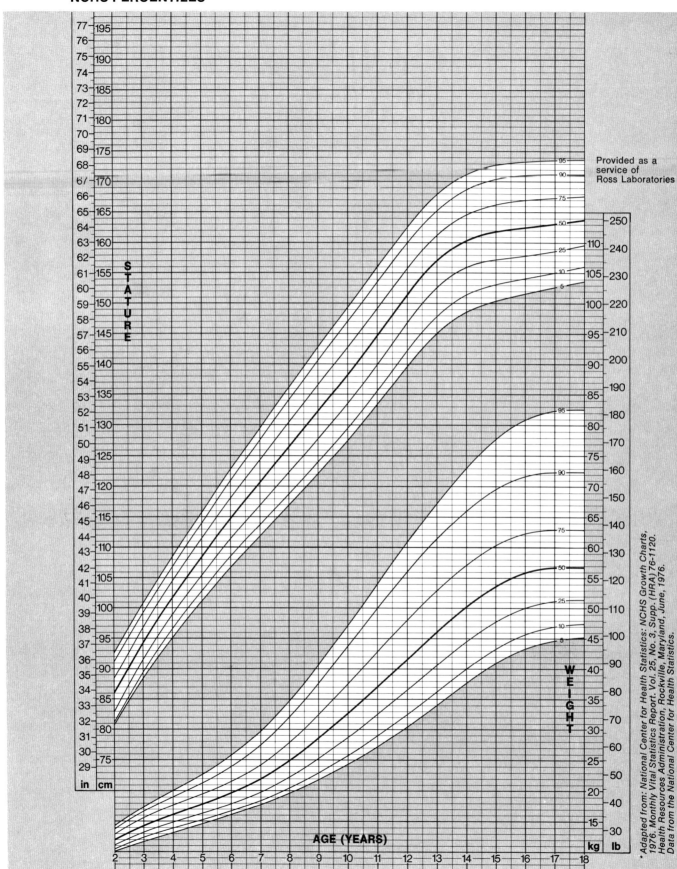

* Adapted from: National Center for Health Statistics: NCHS Growth Charts, 1976. Monthly Vital Statistics Report. Vol. 25, No. 3, Supp. (HRA) 76-1120. Health Resources Administration, Rockville, Maryland, June, 1976. Data from the National Center for Health Statistics.

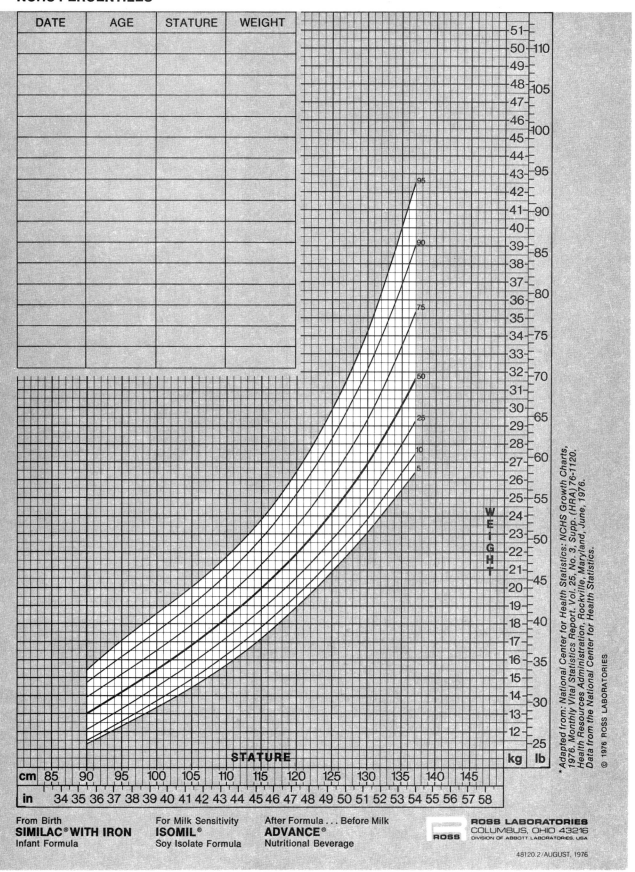

DATE	AGE	STATURE	WEIGHT

STATURE

cm 85 90 95 100 105 110 115 120 125 130 135 140 145

in 34 35 36 37 38 39 40 41 42 43 44 45 46 47 48 49 50 51 52 53 54 55 56 57 58

WEIGHT

*Adapted from: National Center for Health Statistics: NCHS Growth Charts, 1976. Monthly Vital Statistics Report. Vol. 25, No. 3, Supp. (HRA) 76-1120. Health Resources Administration, Rockville, Maryland, June, 1976. Data from the National Center for Health Statistics.

© 1976 ROSS LABORATORIES

From Birth
SIMILAC® WITH IRON
Infant Formula

For Milk Sensitivity
ISOMIL®
Soy Isolate Formula

After Formula . . . Before Milk
ADVANCE®
Nutritional Beverage

ROSS LABORATORIES
COLUMBUS, OHIO 43216
DIVISION OF ABBOTT LABORATORIES, USA

48120.2/AUGUST, 1976

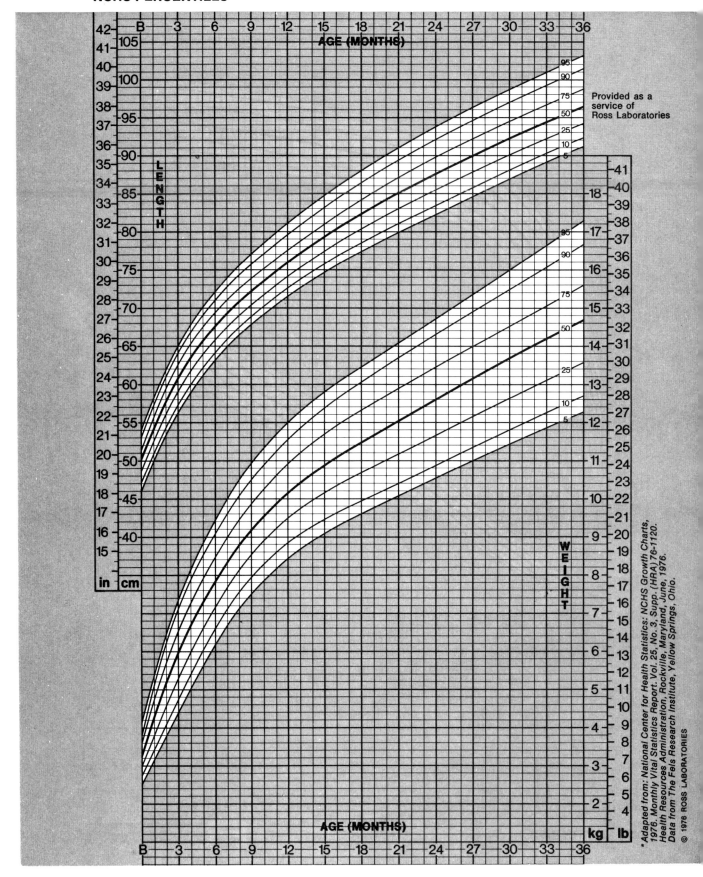

Provided as a
service of
Ross Laboratories

*Adapted from: National Center for Health Statistics: NCHS Growth Charts,
1976. Monthly Vital Statistics Report. Vol. 25, No. 3, Supp. (HRA) 76-1120.
Health Resources Administration, Rockville, Maryland, June, 1976.
Data from The Fels Research Institute, Yellow Springs, Ohio.

© 1976 ROSS LABORATORIES

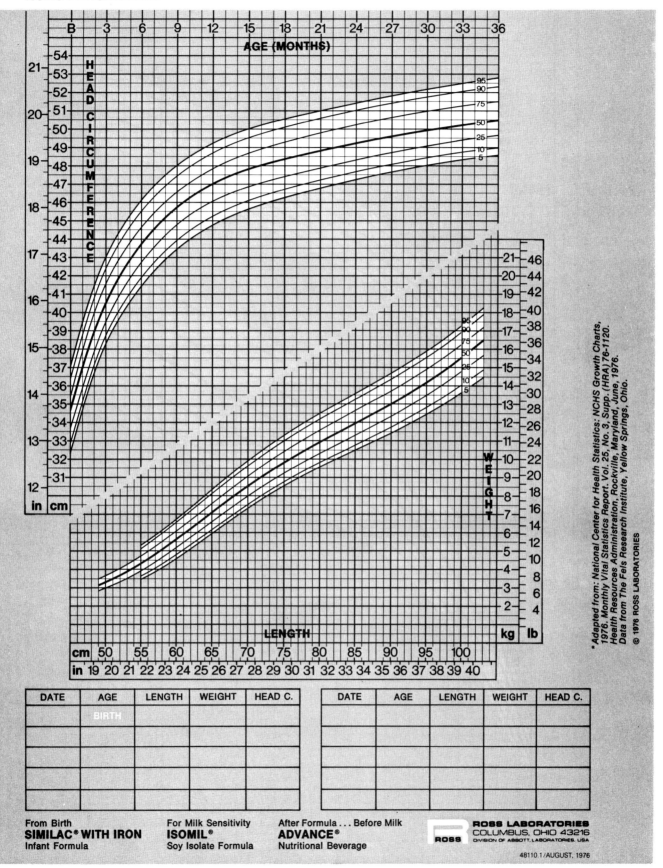

*Adapted from: National Center for Health Statistics: NCHS Growth Charts, 1976. Monthly Vital Statistics Report, Vol. 25, No. 3, Supp. (HRA) 76-1120. Health Resources Administration, Rockville, Maryland, June, 1976. Data from The Fels Research Institute, Yellow Springs, Ohio.
© 1976 ROSS LABORATORIES

DATE	AGE	LENGTH	WEIGHT	HEAD C.
	BIRTH			

DATE	AGE	LENGTH	WEIGHT	HEAD C.

From Birth
SIMILAC® WITH IRON
Infant Formula

For Milk Sensitivity
ISOMIL®
Soy Isolate Formula

After Formula . . . Before Milk
ADVANCE®
Nutritional Beverage

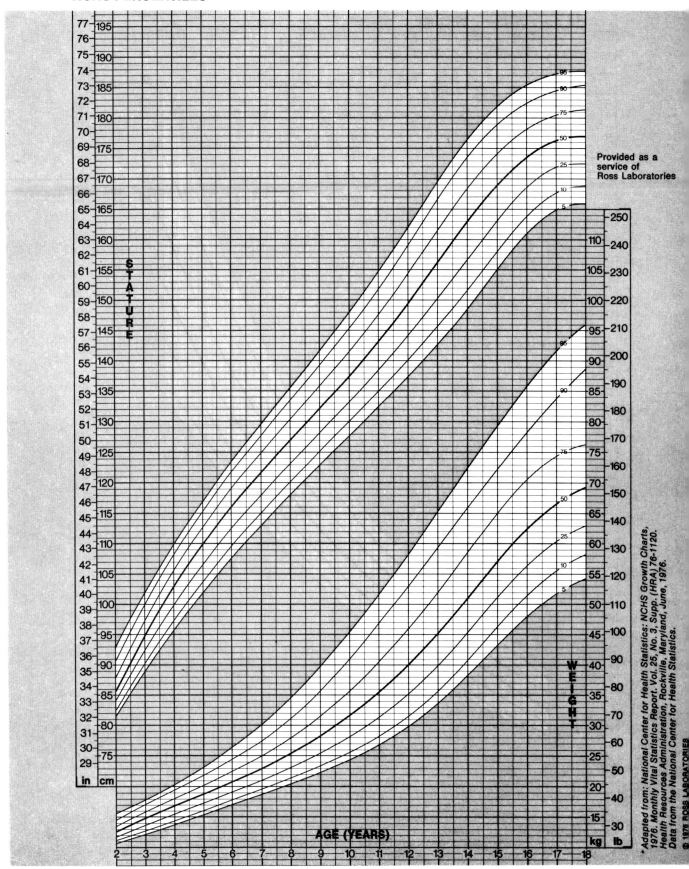

Provided as a
service of
Ross Laboratories

STATURE

WEIGHT

AGE (YEARS)

in cm

kg lb

* Adapted from: National Center for Health Statistics: NCHS Growth Charts,
1976. Monthly Vital Statistics Report. Vol. 25, No. 3, Supp. (HRA) 76-1120.
Health Resources Administration, Rockville, Maryland, June, 1976.
Data from the National Center for Health Statistics.

© 1976 ROSS LABORATORIES

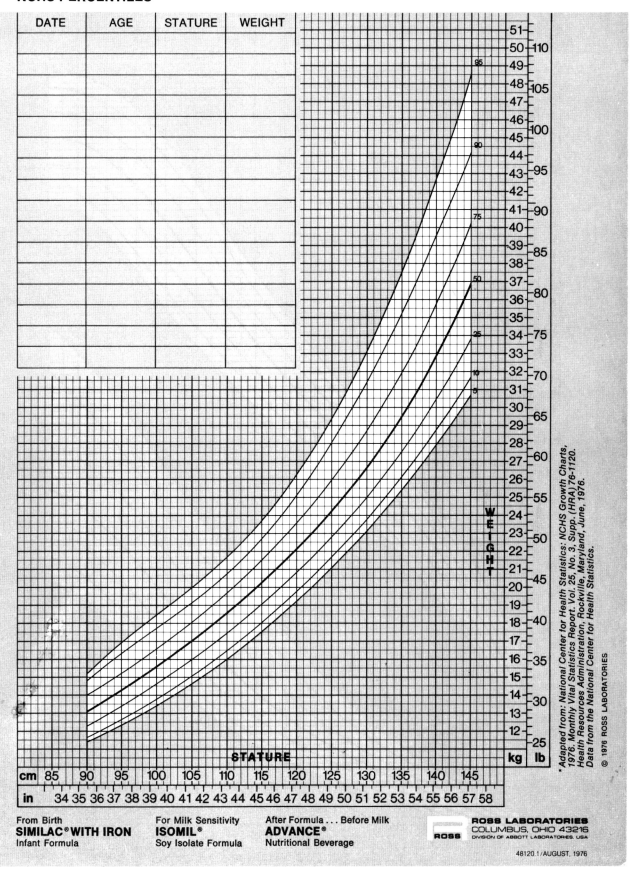

DATE	AGE	STATURE	WEIGHT

* Adapted from: National Center for Health Statistics: NCHS Growth Charts, 1976. Monthly Vital Statistics Report. Vol. 25, No. 3, Supp. (HRA) 76-1120. Health Resources Administration, Rockville, Maryland, June, 1976. Data from the National Center for Health Statistics.

© 1976 ROSS LABORATORIES

From Birth
SIMILAC® WITH IRON
Infant Formula

For Milk Sensitivity
ISOMIL®
Soy Isolate Formula

After Formula . . . Before Milk
ADVANCE®
Nutritional Beverage

ROSS LABORATORIES
COLUMBUS, OHIO 43216
DIVISION OF ABBOTT LABORATORIES, USA

48120.1/AUGUST, 1976

Occasionally, a rapid increase in growth occurs between 6 and 7 years of age. This period of rapid growth is termed the mid-growth spurt. Figure 16-11(a) through (h) illustrates growth curves from birth to 18 years of age for males and females. This type of growth chart is frequently used to record the growth of individuals, thus providing longitudinal data about growth characteristics.

During adolescence, a major growth spurt is encountered. For the female it generally occurs between the ages of 10 and 11; for the male it occurs between the ages of 12 and 13. Growth during this time may be up to 20 cm. By the age of 18 in females and 20 in males, longitudinal growth ceases and adult height is reached. Bone maturation and molding continue until approximately 21 years of age for both sexes. The adult height gradually decreases as aging occurs. The vertebral column becomes shorter as the intervertebral discs narrow, and the individual vertebra decrease in height. Kyphosis of the upper thoracic spine and flexion of the hips and knees also decreases the longitudinal height of the elderly adult (Figure 16-12).

Other factors that affect longitudinal height are vertebral compression and muscle tension. At any time during the life span, an individual's height is dependent upon the time of day at which the measurement is taken, unless the individual is bedridden. The pull of gravity and the compression of the intervertebral discs supporting the body's weight decreases the total height as the day progresses. Muscle tension controls the tilt of the pelvis and vertebral column, thus affecting posture and height.

Skeletal maturation also produces varied changes in body structure. In the newborn and during childhood, bones possess a greater ratio of collagen to mineral salts. As a result, bones are more pliable. Following childhood, bones contain mostly mineral substances, leading to decreased pliability. In the elderly, bone structure is brittle owing to reduced amounts of both collagenous and mineral substances.

In the newborn, the cranium seems more prominent than the facial features, which appear almost as compressed, small, underdeveloped structures underlying the cranium. The skull appears large in comparison to the rest of the body structures. The bony structures of the face grow more rapidly than those of the cranium, espe-

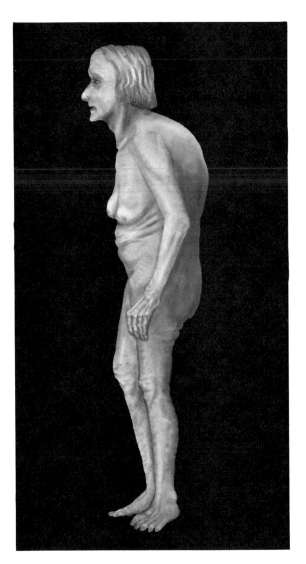

FIGURE 16-12
Observed changes resulting from the aging process that affect height.

cially the maxilla and mandible. The mandible is often receded during infancy. At the completion of adolescence, as the length and breadth of the facial bones increase, the facial features become more proportional to the rest of the skull. In the elderly, with the loss of teeth and subsequent atrophy of the jawbone, the lower jaw may appear receded. The face appears more angular and the nose more prominent in later years.

The neck is short, almost nonexistent in the newborn. The chest appears rounded or barrel-shaped. As growth takes place throughout the body, the trunk elongates and more room is created in both the thoracic and abdominal cavities. Some of the abdominal organs descend into the pelvis, decreasing the organ pressure within the thoracic cavity. At this time, about the age of 2 years, the ribs descend and the neck is more visible.

In the neonate and infant, the arm length appears short in relation to total body length. This disproportion decreases with growth. In the elderly, the decrease in height of the spinal column gives the arms an appearance of being longer, so the proportion is again changed. Relative to height, the forearm is longer in the male than in the female. The ratio of the lower extremities to body height in the newborn is 1:3; in the adult it is 1:2. Another sexual difference is bone growth between the shoulders and pelvis. In the female, the breadth of pelvic skeletal structure growth is greater than in the male; however, in men, the breadth of the shoulder skeletal growth is greater than in women.

The spinal column undergoes changes from birth to old age. In the newborn, two primary curvatures exist. These curvatures are the thoracic and sacral areas of the spine and are convex in nature. As the infant develops sufficient muscle strength to hold up the head, generally by 3 months of age, a secondary concave curvature develops in the cervical segment of the spine. At approximately 6 months, when the infant is able to sit up, another secondary curvature is created. This one is in the lumbar area and is also concave in nature. Thus, throughout childhood and adulthood, the spinal column possesses four curvatures: cervical, thoracic, lumbar, and sacral (Figure 16-13). In the elderly, the aging process may result in an exaggerated thoracic curve known as **kyphosis**.

The posture of the body dictates where the individual's center of gravity lies. From the time an infant begins to walk to approximately 4 years of age, the center of gravity is relatively high. As a result of this, when the infant learns to walk, and in the succeeding 3 years, balance is maintained with the legs spread widely. This posture is also accompanied by an increase in the lumbar spinal curvature. In the adult, the center of gravity is approximately at the crest of the pelvis. The line or level of gravity changes with the posture a person assumes or with a particular posture created by aging, pregnancy, or pathological processes.

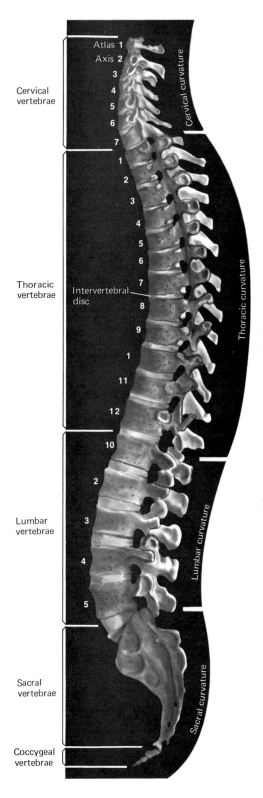

FIGURE 16-13

Regions, curvatures, and vertebrae of the spinal column.

The muscular structures of the body also undergo maturational changes. In the infant, the muscle mass comprises approximately 25 percent of the body weight; in the adult it comprises 40 percent of body weight. Muscle fibers continue to grow from infancy to approximately 10 years of age in the female and 14 years of age in the male. Marked muscle growth occurs in adolescence when development of increased muscle mass is readily evident. This muscle mass development corresponds to the increased body weight, but it is not the only factor contributing to additional body weight. Maximal muscular strength is generally achieved and maintained between the ages of 25 to 30 years, with a subsequent gradual decrease. Following the age of 50 years, muscle mass begins to decrease in size. Unless the individual is obese, the loss of subcutaneous tissue with aging may increase the prominence of muscle masses and tendons.

HEALTH ASSESSMENT OF THE MUSCULOSKELETAL SYSTEM

Part 2

Assessment of the musculoskeletal system proceeds systematically, although the approach varies with examiners and the age of the client. Frequently, the data are collected as the examiner assesses each body region, such as the trapezius and sternocleidomastoid muscles being assessed while the neck is examined, or the muscles of the back being assessed at some point during the examination of the posterior chest and thoracic wall. Other examiners assess the musculoskeletal system separately. In this chapter, the assessment will proceed from the neck to the upper extremities, back, and finally, the lower extremities, and will be concerned with major muscular, bony, and vascular structures. Assessment of range of motion will be covered separately and not integrated into the aforementioned approach.

The skills of inspection and palpation are of greatest value in the collection of objective data. The skills of percussion and auscultation are rarely used; however, auscultation may be utilized to ascertain data about the major vascular structures and bone crepitation. Percussion may be used to determine the presence of fluid within joint regions or to elicit tenderness.

Assessment of each region of the musculoskeletal system is preceded by the assessment of the integument overlying the muscular, cartilaginous, and bony structures. The integument as described in Chapter 3 is assessed for the characteristics of color, pigmentation, smoothness, elasticity, and hair pattern and distribution.

As each muscular region is inspected, it is observed for involuntary movement. Fasciculations are localized contractions of small muscle units and are observed as a quivering type of motion. Tics frequently begin voluntarily and may eventuate into reflex activity. Spasm may also be noted, and it can be one of two basic types. Spasm is the involuntary contraction of a muscle or group of muscles that interferes with normal function of that particular muscle group. Tonic spasms are those in which the rigidity of the contraction exists for a marked period of time; clonic spasms are characterized by a sudden contraction followed immediately by relaxation of the contraction.

INSPECTION AND PALPATION OF THE NECK

The contour of the neck is variable from infancy through elderly years, dependent upon the amount of fatty tissue. Numerous fat folds may make the neck appear asymmetrical and occasionally shortened. Bilaterally, muscular structures and skin folds should appear symmetrical in structure. Hypertrophy, atrophy, masses, or tumorous growths will give the neck an asymmetrical appearance unilaterally or bilaterally.

The strength of muscles is assessed and recorded using a muscle-strength grading system. This scale ranges from 0 to 5, with zero indicating no muscle contraction and 5 indicating full range of motion against full gravitational resistance and additional resistance applied by the examiner. A score of 4 indicates that the individual is able to utilize a particular muscle in a full range of motion against gravity and with minimal added resistance applied by the examiner. Grade 3 is the full range of motion against gravity only, and grade 2 is the ability to perform the complete range of motion with gravitational resistance removed. A grade of 1 indicates that evidence of muscular contraction is present, but no motion is evident through joint activity.

The strength of the sternocleidomastoid mus-cle is assessed using the grading system described. The client is requested to actively turn the head from midline to the right side and then to the left side. Each time, the head should be brought back to midline before the turn to the opposite side is made (Figure 16-14).

Determination of the sternocleidomastoid muscle strength with additional resistance is done in several steps.

1. With the client's head in midline, the examiner places the right hand on the left side of the client's mandible and requests the client to turn the head to the left with the examiner resisting this movement. This procedure is repeated on the opposite side.
2. With the client's head turned to the right side, the examiner places one hand on the left side of the client's mandible and resists the motion of the client to return the head to midline. The client is instructed to turn the head back to the midline position while resistance is being applied.

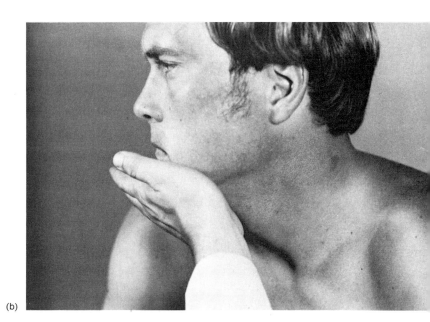

FIGURE 16-14

Assessment of sternocleidomastoid muscle strength: (a) the client attempts to turn his head against the examiner's resistance; (b) the client attempts to return his head to the midline against the examiner's resistance.

(a)

(b)

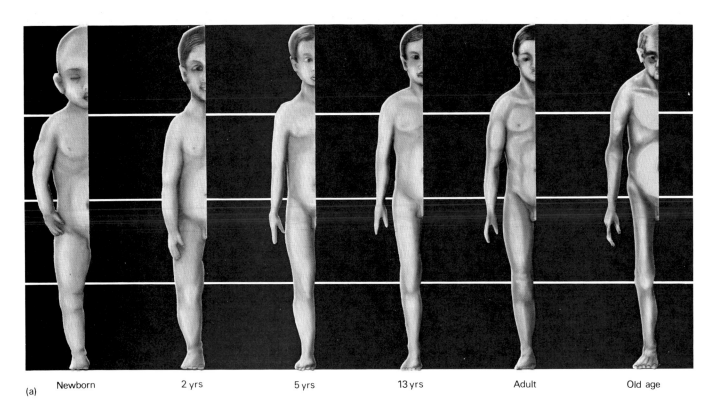

(a) Newborn   2 yrs   5 yrs   13 yrs   Adult   Old age

FIGURE 16-15

Proportions of extremities to body height. In (a) the stature is shown constant and the body is divided in quarters; in (b) body sizes and proportions are shown relative to growth.

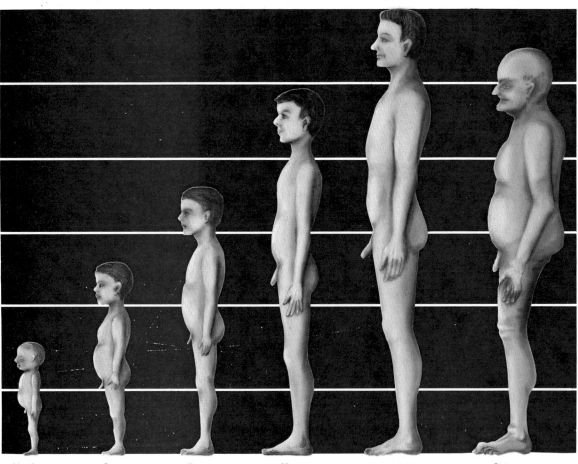

(b) Newborn   2 yrs   5 yrs   13 yrs   Adult   Old age

INSPECTION AND PALPATION OF THE UPPER EXTREMITIES

The upper extremities are assessed by making bilateral comparisons and progressing from the shoulders to the hands. Normally, these structures are symmetrical in size, shape, and position. In the newborn, the upper extremities appear to have an exaggerated length in comparison to the rest of the body trunk. As growth occurs, the upper extremities become more proportional to the trunk of the body. In the elderly, the upper extremities frequently appear longer and out of proportion to the remainder of the body as longitudinal height has decreased (Figure 16-15).

At birth, and for several succeeding months, the arms are held close to the body in a flexed position. In the older child and adult, the arms normally lie in close approximation to the body. Abnormally, the arms may be in an internally or externally rotated position, or they may be abducted or adducted. Splinting of the arm also results as a deviation of the normal resting or carrying position. Drooping or contracture of the shoulder (Figure 16-16) may produce what appears to be asymmetrical arm length and/or asymmetrical contour of the shoulder.

The shoulder normally is rounded and smooth. The biceps muscle presents a longitudinal rounding on the anterior surface of the arm; the triceps presents a similar, often less pronounced, rounding of the posterior arm surface. The contour of the biceps muscle can deviate from normal with rupture of the muscle or its associated structures, forming a localized bulging mass in the middle of the arm during muscle contraction (Figure 16-17). The forearm is greater in diameter at the cubital region and smaller in diameter at the radial and ulnar prominences.

Palpation of the upper extremities is initiated at the shoulder, using the palmar surface of the fingers, and is completed with the hand. It is important to palpate all aspects of the extremity. In all age groups, muscles of the upper extremities should be firm. The size of the muscle mass varies with the individual's genetic composition and activities, but can also be affected by disruption of the nerves supplying a particular muscle group. Disruption of the innervating nerves may result in atrophy, a condition that is characterized by a decrease in muscle size and by atonia or flabby musculature.

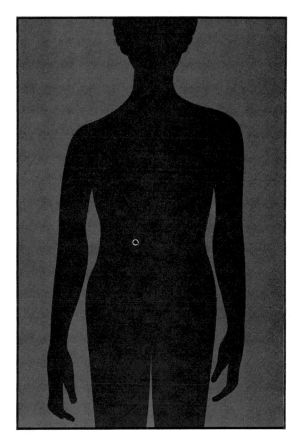

FIGURE 16-16
Deviation in shoulder contour resulting in asymmetrical arm length.

FIGURE 16-17
Contour of the biceps muscle: (a) normal contour; (b) rupture of the biceps muscle resulting in a localized bulging mass.

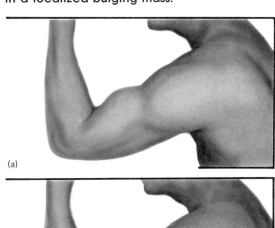

(a)

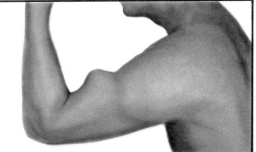

(b)

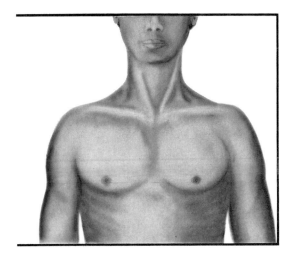

FIGURE 16-18
Inspection of the integrity
of the clavicle from the manubrium
to the shoulder.

The clavicle is inspected and palpated. Upon inspection, the clavicle presents as a bony prominence crossing the superior aspect of the chest from the manubrium to the shoulder (Figure 16-18). Disruption of this continuous prominence may occur with a fracture when the bony ends are not in alignment. Palpation of this structure is accomplished by beginning at the distal or proximal ends and gliding the palmar aspect of the fingers along its surfaces until reaching the opposite juncture. Palpation of the clavicle normally

FIGURE 16-19
Assessment of trapezius muscle strength.

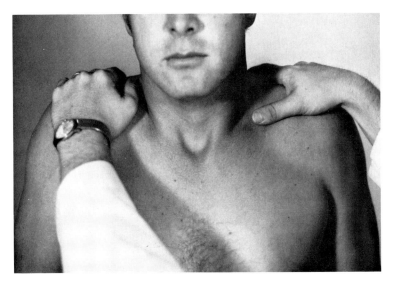

yields a smooth and firm surface; a complete fracture of the clavicle generally yields an interrupted surface as well as bony crepitus. A fracture of the clavicle is common in young children as a result of falling on the shoulder.

The strength of the trapezius muscle is assessed by standing in front of or behind the client and placing the hands on the shoulders. The client is then requested to shrug the shoulders while application of a resisting force is made (Figure 16-19). The strength of this muscle is compared bilaterally for equality, and the results are recorded using the muscle-strength grading criteria.

Bilaterally, the contour of the deltoid muscle appears full and round. The normal characteristics of this muscle can be disrupted by unilateral swelling, hypertrophy, atrophy, and dislocation of the shoulder. In the presence of atrophy of the deltoid, the greater tuberosity of the humerus increases in prominence. With dislocation of the shoulder, the structure is displaced and the rounding contour may possess hollows (Figure 16-20).

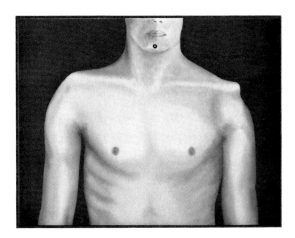

FIGURE 16-20
Observed contour changes with
dislocation of the shoulder.

The rotator cuff of the shoulder is also assessed. This structure is composed of four muscles. Extension of the shoulder enables palpation of the rotator cuff proximal and inferior to the anterior border of the acromion (Figure 16-21). Normally, this structure is firm and nontender.

The triangular scapulae are symmetrical in size and shape and are generally well defined on the posterior chest wall with the arms in extension.

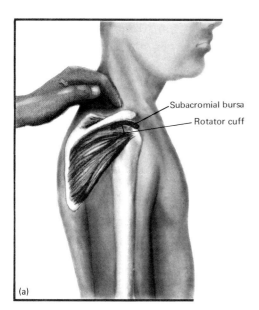

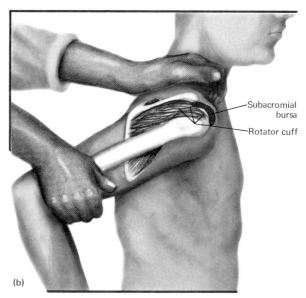

FIGURE 16-21

Assessment of the rotator cuff of the shoulder:
(a) position of the rotator cuff with arm in extension;
(b) positioning of the arm and shoulder to enable palpation of the rotator cuff.

This structure can be made more pronounced by requesting the client to sit up straight and push the shoulders backward. The scapulae are divided into regions or areas called the medial, lateral, superior, and inferior regions. These regions are frequently used as landmarks for the purpose of identifying the location of findings. Bilaterally, each scapula rests an equal distance from the mid-spinal column and is anatomically located over thoracic ribs two through seven. Asymmetry of the anatomical location may be the result of weakness or atrophy of the serratus muscle, abnormal spinal curvature, or a congenital state in which the scapula fails to descend (Figure 16-22).

Integrity of the muscles that maintain the scapulae's placement is assessed by requesting the client to stand close to a wall and push against it with the hands. When the muscles and nerves are intact, the scapulae remain closely approximated to the posterior chest wall, whereas with disruption of nerves and muscles, a winging or pushing out of the scapulae results. The presence of this outward prominence is termed a winged scapula (Figure 16-23). Palpation of the scapular body and all its margins normally presents the characteristic of smoothness, while the bordering muscles are firm.

The elbow joint forms an angle between the arm and the forearm (Figure 16-24). This angle is called the carrying angle and is assessed with the arm in passive extension. The carrying angle is normally between 5 and 15 degrees in the adult and approximately 5 degrees in children. Abnor-

FIGURE 16-22

Asymmetrical position of the scapula.

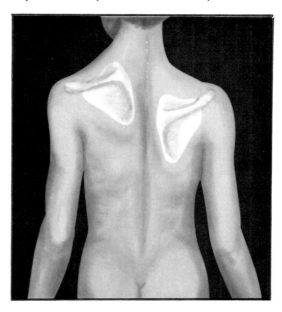

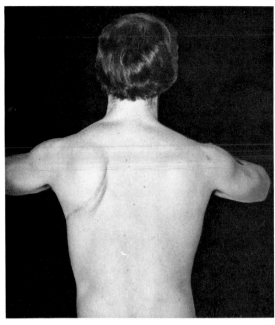

(a)

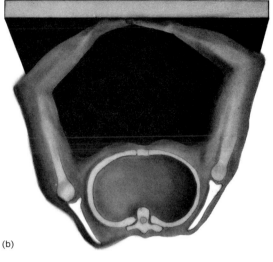

(b)

FIGURE 16-23
Scapular winging:
(a) as present in a client;
(b) internal skeletal displacement.

FIGURE 16-24
Carrying angle of the arm.

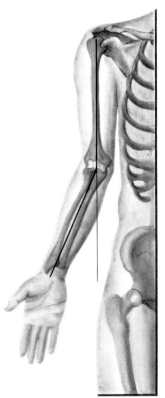

FIGURE 16-25
Deviations in the carrying angle of the arm:
(a) cubitus valgus; (b) cubitus varus.

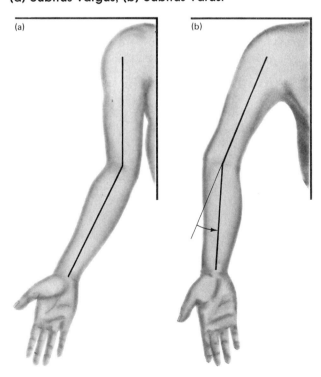

(a)   (b)

mally, this angle can be increased or decreased; these conditions are respectively termed cubitus valgus and cubitus varus (Figure 16-25). Subluxation of the radial head is a common deviation in children 4 years of age and younger. Frequently, in trying to prevent a young child's fall, an adult will pull on the child's hand. This results in a disturbance in the carrying angle, a partially flexed elbow, a pronated forearm, and a refusal to utilize or move the arm.

The cubital region is more prominent and rounded during flexion than in extension. Disruptions in the skin's characteristics and cubital contour are a result of inflammation, localized or diffuse fluid accumulation, nodule formation, fractures, and dislocations.

Localized accumulation of fluid or effusion may exist over the olecranon process, yielding a bogginess to palpation. Generally, this is indicative of inflammation of the olecranon bursa. Effusions that change the contour of the regions medial and lateral to the olecranon process are generalized in the joint.

Contour changes also result from the development of firm, nontender nodules just distal to the olecranon process (Figure 16-26). Nodular development anterior to the olecranon bursa can also occur. Both of these nodular protrusions may be due to arthritic changes; the latter also occurs with inflammation of the olecranon bursa (Figure 16-26).

Immediately superior to the epicondyles are the supracondylar lymph nodes, which are normally not palpable. An infectious process in the regions below the elbow may cause enlargement of these nodes, making them palpable.

Subsequent to assessing the elbow, the examiner proceeds to the wrist. The contour, position, and symmetry of the radial and styloid processes are observed. The radial styloid process is less prominent than the ulnar, with both the radial and ulnar processes having a rounded contour. These processes are palpated using the palmar surface of the fingers moving in a circular motion and by gliding over the structures in both a horizontal and vertical plane. Normally, these structures are smooth, firm, and nontender.

A hollow, bordered by tendinous structures located on the radial side of the wrist, is termed the anatomic snuff box (Figure 16-27). Pronouncement of this structure occurs with extension of the thumb away from the fingers. The anatomic snuff box is palpated to determine the

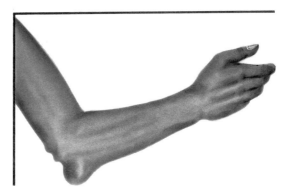

FIGURE 16-26
Contour changes of the olecranon process.

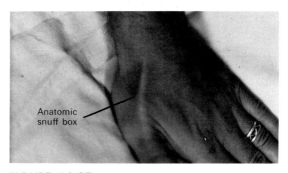

Anatomic
snuff box

FIGURE 16-27
Anatomic snuff box.

presence or absence of tenderness. Tenderness elicited in this region is indicative of underlying pathology.

The hands and fingers are the last structures of the upper extremities to be assessed. Observe the symmetry, size, position, and shape. The hands are normally symmetrical in size; deviations of hypertrophy or atrophy may be either unilateral or bilateral. The hands may also be enlarged and proportional, as in acromegaly, short, thick, and fat, as in cretinism, or slender and elongated. Frequently, the latter finding is associated with hyperextensible joints termed spider fingers.

In the neonate, the hand is held fisted close to the body, especially to the chest. By 15 months of age, the arms and hands are carried at the individual's sides, with the hands in an open, but slightly flexed, position. These features are carried throughout the remainder of the life cycle. In rheumatoid arthritis, the digits may be deviated toward the ulnar side of the hand, or there may exist hyperextension of the metacarpophalangeal joints and flexion of the interphalangeal joints

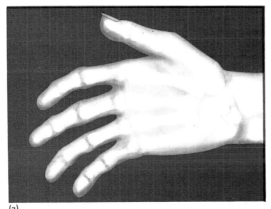

(a)

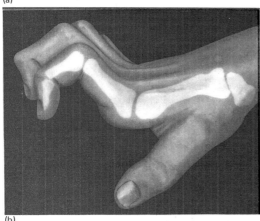

(b)

FIGURE 16-28

Changes in the contour of the hand:
(a) digital deviation toward
the ulnar side of the hand;
(b) hyperextension of the metacarpal
phalangeal joints and flexion of
the interphalangeal joints.

FIGURE 16-29

Location of Heberden's nodes.

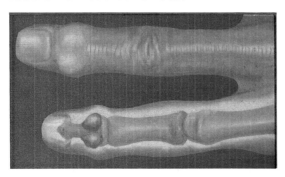

(claw hand). These changes in hand shape are indicative of underlying pathology (Figure 16-28).

The position, shape, number, and completeness of the digits is observed, as well as the symmetry. In all age groups, the fingers are held in close approximation, are straight, and possess minimal enlargement in the joint areas. The third digit is normally longer than the other fingers. When palpated, joint surfaces are smooth, with the lateral surface possessing an additional quality of tapering. Abnormally, the joints may feel roughened, nodular, boggy, or tensely swollen.

Hard nodules, which are nontender, approximately 2 to 3 mm in diameter, and located on either side of the midline of the distal joints are Heberden's nodes (Figure 16-29). Haygarth's nodes (Figure 16-30) create changes in the fingers' shape, increasing the size of the middle and proximal joints, and are associated with the inflammatory process of rheumatoid arthritis.

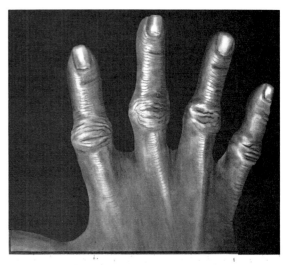

FIGURE 16-30

Location of Haygarth's nodes.

When present, these nodes interfere with joint mobility.

A missing digit or missing section of a digit resulting from trauma or congenital anomaly may not be readily observed by a brief, cursory inspection process, as the client's hand posture may hide this disfigurement. In the newborn and infant, additional or supernumerary digits, found most often on the ulnar portion of the hand, may be observed. Frequently, polydactyly or a super-

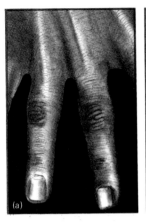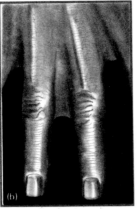

FIGURE 16-31
Interdigital webbing: (a) normal;
(b) syndactyly.

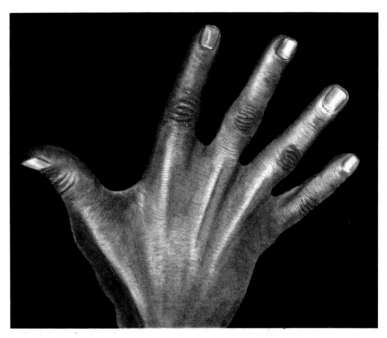

FIGURE 16-32
Characteristics of the dorsal hand surface.

numerary digit is no longer present in the older child, adolescent, adult, or the elderly because of previous surgical intervention for cosmetic and other reasons.

Between each finger, closely approximated to the metacarpophalangeal joint, is a minimal amount of webbing, most notable with the fingers spread apart (Figure 16-31). Abnormal extension of the interdigital webbing to a higher plane on the fingers is called syndactyly and may be congenital in nature or due to trauma that results in the formation of scar tissue. Inflammation of the interdigital webbing may result in increased distance between two bordering fingers, decreased mobility, and protective splinting.

The dorsal surface of the hand is smooth in appearance, with prominent vascular structures and tendons creating ridges (Figure 16-32). Palpation of the dorsal hand surface is accomplished using one of two methods. The first is to support the client's hand by resting it on one of the examiner's, palmar surface to palmar surface. The fingers of the examiner's other hand are then free to palpate the dorsal surface. The second method is to support the client's hand with the palmar surfaces of the fingers from both hands and palpate the dorsal surface with the thumbs. When palpating the dorsal hand surface, the underlying bony structures can be felt. Each should be smooth and nontender. Hollows present between the tendons that are soft to palpation are indicative of muscle atrophy. Localized swelling may be a sign of a local or systemic deviation.

The metacarpophalangeal joints are round and raised in appearance and smooth to palpation. There are three depressions or valleys, one between each joint (Figure 16-33). Abnormally, these depressions may lose their depth or disappear entirely.

FIGURE 16-33
Contour of the metacarpophalangeal joints:
(a) normal contour of joint with flexed hand;
(b) normal contour of joint with clenched fist.

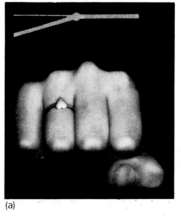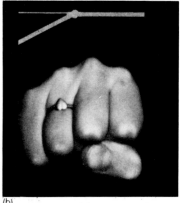

(a)   (b)

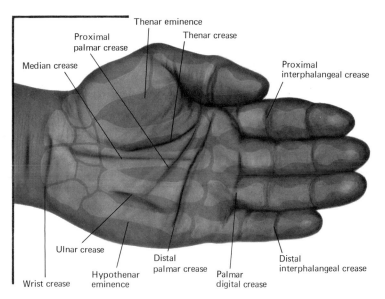

FIGURE 16-34

Normal characteristics of the palmar or flexor surface of the hand.

When inspected, a central depression is evident on the palmar or flexor surface of the hand. The presence or absence of this depression is generally dependent upon the bordering structures; the prominent, rounded thenar eminence on the side of the first digit, the less prominent hypothenar eminence on the fifth digit side, and the slightly raised area extending across the metacarpophalangeal joints (Figure 16-34).

FIGURE 16-35

Simian crease.

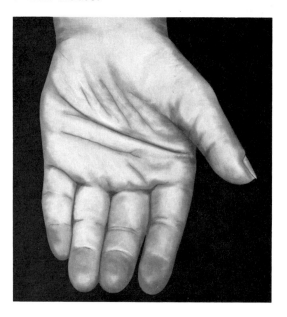

Compression or destruction of the innervation to any of these areas results in muscle atrophy, which, in turn, results in a decreased depth or total loss of the palmar depression.

Especially in the newborn and infant, the palmar creases are observed. Normally, there are two prominent creases located in the proximal and distal areas of the palm. Abnormally, there may exist only a single transverse crease (Figure 16-35). This single crease is called a **simian crease** or simian line and is frequently associated with Down's syndrome (trisomy 21).

The vascular structures of the upper extremities are assessed through palpation. The palmar surface of the fingers is used to elicit the pulsatile sensations. Generally, digits two through four are used and positioned longitudinally over the artery. A gentle pressure is exerted, compressing the artery over the underlying bony structures. The major arteries assessed are the axillary, located in the lateral region of the axilla; the brachial, located in the medial aspect of the cubital fossa; the radial, located immediately proximal to the thumb in the wrist; and the ulnar, located in the wrist aligning with the little finger. The pulsations produced by blood flow through the arteries are the same bilaterally in rate, rhythm, and quality.

INSPECTION AND PALPATION OF THE BACK

Assessment of the back is performed while the client's back, from the shoulders to the buttocks, is exposed. The skills of inspection and palpation are used sequentially, and the client is requested to assume the various positions of sitting, standing, and supination.

Inspect the curvature of the spinal column with the client standing. Observe first from a lateral position to obtain an oblique view; then observe directly posterior to the client (Figure 16-36). The spinal curvature of the neonate is assessed while supporting the infant under the arms and holding the child erect and in a prone position. In the term newborn, the spinal curvature is C shaped but more righted than in the preterm infant. Cervical curvature begins its formation when the infant learns to hold its head in midline, and the lumbar curvature originates with sitting up. It is normal for the lumbar curvature to be accentuated in the infant learning to walk, the toddler, and the preschooler up to the age of 4 years. At this time, the normal spinal column has four basic curvatures: the concave cervical curve, the convex thoracic curve, the concave lumbar curve, and the convex pelvic curve (Figure 16-12). The cervical curve extends from C2 to T2, followed by the thoracic curve, which extends from T2 to T12. The lumbar curve encompasses the vertebrae from T12 to the lumbosacral joint; the pelvic curve extends from the lumbosacral joint to the end of the coccyx.

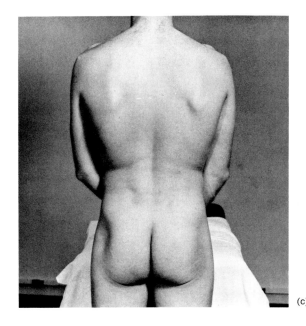

(c)

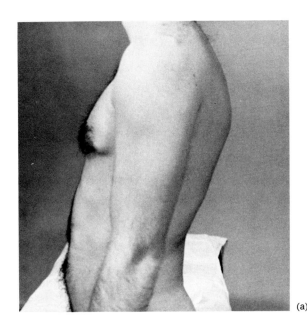

(a)

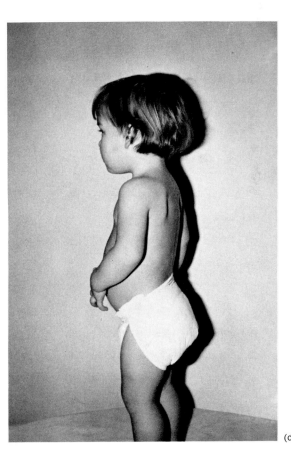

(d)

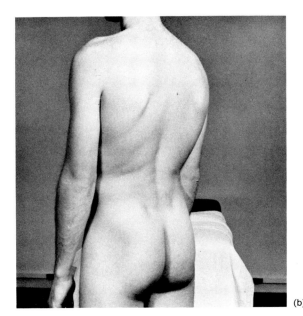

(b)

FIGURE 16-36

Characteristics of normal spinal curvature:
(a) lateral view; (b) oblique view;
(c) posterior view;
(d) lateral view of child.

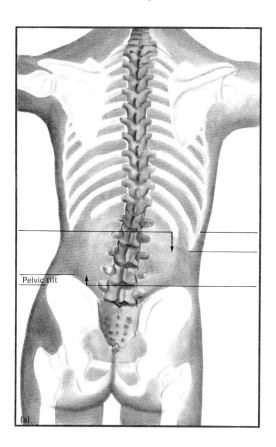

Pelvic tilt

Deviations in the normal spinal curvature include scoliosis, kyphosis, lordosis, and loss of curvature (Figure 16-37). Scoliosis is the lateral deviation of the spinal column. Minimal lateral deviation is not always immediately apparent during inspection. Several techniques may be utilized to facilitate the examiner's use of inspection while assessing for lateral spinal deviation. A water-soluble pen may be used to mark each vertebral process while the client is standing. Once completed, these markings will readily outline the shape of the spinal column (Figure 16-38). Another method is to request the client to lean forward and attempt to touch the toes. With the client in this position, the muscular structures lateral to the spine are observed. Normally, they are symmetrical in size, contour, and position.

FIGURE 16-37

Deviations of spinal column curvature: (a) scoliosis with pelvic tilt; (b) kyphosis; (c) lordosis; (d) loss of curvature.

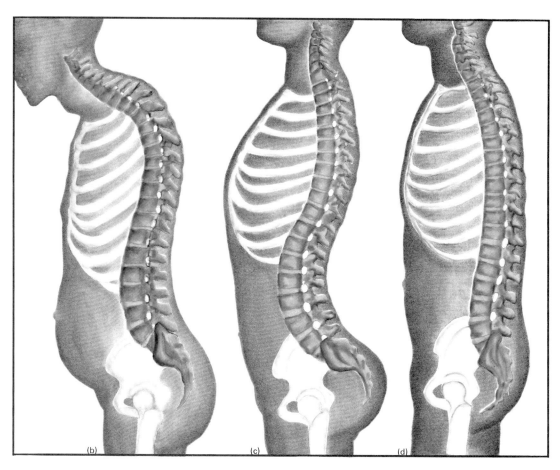

Abnormally, these muscles are asymmetrical, with the muscle mass on one side being more prominent, and positioned higher than those of the opposite side (Figure 16-39).

With the progression of a scoliotic condition, its effects on other parts of the musculoskeletal system become apparent. The anterior chest on the side of the lateral deviation flattens, while the structures on the opposite side become pronounced. The shoulders lose the symmetrical horizontal plane in which they reside, and the shoulder on the deviated side assumes a higher plane. The scapular position also changes from its normal anatomical location and from being on a horizontal plane to one of a lateral and forward position. Any indications of the existence of scoliosis demand referral for further evaluation, as early medical intervention can prevent the onset of chronic pain and alterations in cardiopulmonary functions.

Kyphosis is the accentuation of the convex thoracic curve. Kyphosis, resulting from poor posture habits, will spontaneously disappear when the client is requested to bend over and touch the toes. Rigid kyphosis and senile kyphosis, also termed dorsum rotundum, remain during flexion of the spine and are indicative of underlying pathology.

Lordosis, an exaggeration of the lumbar curvature, is frequently present during the later stages of pregnancy and with obesity when the abdomen is protuberant or when weak abdominal musculature is present.

Loss of spinal curvature can be generalized or localized. In a generalized loss, the spine becomes straight, and, frequently, loses its range of motion. This is termed poker spine and may result from an arthritic state. Localized loss of the lumbar curvature may result from muscle spasms.

Any deviation in the spinal curvature results in compensatory changes in the remainder of the musculoskeletal system. It is, therefore, essential to consult someone with expertise who can intervene and prevent continued deterioration of the involved area and secondary complications.

The integrity of the spinal column can be affected by congenital anomalies such as the three types of spina bifida. Spina bifida occulta may present a dimpling of the skin over the spinal column, a hairy patch of skin, or a nevus. A sacral coccygeal dimple in midline of the spine, at approximately 2 to 3 cm above the superior-most limits of the gluteal cleft, may be an embry-

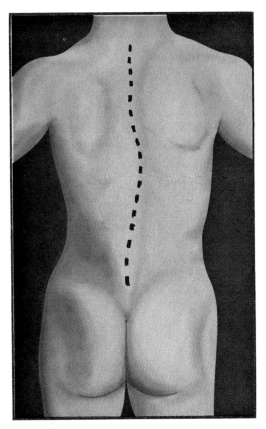

FIGURE 16-38

Assessment of spinal column curvature by marking the vertebral processes.

FIGURE 16-39

Assessment of spinal column curvature with the client flexed at the hips and touching the toes: (a) lateral view; (b) posterior view with symmetrical musculoskeletal characteristics; (c) posterior view with asymmetrical musculoskeletal characteristics.

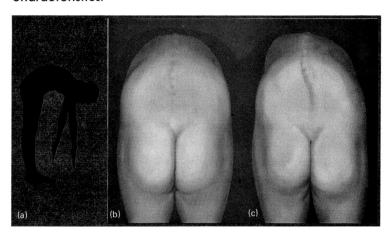

ological developmental remnant, which disappears during infancy, but must be evaluated to differentiate it from an occult spina bifida or a sacral sinus. To evaluate dimpling in the sacral area, grasp the lateral margins of the dimple and spread them apart. The area is then observed for the presence of a sinus opening and/or secretion. Normally, palpation should yield a firm area; abnormally, a soft hollow or indentation will be noted.

When a congenital defect of the spinal column permits the meninges to protrude into the saclike structure, it is termed a **meningocele.** This anomaly is translucent when inspected and fluctuant to palpation. A myelomeningocele contains the spinal cord, and, when transilluminated, the nerve fibers may be visible. Transillumination of the protruding sac is accomplished in a dark room with a bright light directed into the structure from its base.

After assessing the spinal column's contour, the characteristics of the bony structures and muscle masses are ascertained. The spinal column appears set in a valley, laterally bordered by the rounded musculature of the paraspinal muscles. Using the palmar surface of the fingers, the vertebrae are palpated with a firm and gentle gliding motion, first in a horizontal plane and then in a vertical plane. These bony structures are smooth and yield a sensation of alignment. Deviations in the surface characteristics include nodularity, gapping between vertebral bodies, and protrusion of one or several spinous processes.

The paraspinous muscles are palpated using the palmar surface of the fingers in a circular motion. These muscles are firm, and the overlying skin has minimal mobility. Abnormally, the muscles may be rigid or boardlike during a continuous state of contraction or soft and atonic with neuromuscular impairment.

INSPECTION AND PALPATION OF THE LOWER EXTREMITIES

The lower extremities are initially examined by assessing the gait, which consists of the stance phase and the swing phase. The stance phase consists of that portion of the gait when the foot is in contact with the floor or ground; the swing phase is subdivided into acceleration, midswing, and deceleration (Figure 16-40).

The gait is observed, noting each phase and its subcomponents, by requesting the client to walk toward a designated area and then return to the original starting point. The gait is observed in positions anterior, posterior, and lateral to the client. The gait is normally smooth and coordinated, with a base width of 2 to 4 in. between the heels and an approximate stride length of 15 in.; variations, dependent upon the individual's height, exist. Table 16-1 presents normal characteristics and deviations of gait and some possible associated causes.

Next, the general shape and contour of the lower extremities, from the pelvic crest to the feet, are assessed using a proximal-to-distal approach. It is important for the examiner to be in the same plane as the lower extremities, which can be accomplished by sitting on an examination stool or chair. The client is requested to stand straight with both feet flat on the floor while the examiner carries out a generalized inspection of the anterior and posterior structures (Figure 16-41).

While posterior to the client, the plane in which the pelvis lies can be assessed using two techniques. The sacral triangle is imaginary and superimposed upon the structures of the sacral area. The tip of the triangle is at the top of the gluteal cleft, and the base is bordered laterally by the posterior superior iliac spines. Frequently, the lateral borders are marked by dimples, one over each of the iliac spines. The base of this triangle normally forms a straight, level line (Figure 16-42). The plane in which the iliac crest resides can also be assessed. The examiner's fingers are placed on the iliac crest, and the thumbs are extended across the back in a straight line from the crest. An imaginary line is then drawn from crest to crest using the thumbs as a guide. This imaginary line should be on a level, horizontal plane (Figure 16-43). Tilting of these superimposed lines is abnormal and may be the result of abnormal spinal curvatures, impaired muscle function, or discrepant leg length.

The rounding muscle mass of the buttocks varies in size from client to client. The buttocks are divided in the midline by the gluteal cleft. A lower border is formed by the gluteal fold. The size, shape, and plane in which the buttocks and gluteal folds reside is symmetrical (Figure 16-44). Deviations from a symmetrical appearance may be due to congenital hip dislocation, leg length inequality, or atrophy of muscular structures.

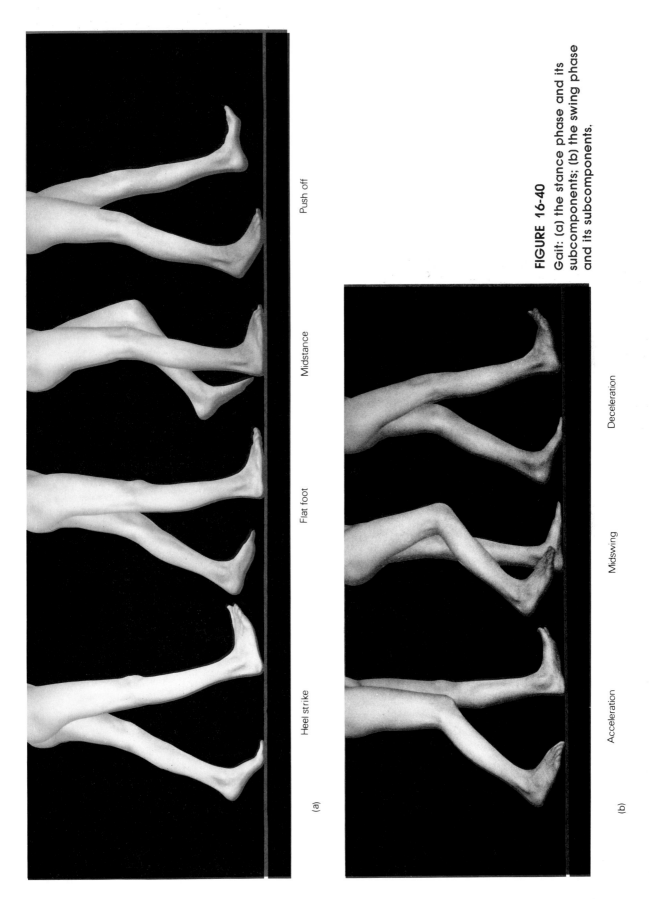

Heel strike   Flat foot   Midstance   Push off

(a)

Acceleration   Midswing   Deceleration

(b)

FIGURE 16-40

Gait: (a) the stance phase and its subcomponents; (b) the swing phase and its subcomponents.

TABLE 16-1

Phases of the Normal Gait and Some Associated Descriptions

PHASE	COMPONENT	NORMAL MOVEMENT	DEVIATED MOVEMENT	POSSIBLE CAUSE(S)
STANCE	Heel strike	Quiet, controlled Smooth, coordinated	Avoidance of heel strike, producing a hoppinglike motion or placement of foot on underlying surface, stepping on ball of foot	Heel spur Bursitis Sharp objects in shoe
		Knee is in extension	Inability to extend knee	Weak quadriceps Fusion of knee joint in flexed position
	Foot flat	Foot flattens over undersurface smoothly	Slapping of the foot following heel strike	Muscles of dorsiflexion are weak or nonfunctional
			Inability to flatten foot on undersurface until mid-stance	Fusion of the ankle
	Mid-stance	2.5-cm lateral displacement of the hip to weight-bearing side	Lurching movement toward side of muscle weakness	Weak gluteus medius muscle
			Hip extension maintained by thrusting thorax posteriorly	Weak gluteus maximus muscle
		Knee in flexion	Excessive flexion of knee resulting in instability	Weak quadriceps Dislocating kneecaps Torn menisci Torn collateral ligaments
		Weight is borne evenly over all aspects of the foot	Inability to bear weight evenly over entire foot	Rigid pes planus Fallen transverse arches Corns rubbing on shoes Objects in shoes
	Push off	Smooth, coordinated push off with hyperextension of metatarsophalangeal joint	Push off from lateral or medial side of foot	Osteoarthritis of single or multiple metatarsophalangeal joints Fusion of metatarsophalangeal joint(s)
			Flat-footed gait	Weak gastrocnemius, soleus, and flexor hallucis longus muscles
SWING	Acceleration	Quadriceps contract and initiate forward swing of leg	Exaggerated anterior rotation of pelvis facilitating forward thrust of the leg	Weak quadriceps
		Leg shortens through flexion of knee, permitting ground clearance	Inability to flex knee	Fusion of knee Limited flexion
		Ankle dorsiflexes, permitting ground clearance	Lack of dorsiflexion	Ankle fusion Impairment of muscles, producing dorsiflexion
	Midswing	Ankle is in dorsiflexion while leg is moving forward	Scraping of toes on walking surface	Impairment of muscles, producing dorsiflexion
			Steppage gate: excessive flexion of hip characterized by high stepping	Impairment of muscles, producing dorsiflexion
	Deceleration	Contraction of hamstring muscles decelerate the forward swing just prior to heel strike	Sharp, harsh heel striking with hyperextension of knee	Weak hamstring muscle

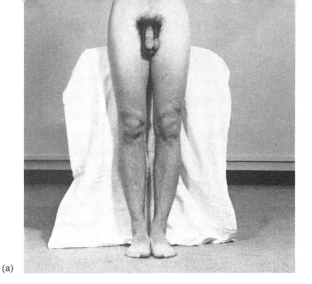

(a)

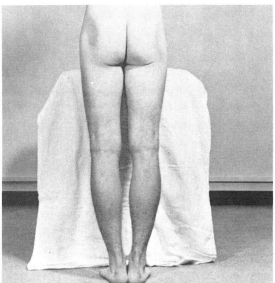

(b)

FIGURE 16-41

Contour of the lower extremities:
(a) anterior view; (b) posterior view.

FIGURE 16-42

The sacral triangle.

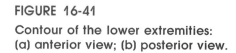

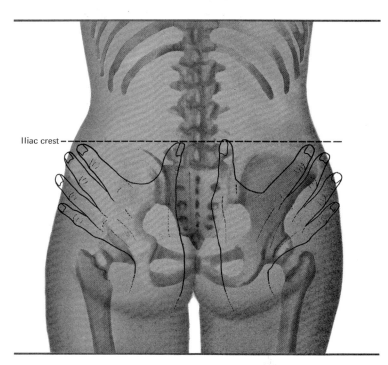

FIGURE 16-43

The horizontal plane of the iliac crest.

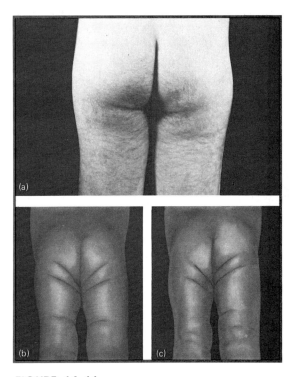

FIGURE 16-44

Inspection of symmetry, size, shape, and planes of the buttocks and gluteal folds: (a) in the normal adult; (b) in the normal newborn; (c) abnormal asymmetry of the gluteal folds.

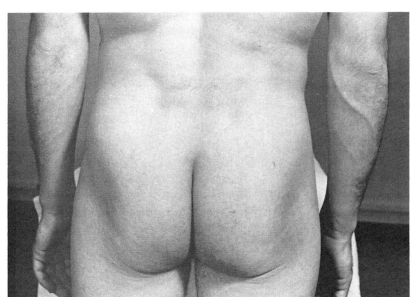

285

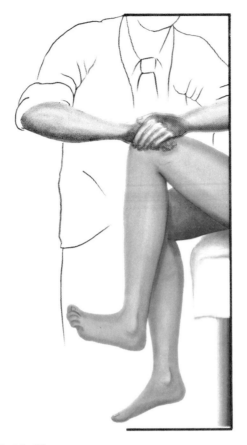

FIGURE 16-45
Assessment of the hip's muscular strength with the client in a sitting position.

FIGURE 16-46
Assessment of the hip's muscular strength with the client in a prone position.

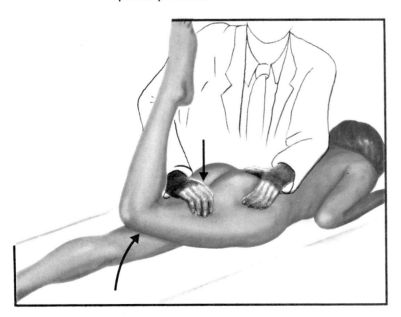

Muscular strength of the hip is assessed and recorded using the previously described grading scale. Muscular strength is first determined by utilizing an added resistant force. If the client is unable to overcome the additional resistance, the examiner gradually decreases the amount of resistance, including gravity if necessary. Three techniques used to assess the strength of the hip muscles are as follows:

1. The client is in a sitting position with the legs dangling over the edge of the examining table or bed. The examiner places one hand on the iliac crest to stabilize the pelvis. Upon request, the client raises the flexed leg off the supporting surface; and once the leg is raised, the examiner applies a resisting pressure on the distal segment of the thigh. The amount of resistance that the client is able to overcome is determined and recorded (Figure 16-45).

2. The client is in a prone position with the knees flexed. The examiner stabilizes the pelvis by placing the forearm over the iliac crest on the side being tested. The client raises the leg off from the supporting surface upon request, and the examiner applies an additional resisting force in a downward direction. The hand applying the additional resistance is placed immediately in front of the poples (Figure 16-46). Again, the amount of resistance that the client is able to overcome is graded and recorded.

3. A third technique of assessing muscle strength is the Trendelenburg test. The client is in a standing position with feet flat on the floor. The examiner determines the level of the sacral dimples, the crest of the ilium, and the gluteal folds and uses this in determining changes in the pelvic level. The client is then requested to stand on one leg. In this position the pelvis on the side opposite the leg support will rise (Figure 16-47). Abnormally, the pelvis opposite the leg support will remain at the same level or drop to a lower level. This is termed a **positive Trendelenburg.**

The skeletal structures of the newborn and infant's hips are assessed for congenital dislocation. With the infant in a supine position, the examiner flexes the infant's legs and abducts and externally rotates the extremities (Figure 16-48).

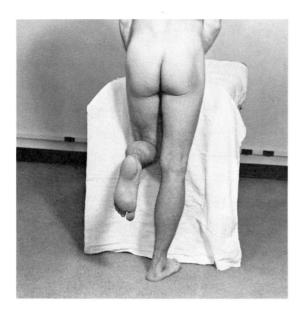

FIGURE 16-47
The Trendelenburg test, used to assess muscle strength.

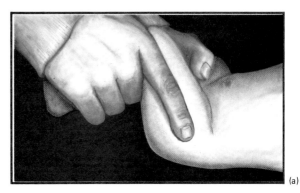

(a)

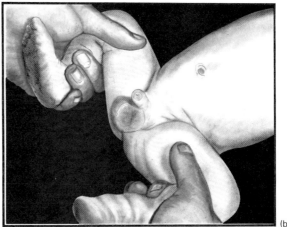

(b)

FIGURE 16-48
Assessment of the infant's hips for dislocation (Ortolani's sign).

FIGURE 16-49
Measurement of thigh circumference.

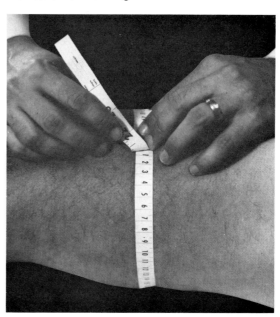

Deviations are produced when the femoral head slides over the acetabular rim, producing a palpable and often audible click. This click is termed **Ortolani's sign.** Normally, there is no audible or palpable sign.

Subsequent to hip assessment is the examination of the thigh and knee. The thighs are inspected, comparing the symmetry of contour and size. Generally, the muscle contour is symmetrical, tapering from the uppermost thigh to the knee. If the muscle masses appear asymmetrical, the thigh is measured at discrete intervals using a paper or metal tape measure. The examiner measures the thigh longitudinally first, marking the skin with a pen (ensuring that the same horizontal area on each thigh is measured); if necessary, subsequent measurements can then be obtained in the same region. It is also necessary to ensure that the measurement is taken on a horizontal plane (Figure 16-49). The results of the bilateral measurements should be equal: a difference of up to 1 cm is considered normal. The dominant side is usually slightly larger than the opposite.

The muscle structures of the thigh are palpated with the palmar surface of the fingers using a circular motion and moving in a longitudinal direction, starting from the uppermost aspect of the thigh. It is essential that all aspects of the thigh—anterior, posterior, medial, and lateral—be palpated. Generally, the consistency of the

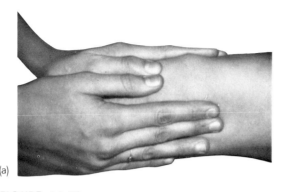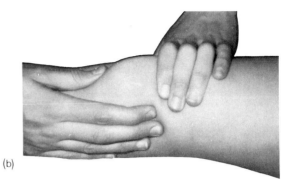

FIGURE 16-50
Palpation of the knee: (a) bilateral palpation; (b) palpation of the knee with suprapatellar compression applied.

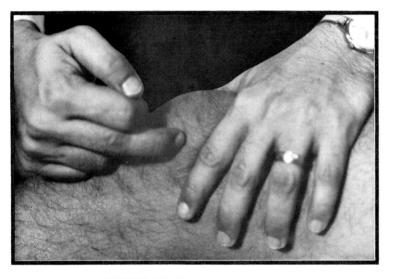

FIGURE 16-51
Direct percussion of the lateral hollow of the knee following upward stroking of the medial patellar hollow.

FIGURE 16-52
Assessment for evidence of effusion by suprapatellar compression and direct patellar tapping.

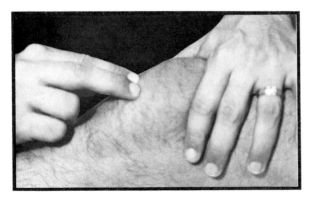

muscles is one of firmness, and there is total continuity from origin to insertion. Abnormally, the muscles may be soft, flabby, or possess a gapping characteristic. Occasionally, localized atrophic or nodular areas in the upper thigh region may be found in insulin-dependent diabetics who use the thigh as the only site for injection.

The contour of the knee and angle of the lower leg are observed next. The patellae are prominent and encircled by valleys or hollows. These hollows are most prominent when the knee is extended. Bony growth, swelling, fluid in the knee joint, cyst or abscess formation, and displacement of the patella will change the contours of the knee. These changes may be anterior to the patella, or they may be superiorly, inferiorly, laterally, or medially located, and may be contained within a single area or encompass several areas. The major deviation affecting the contour of the knee is loss of the hollows surrounding the patella.

The suprapatellar pouch, lateral and medial hollows, and the tibiofemoral joint space are palpated with the thumb and fingers of one hand or the fingers of both hands. They are also palpated with compression applied over the suprapatellar pouch by means of the opposite hand (Figure 16-50). Normally, these spaces are firm and smooth. When the sensations of bogginess or doughiness are ascertained, an inflammatory process or joint effusion may be present.

Determination of the presence of fluid can be accomplished using several techniques. With the client supine and the knee extended, the medial side of the patella is stroked or milked in an upward direction, displacing any existing fluid. Next, using direct percussion, a single tap is made on the lateral hollow immediately adjacent to the patella. The medial side of the patella is then observed for bulging, again as a result of the fluid displacement (Figure 16-51). Another technique to assess knee joint integrity with the client supine and the knee extended is to firmly grasp the thigh immediately above the knee. This displaces fluid in the suprapatellar pouch into the area between the patella and femur. With the second and third digits of the opposite hand, briskly push the patella against the femur (Figure 16-52). If fluid is present, this maneuver generally results in a palpable tapping or clicking sensation.

The contour or angulation of the lower leg deviates from what is considered normal in the older child and adult during the early weight-bearing stages of walking. This deviation may also occur with underlying disease processes. The two major types of deviated angulation are genu valgum and genu varum (Figure 16-53). Genu valgum, also called knock-knee, is most evident when the knees are in full extension. Normally, an imaginary line drawn from the anterior iliac spine to the base of the second toe will bisect the patella. With the presence of genu valgum, the patella is located medially to the dissecting line.

Genu varum, also called bowleg, is the outward bowing of the legs. Again, as in genu valgum, it is most evident when standing. When genu varum is present, an imaginary line drawn from the anterior iliac spine to the base of the second toe will be located medially to the patella.

Generally, stability of the knee joint is not assessed unless pain or buckling sensations are experienced by the client or when sports activities are anticipated. The collateral ligaments are assessed while the client assumes the supine position with slight flexion of the knee. The examiner places one hand on the fibular head and the other over the medial aspect of the lower leg, and pushes laterally with the hand positioned over the lower leg while the upper hand applies pressure in a medial direction (Figure 16-54). These opposing forces stress the joint. If stability problems involving the collateral ligament exist, a palpable gap in the medial joint may be elicited.

The cruciate ligaments are assessed for a draw sign. The anterior and posterior ligaments are examined with the client in a supine or sitting position with the knees flexed at 90 degrees. Sta-

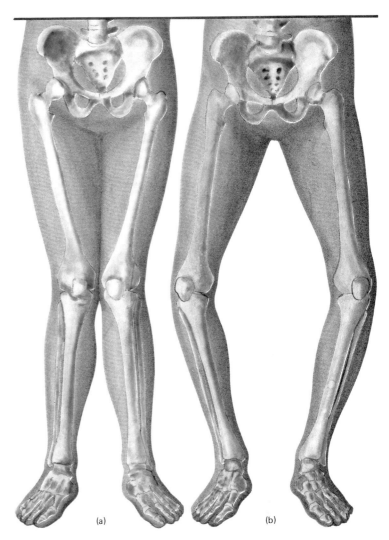

FIGURE 16-53
Deviations of lower leg angulation:
(a) genu valgum; (b) genu varum.

bilization of the client's foot is achieved by holding it between the examiner's knees when the client is sitting, or gently sitting on the client's foot when a supine position is used. The examiner then grasps the knee and draws it forward (Figure 16-55). Commonly, there is a minimal forward gliding of the knee; a distinct forward motion is abnormal. The posterior ligament is assessed in the same position, only the examiner pushes posteriorly on the knee. Absence of motion in this direction is normal.

Assessment of the ankle is initiated by inspection of the medial and more prominent lateral

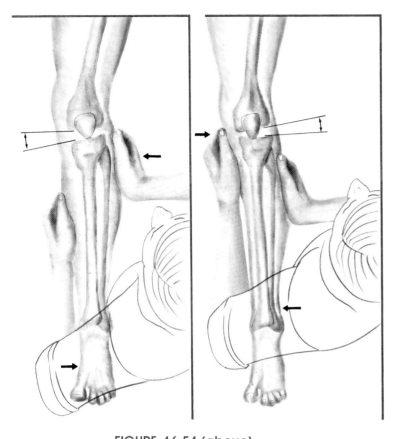

FIGURE 16-54 (above)

Assessment of the medial and lateral knee for stability with the client sitting and the examiner stabilizing the lower leg between the arm and body.

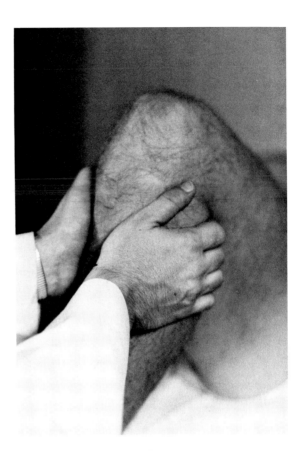

FIGURE 16-55 (above)

Assessment of the cruciate ligaments for a draw sign.

FIGURE 16-56 (left)

Assessment of ankle-joint stability.

FIGURE 16-57 (below)

Hallux valgus.

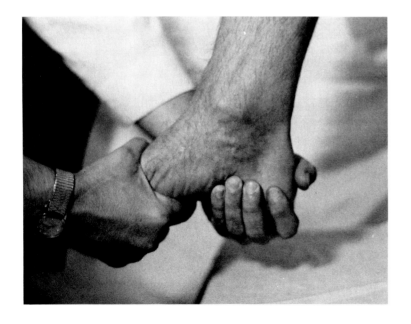

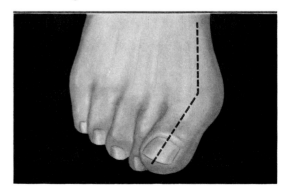

malleoli. These malleolar prominences are smooth and rounded when inspected and palpated. Loss of the malleolar prominence may be due to subcutaneous edema or inflammatory processes.

Stability of the ankle joint is not a routine component of an assessment but is performed if the client has experienced pain, frequent sprains, or intends to participate in athletic activities. With the client supine or sitting, the examiner stabilizes the lower leg with one hand while the other hand grasps the heel. The foot is then everted, and any notable gapping is indicative of damage to the ligaments (Figure 16-56).

The foot and its digits are assessed, determining size, contour, and number of digits present. Normally, when inspected, the toes are straight and flat, and extend from the distal end of the rounded dorsal surface. Several common contour deviations of the toes are the following:

1. Hallux valgus: lateral deviation of great toe; if marked, may overlap second toe (Figure 16-57)
2. Claw toe: hyperextension of metatarsophalangeal joint with flexion of the proximal and interphalangeal joint (Figure 16-58)
3. Hammer toe: hyperextension of metatarsophalangeal joint and distal interphalangeal joint with flexion of the proximal interphalangeal joint; hammer toe generally involves the second digit (Figure 16-59)

Upon inspection, the plantar surface of the foot presents a medial longitudinal arch, a prominent heel, and prominent metatarsophalangeal joints or ball of the foot. If the medial arch is excessively high, it is termed pes cavus (high instep); its absence is termed pes planus (flat feet) (Figure 16-60(a), (b), and (c)). Pes cavus may be normal or a sign of spinocerebellar pathway degeneration. In the newborn, the feet are flat due to the presence of plantar surface fat pads, which gradually involute after walking for a period of time.

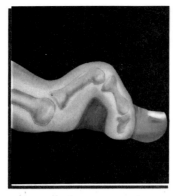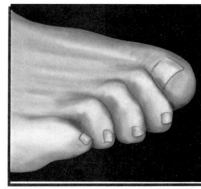

FIGURE 16-58
Claw toe.

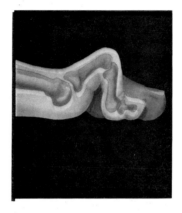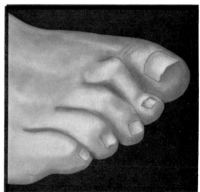

FIGURE 16-59
Hammer toe.

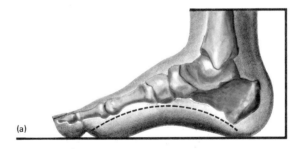

(a)

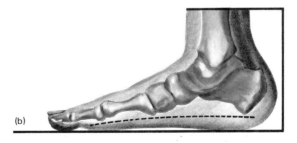

(b)

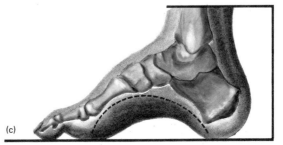

(c)

FIGURE 16-60 (right)
Medial longitudinal arch variations:
(a) normal longitudinal arch;
(b) pes planus; (c) pes cavus.

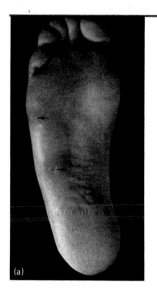
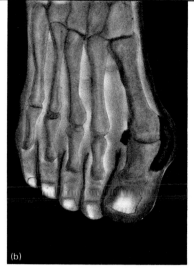
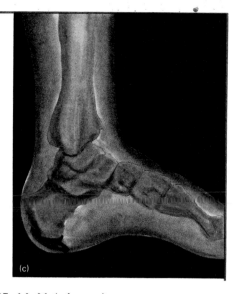

FIGURE 16-61 (above)
Deviations of the foot's plantar-surface characteristics: (a) plantar warts; (b) bunions; (c) heel spur.

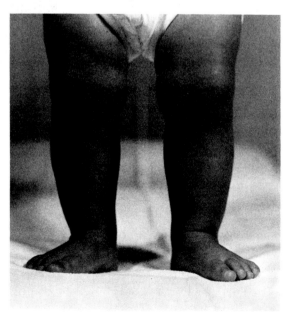

FIGURE 16-62 (left)
Pes varus, or toeing in.

FIGURE 16-63 (below)
Pes valgus, or toeing out.

Palpation of the plantar surface of the foot yields a smooth, firm, fleshy surface. The presence of plantar warts, bunions, and heel spurs will change the plantar surface characteristics (Figure 16-61(a), (b), and (c)).

It is important in all age groups to assess the alignment of the foot, but particular care is taken in assessing this aspect in the newborn and young child. Normally, the foot is straight. If the feet are toeing in, that is, the entire foot turns inward, it is termed pes varus (Figure 16-62) and may be caused by tibial torsion. In toeing out or pes valgus (Figure 16-63), the entire foot is directed outward and may cause tibial torsion. Other deviations of the foot alignment may occur, with the heel remaining straight and the forefoot in abduction, called metatarsus varus (Figure 16-64(a), (b), and (c)), or the forefoot in adduction, called metatarsus valgus.

The vascular structures of the lower extremities are assessed through palpation. The same techniques used to elicit pulsations in the upper extremities are used in the lower extremities. The major arteries assessed are the femoral, located in the upper aspect of the femoral triangle; the popliteal, located in the medial aspect of the popliteal fossa; the posterior tibialis, located immediately posterior to the medial malleolus; and the dorsalis pedis, located on the dorsal surface of the foot just above the longitudinal arch (Figure 16-65). The dorsalis pedis pulse is more readily located by drawing an imaginary straight line on the dorsal surface of the foot from the interspace between the first and second digit of the foot to the midpoint between the lateral and medial malleoli. The popliteal artery is made palpable by flexing the knee, thus relaxing the muscular structures of the area.

To assess adequacy of arterial blood supply in the lower extremities, request the client to assume a supine position. The legs should be extended, should be elevated from the surface at a 45 degree angle, and should be supported in this position for several minutes. While the legs are elevated, the plantar and dorsal surfaces of the foot are observed for color, as well as for the appearance of the superficial prominent veins. Normally, there is little color change and the veins are flush with the skin's surface. After the extremity has been elevated for several minutes, the client is requested to sit up with the legs dangling. Normally, the foot color returns and the veins fill and become prominent within 10 seconds. Abnormally, with the legs in the elevated position, the foot color becomes pale and the prominent superficial veins become hollowed. In the position of sitting with the legs dangling, a cyanotic color occurs within 1 to 2 minutes and vein filling takes 1 to 2 minutes. This assessment procedure is called Buerger's test.

Assessment of the venous system of the lower extremities is important. Normal superficial veins that are prominent possess a smooth course and are full. Deviations from these normal characteristics are dilation and tortuosity. Veins that possess these characteristics are termed varicose (Figure 16-66).

In further assessing the venous structures of the lower extremities, it is important to remember that the greater saphenous and lesser saphenous veins communicate with the deep femoral venous system through communicating veins. The leg

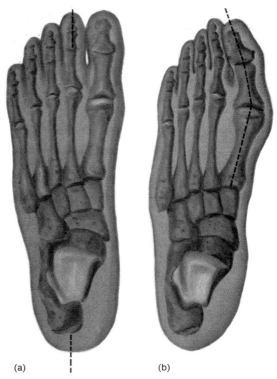

(a)   (b)

FIGURE 16-64

Metatarsal alignment: (a) normal;
(b) metatarsus varus;
(c) metatarsus valgus.

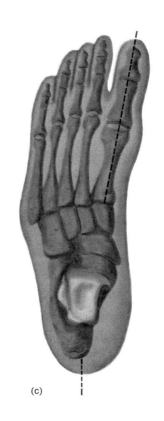

(c)

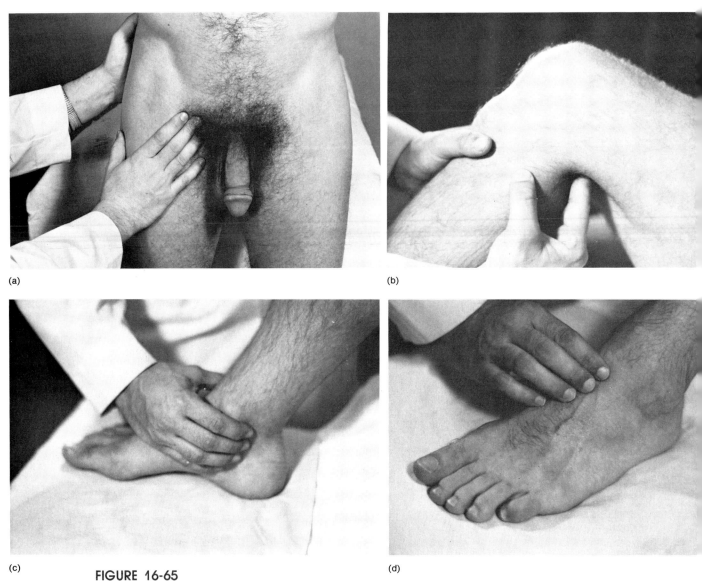

(a)

(b)

(c)

(d)

FIGURE 16-65
Pulses of the lower extremities: (a) femoral; (b) popliteal; (c) posterior tibial;
(d) dorsalis pedis.

veins also possess valves that ensure unidirectional flow of blood.

The Brodie–Trendelenburg test is used to assess the competency of the communicating veins. With the client in a supine position, the leg is elevated, and a tourniquet is applied to the thigh with enough pressure to occlude venous flow but not arterial flow. The client is then requested to stand, and the veins are observed. If the valves of the communicating veins are incompetent, the veins fill from below. Normally, the veins remain collapsed. Removal of the tourniquet in a standing position enables further assessment as the direction of vein filling can be observed. Normally, filling occurs from below and moves in an upward direction. Abnormally, venous filling that

occurs quickly in a downward direction is indicative of incompetent saphenous valves.

Perthes' test is used to assess the patency of the deep veins. A tourniquet is applied to the thigh, occluding the superficial venous circulation. The superficial veins are observed, noting their characteristics. The client is then requested to walk at a quick pace for approximately 5 minutes. Varices that remain prominent and dilated are indicative of saphenous and communicating vein incompetency. Increased distention of the veins while walking is indicative of obstruction with the deep veins, as well as incompetent valves in the communicating veins.

To assess deep vein thrombosis, the foot is quickly and forcefully dorsiflexed at the ankle.

This dorsiflexion is accomplished by stabilizing the heel with one hand and grasping the forefoot with the opposite hand (Figure 16-67). When this activity produces pain in the calf or popliteal area, it is termed a positive Homans's sign.

Chronic venous stasis produces brownish pigmentary changes in the skin. Ulcerations resulting from venous problems are shallow and are frequently covered with exudate. Arterial ulcers possess irregular edges, pale and boggy granulation tissue, and frequently have an eschar covering. Arterial problems in the lower leg are frequently accompanied by hair loss on the involved extremity at or below the origin of the problem. These changes in the integument reflect vascular deviations and are readily seen upon inspection.

RANGE OF MOTION

Performance of the range of motion of the musculoskeletal system can be used to assess the degree of motion that the client can produce and can serve as an intervention to restore, maintain, and promote the degree of mobility. The purpose of this description of range of motion is for assessment, not intervention.

Generally, the range of motion is assessed actively or by requesting the client to perform specific motions. Passive range of motion or those motions performed for the client in a relaxed state by the examiner are implemented when deviations from the normal degree of mobility exist or when the client for some reason is unable to perform the motions. Passive range of motion is performed in the neonate and child who is unable to cooperate as a result of inability to understand the request being made. During passive range of motion assessment, the extremity is not forced beyond a point of resistance or past the point where tenderness is elicited. When the degree of mobility is determined and resistance is encountered, it is recorded in the following manner: "Left arm abduction, 90 degrees resistance encountered."

Do not move the area being assessed in an unnatural plane. For example, abducting the arm in the wrong plane can initiate or aggravate brachial plexus problems. Refer to Table 16-2 for a detailed description of active and passive range of motion maneuvers. The normal range of motion frequently decreases with age. Deviations exist when daily functional activities are interrupted by pain or limited mobility.

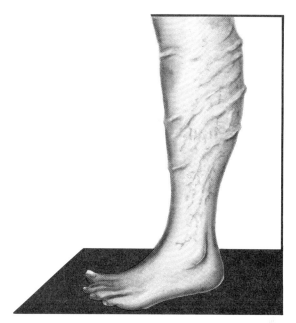

FIGURE 16-66
Varicose veins.

FIGURE 16-67
Dorsiflexion of the foot to assess Homans's sign.

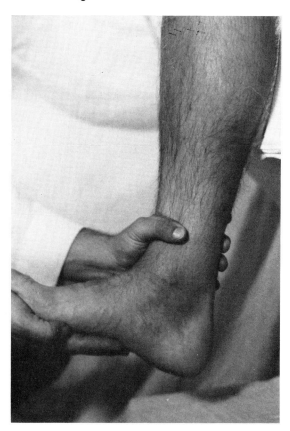

TABLE 16-2

Active and Passive Range of Motion Maneuvers*

STRUCTURE AND RANGE OF MOTION	ILLUSTRATION	METHODOLOGY OF ACTIVE AND PASSIVE RANGE OF MOTION
HEAD AND NECK 1. Flexion 45°		A: client bends the head and attempts to touch the chin on the chest P: place one hand on each side of the head and bend it forward, attempting to touch the chin on the chest
2. Extension 0° or neutral	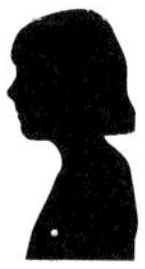	A: client returns the head back to midline following flexion and holds it in that position P: placing one hand on each side of the head, it is returned from a flexed position to one of midline
3. Hyperextension 45°	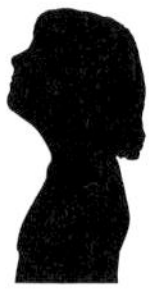	A: client bends the head backward or looks up at the ceiling P: with one hand on each side of the head, gently tilt it backward
4. Lateral bending 45°	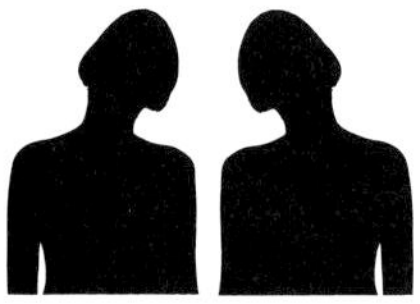	A: client bends the head toward the shoulder with the shoulders in a horizontal plane P: place one hand on each side of the head and bend it in a lateral direction toward the shoulder
5. Lateral rotation 45°	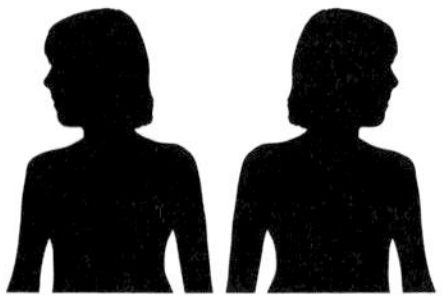	A: client turns the head to the right and to the left as far as possible P: with one hand on each side of the head, the head is turned laterally to the right and left
SHOULDER 1. Flexion 90°		A: with arm first at the side, client brings the arm forward, keeping the elbow straight and raising the arm above the head P: place one hand over the acromion, applying gentle pressure while the other hand supports and moves the arm above the head
2. Extension 0° or neutral	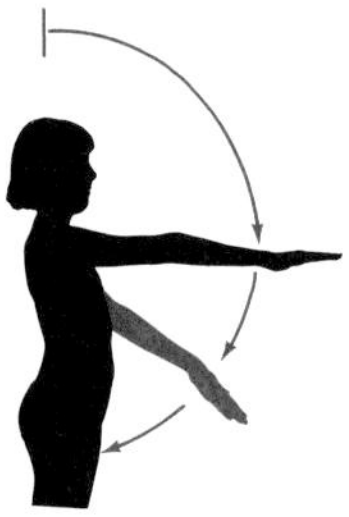	A: after the shoulder has been flexed, client returns the arm to the side, keeping the elbow straight P: place one hand over the acromion; support the extremity at the elbow and move the entire arm from a flexed position to the side

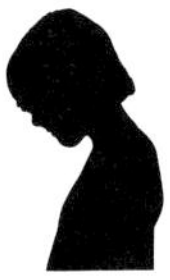

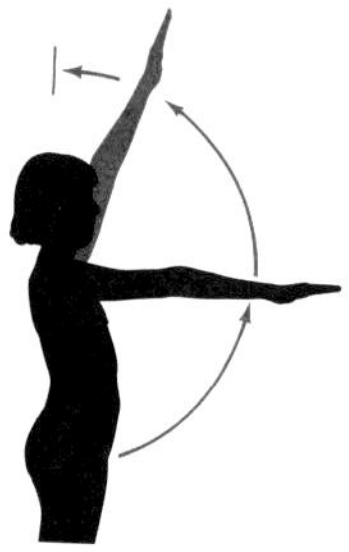

296

TABLE 16-2 CONTINUED

STRUCTURE AND RANGE OF MOTION	ILLUSTRATION	METHODOLOGY OF ACTIVE AND PASSIVE RANGE OF MOTION
SHOULDER (cont.)		
3. Hyperextension 45°	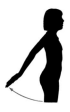	A: with the elbow straight, client moves the arm in a straight line directly behind the body P: with client in a sitting, lateral, or prone position, place one hand on the acromion, and with the other hand, move the extremity directly behind the client
4. Internal rotation 55°	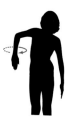	A: client raises the arm to shoulder level with the elbow flexed, the fingers pointed toward the floor, and the palmar surface of the hand facing posteriorly; the forearm is then rotated by the client posteriorly P: holding client's arm immediately proximal to elbow, allowing it to flex, raise the arm to shoulder level; grasp the wrist and hand and rotate the forearm posteriorly
5. External rotation 40° to 45°	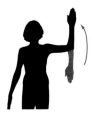	A: client rotates the forearm anteriorly while the arm is at the shoulder level, with the elbow bent and fingers pointed toward the floor P: grasp client's arm immediately proximal to elbow, allowing it to flex, and raise it to shoulder level; grasp the wrist and hand and rotate the forearm anteriorly until the palmar surface faces anteriorly
6. Abduction 180°	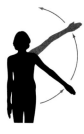	A: with the elbow straight, client moves the arm from the side directly away from the body P: grasp the extremity with one hand supporting the elbow joint and the other hand supporting the wrist and hand; then move the arm from the client's side directly away from the body
7. Adduction 45°	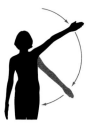	A: with the elbow straight, client moves the arm across the front of the chest P: grasp the arm with one hand supporting the elbow joint and the other hand supporting the wrist and hand; then move the arm from the client's side directly across the midline of the anterior chest

TABLE 16-2 CONTINUED

STRUCTURE AND RANGE OF MOTION	ILLUSTRATION	METHODOLOGY OF ACTIVE AND PASSIVE RANGE OF MOTION
ELBOW		
1. Flexion 135°+		A: with the wrist straight, client bends the elbow and attempts to touch the hand to the shoulder P: supporting the arm at the elbow with one hand, grasp the wrist with the other hand and move the forearm toward the shoulder
2. Extension 0° or neutral		A: from a flexed position, client straightens the elbow P: after the elbow has been flexed, move the forearm in a posterior direction to straighten the elbow
3. Supination 90°		A: with the elbow flexed and the hand held palmar surface down, client rotates the hand until palmar surface faces up P: cup client's elbow with one hand while the other hand grasps the client's hand, palmar surface to palmar surface; flex the elbow 90° and then rotate the palmar surface of client's hand until it is upward
4. Pronation 90°		A: with the elbow flexed 90° and the hand held palmar surface up, client rotates the hand until palmar surface faces down P: cup client's elbow with one hand while the other hand grasps the client's hand, palmar surface to palmar surface; flex the elbow 90° and then rotate palmar surface of client's hand until it faces down
WRIST		
1. Flexion 80°+	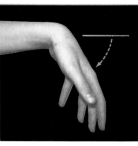	A: client bends the wrist downward from a straight position P: flex client's arm at the elbow, grasp the wrist, and bend the wrist down
2. Extension 0° or neutral	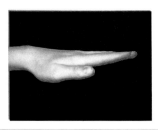	A: from a flexed position, client moves the hand to straight alignment with the forearm P: flex client's arm at the elbow, grasp the wrist, and move the wrist from a flexed position to one of straight alignment with the forearm

TABLE 16-2 CONTINUED

STRUCTURE AND RANGE OF MOTION	ILLUSTRATION	METHODOLOGY OF ACTIVE AND PASSIVE RANGE OF MOTION

WRIST (cont.)

3. Dorsiflexion
   70°

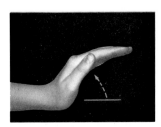

A: client bends the wrist from a straight position upward

P: support client's forearm with one hand, grasp client's wrist and hand firmly, and bend in an upward direction

4. Ulnar deviation
   30°

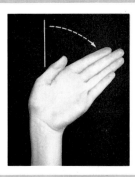

A: client moves the wrist from a straight position toward the ulnar side

P: support client's forearm with one hand, grasp client's hand firmly, move the wrist toward the ulnar side

5. Radial deviation
   20°

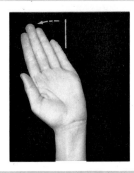

A: client moves the wrist from a straight position toward the thumb side

P: support client's forearm with one hand, grasp client's hand firmly, and deviate the wrist toward the radial side

FINGERS

1. Flexion
   a. Metacarpophalangeal joint, 90°
   b. Proximal interphalangeal joint, 100°
   c. Distal interphalangeal joint, 90°

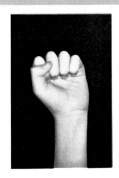

A: client makes a tight fist

P: support the client's forearm and place the palmar surface of the other hand onto the client's dorsal hand surface; move client's fingers into a fisted position

2. Extension
   0° or neutral

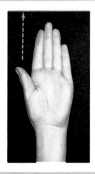

A: after flexing the fingers, client straightens the fingers

P: after flexing fingers, grasp fingers and return them to straight alignment with hand and wrist

TABLE 16-2 CONTINUED

STRUCTURE AND RANGE OF MOTION	ILLUSTRATION	METHODOLOGY OF ACTIVE AND PASSIVE RANGE OF MOTION
FINGERS (cont.) 3. Hyperextension 30° to 45°	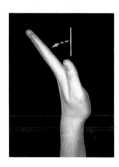	A: with fingers straight forward, client moves the fingers backward as a total unit P: support forearm with one hand; with the other hand, palmar surface to palmar surface in client's hand, gently move fingers upward
4. Abduction 20°	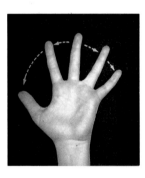	A: with fingers straight forward, the client spreads fingers apart P: support client's hand; deviate each finger away from midline by grasping each one on its lateral and medial sides
5. Adduction 0°	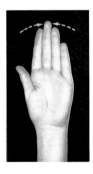	A: after abducting the fingers, client brings the fingers together in close approximation P: after deviating each finger away from midline, continue to support hand and return each finger to the midline

THUMB
 	
1. Flexion
  a. Metacarpophalangeal joint 50°
  b. Interphalangeal joint 90°
	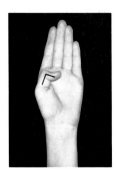	A: client bends the thumb
		
		P: supporting client's hand, bend the metacarpophalangeal and interphalangeal joints

TABLE 16-2 CONTINUED

STRUCTURE AND RANGE OF MOTION	ILLUSTRATION	METHODOLOGY OF ACTIVE AND PASSIVE RANGE OF MOTION
THUMB (cont.)		
2. Extension 0° or neutral	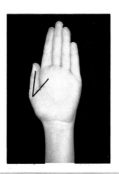	A: client straightens the thumb from a flexed position P: grasp flexed thumb and straighten
3. Hyperextension: interphalangeal joint, 20°	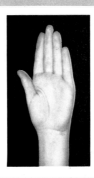	A: client extends thumb backward as far as possible P: grasp the lateral and medial aspect of the distal portion of the thumb and extend it backward
4. Palmar abduction 70°	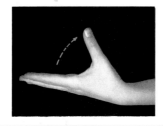	A: client moves the thumb in a horizontal plane away from the palm of the hand P: support client's hand and move the thumb in a horizontal plane away from the palm by grasping the thumb over the interphalangeal joint.
5. Palmar adduction 0°	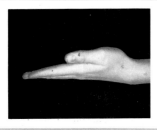	A: after abducting the thumb, client approximates it to the index finger P: after abducting the thumb, bring it in approximation with the index finger
6. Opposition	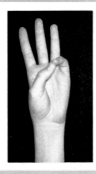	A: client touches the thumb to each of the fingertips P: supporting the hand, move the thumb anteriorly and around toward the little finger

301

TABLE 16-2 CONTINUED

STRUCTURE AND RANGE OF MOTION	ILLUSTRATION	METHODOLOGY OF ACTIVE AND PASSIVE RANGE OF MOTION
TRUNK/SPINAL COLUMN		
1. Flexion 75–90°	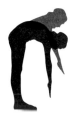	A: client bends over in an attempt to touch the toes, keeping the knees straight P: seldom done
2. Extension 0°		A: client stands up straight P: seldom done
3. Hyperextension 30°	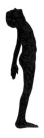	A: client bends backward P: seldom done
4. Lateral bending 35°	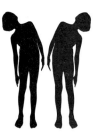	A: with the client standing, the examiner places one hand on the iliac crest; client then bends laterally in a direction opposite the hand placement P: with client standing, place one hand on the iliac crest to stabilize the pelvis; with the opposite hand placed on the ipsilateral shoulder, bend the trunk laterally
5. Rotation 30°	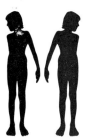	A: holding the legs and pelvis straight, turn first to one side and then the other P: with client standing, place one hand on the iliac crest and the other on the contralateral shoulder; both hands pull in a posterior direction

TABLE 16-2 CONTINUED

STRUCTURE AND RANGE OF MOTION	ILLUSTRATION	METHODOLOGY OF ACTIVE AND PASSIVE RANGE OF MOTION
HIP		
1. Flexion 135°		A: client brings the knee as close to the chest as possible without bending the back P: with the client in a supine position, place one hand under the knee and grasp the ankle with the other hand; bring the leg up toward the chest, flexing the knee
2. Extension 0° or neutral		A: after the leg is in a flexed position, client straightens the leg P: after flexing the leg, continue to support it and return the leg to a straight position
3. Abduction 45°		A: while standing or supine, client moves one leg directly away from the other leg P: with the client supine, place one hand under the knee and grasp the ankle with the other hand; then move the leg away from the midline
4. Adduction 20°		A: client brings the leg across the midline and then across the opposite leg as far as possible P: while supporting the extremity, move it from the abducted position toward the midline and then across the midline
5. Rotation a. Internal, 35° b. External, 45°	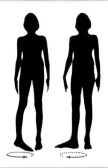	A: while standing or supine, client turns the feet inward and then outward P: with the client supine, place one hand over the knee, the other over the lower leg, and turn the leg inward, then outward

TABLE 16-2 CONTINUED

STRUCTURE AND RANGE OF MOTION	ILLUSTRATION	METHODOLOGY OF ACTIVE AND PASSIVE RANGE OF MOTION
HIP (cont.)		
6. Flexion and adduction		A: client crosses the legs, one thigh over the other P: with the client supine, grasp the ankle supporting the knee, then flex the knee and move the leg across the other
7. Flexion, abduction, and external rotation		A: client places the outside of one foot on the opposite knee P: with client supine, grasp the ankle and support the knee; the leg is flexed at the knee, and the foot is moved to touch the opposite knee
8. Hyperextension 30°		A: while prone or standing, client moves the leg directly behind the body P: with client prone, support the knee and elevate the extremity
KNEE 1. Flexion 130°		A: while supine, client bends the knee and brings the heel up to the buttocks P: with client in a supine position, place one hand under the knee and grasp the ankle with the other hand; bend the leg at the knee, moving the foot toward the buttocks
2. Extension 0° or neutral		A: from a flexed position, client straightens the leg P: once the examiner has flexed the knee, it is returned to a straight position

TABLE 16-2 CONTINUED

STRUCTURE AND RANGE OF MOTION	ILLUSTRATION	METHODOLOGY OF ACTIVE AND PASSIVE RANGE OF MOTION
ANKLE		
1. Dorsiflexion 20°	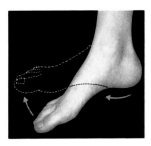	A: while sitting or supine, client brings the foot upward P: with client sitting or supine, grasp the heel with one hand and the foot with the other hand; move the foot in an upward direction
2. Plantarflexion 50°	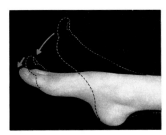	A: while sitting or supine, client bends the foot downward P: with client sitting or supine, grasp the heel with one hand while holding the foot with the other hand and push in a downward direction
3. Inversion 5°	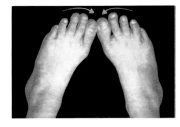	A: while supine or sitting, client tilts the foot inward P: hold the lower leg with one hand, and with the other, grasp the heel and tilt the foot inward
4. Eversion 5°	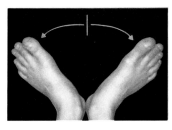	A: while supine or sitting, client tilts the foot outward P: hold the lower leg with one hand, and with the other, grasp the heel and tilt the foot outward
FOREFOOT		
1. Adduction 20°	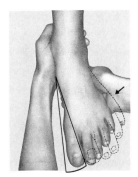	A: client turns the forefoot inward while the examiner stabilizes the heel P: stabilize the heel and turn the forefoot inward

TABLE 16-2 CONTINUED

STRUCTURE AND RANGE OF MOTION	ILLUSTRATION	METHODOLOGY OF ACTIVE AND PASSIVE RANGE OF MOTION

FOREFOOT (cont.)

2. Abduction
10°

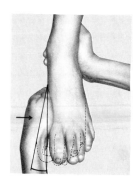

A: client turns the forefoot outward while the examiner stabilizes the heel

P: stabilize the heel and turn the forefoot outward

TOES

1. Flexion: first metatarso-phalangeal joint, 45°

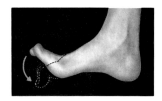

A: client bends the toes

P: with client supine, grasp the first digit and bend it in a downward direction

2. Extension
0° or neutral

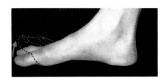

A: client straightens the toes

P: from the flexed position, straighten the toe

3. Abduction

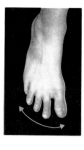

A: client spreads the toes apart

P: grasp each toe and move it away from the midline

4. Adduction
0°

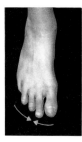

A: after the toes are spread apart, client brings them back together in close approximation

P: grasp each toe and return it to the midline

* After the Sister Kenny Institute, *Range of Motion Exercise: Key to Joint Mobility.* Rehabilitation Publication 703; Patricia Toohey and Corrine W. Larson, 1968.

STUDY GUIDE
QUESTIONS

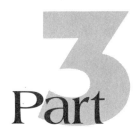

Part

In the following client situations, identify and describe the subjective and objective data to be collected, the specific tools and procedures to be utilized in the collection of those data, and the rationale for the nursing assessment.

1. Joann Woodworth, a 14-year-old female, is brought to clinic by her mother, who states that her spine must be crooked because clothes just don't seem to fit her right.

2. James Karigan, a 17-year-old male, presents at the Free Clinic for a sports physical. You are to assess his musculoskeletal status.

3. John Longsworth, a 60-year-old male, presents with the recent development of "bumps" on his elbow. He has had stiff, aching joints for 2 years.

4. Merna Schwartz, a 30-year-old female, states that her big toe is awful looking, is going toward her other toes, and is extremely painful when wearing shoes.

5. As the nurse in the newborn nursery, you are to assess 1-day-old Jeneal Molar's musculoskeletal status.

6. Pamela Warton brings her 9-month-old son to the well-child clinic, having noted an outward turning of his right foot when attempting to walk.

7. On your home visit to Mrs. Leonard Mier, who is 80 years old, you note an ulcer on her left lower extremity.

SAMPLE FORMAT TO BE USED IN RESPONDING TO THE STUDY GUIDE QUESTIONS

SUBJECTIVE DATA TO BE COLLECTED	OBJECTIVE DATA TO BE COLLECTED	SPECIFIC TOOLS AND PROCEDURES TO BE UTILIZED	RATIONALE FOR NURSING ASSESSMENT

BIBLIOGRAPHY

ALEXANDER, MARY M., and MARIE S. BROWN, *Pediatric Physical Diagnosis for Nurses,* pp. 189–211. New York: McGraw-Hill Book Company, 1974.

DEGOWIN, ELMER, and RICHARD L. DEGOWIN, *Bedside Diagnostic Examination* (3rd ed.), pp. 624–758. New York: Macmillan Publishing Co., Inc., 1976.

EVANS, WILLIAM F., *Anatomy and Physiology* (2nd ed.), pp. 47–143. Englewood Cliffs, N.J.: Prentice-Hall Inc., 1976.

GORDON, EVERETT, J., *Diagnosis and Treatment of Acute Low Back Disorders.* Northridge, California: Riker Laboratories, Inc., 1974.

———, *Diagnosis and Treatment of Common Hip Disorders.* Northridge, California: Riker Laboratories, 1975.

———, *Diagnosis and Treatment of Common Knee Problems.* Northridge, California: Riker Laboratories, 1974.

———, *Diagnosis and Treatment of Common Neck Disorders.* Northridge, California: Riker Laboratories, 1976.

HOCHSTEIN, ELLIOT, and ALBERT L. RUBIN, *Physical Diagnosis,* pp. 304–338. New York: McGraw-Hill Book Company, 1964.

HOLLENSHEAD, W. HENRY, *Textbook of Anatomy* (2nd ed.), pp. 95–111, 147–492. New York: Harper & Row, Inc., 1967.

HOPPENFELD, STANLEY, *Physical Examination of the Spine and Extremities.* New York: Appleton-Century-Crofts, 1976.

LLOYD, G. C., *Orthopedics in Infancy and Childhood.* New York: Appleton-Century-Crofts, 1971.

ROSSE, CORNELIUS, and D. KAY CLAWSON, *Introduction to the Musculoskeletal System.* New York: Harper & Row, 1970.

ROSSMAN, ISADORE, ed., *Clinical Geriatrics,* pp. 3–16. Philadelphia: J. B. Lippincott Company, 1971.

17

The Neurological System

OBJECTIVES

1. Describe the basic functional circuit of the nervous system
2. Describe the function of the primary structures of the brain and spinal cord
3. Identify the function of each division of the peripheral nervous system
4. Compare and contrast the function of the sympathetic and parasympathetic nervous systems
5. Discriminate between function of the upper and lower motor neurons
6. Systematically assess and describe:
   a. General appearance of a client
   b. Facial expression
   c. Level of consciousness
   d. Expression of ideas and thought patterns
   e. Orientation to time, place, and person
   f. Individual's immediate and remote recall
   g. Language and speech
   h. Cranial nerve function
   i. Station and gait
   j. Motor coordination
   k. Symmetry of muscle strength
   l. Muscular movement and tone
   m. Deep tendon, superficial, pathologic, and primitive reflexes
   n. Superficial and deep sensation
   o. Stereognosis and graphesthesia

REVIEW OF STRUCTURE AND FUNCTION

Part 1

dendrites - afferent toward cell body

The central nervous system (CNS) is a highly complex, integrated system that is markedly dependent upon development. The anatomy of the system by no means reflects the complexity of the whole. The functional cell unit of the nervous system is the **neuron** (Figure 17-1). The neuron has a nucleated cell body with protoplasmic arms called **axons** and **dendrites.** The axons are efferent processes directing nerve impulses away from the cell body; dendrites are afferent processes that direct impulses toward the cell body.

Neurons are organized in groups or chains within the nervous system to form nerves, nerve roots, tracts, and pathways through which one or many impulses are conducted. Some of these paths for impulse conduction are afferent, directing impulses away from the brain or spinal cord; others are efferent, directing impulses toward the brain or spinal cord.

The junction between two neurons is called the **synapse.** Impulses from the dendrite of one neuron are conducted through the synapse to the axon of the next neuron by means of chemical electrical messages.

The central structures of the neurological system are the brain and spinal cord.

BRAIN

The brain is located within the skull. It is divided into three major sections, the cerebrum, cerebellum, and the brain stem. The cerebrum is further divided into two hemispheres by the longitudinal fissure. Each hemisphere has five lobes: frontal, parietal, occipital, temporal, and central or insula. The outermost surface of the cerebral hemisphere is the cortex (1.5 to 4.5 mm); then beneath the cortex is the white matter, basal ganglia, and corpus callosum. The corpus callosum and three commissures within the brain unite the right and left cerebral hemispheres by crossing fibers.

Within the cerebrum is the ventricular system from which the cerebrospinal fluid originates. The ventricles include the right and left lateral ventricles, the third ventricle, aqueducts of Sylvius, and the fourth ventricle (Figure 17-2).

The cortex of the cerebrum is convoluted with many sulci (deep creases) and gyri (raised ridges), which permit a cerebral cortex surface area of over 2 ft^2. Although there is much variation in the sulci and gyri of the cerebral surfaces of any two brains, the major creases and ridges form common landmarks (Figure 17-3).

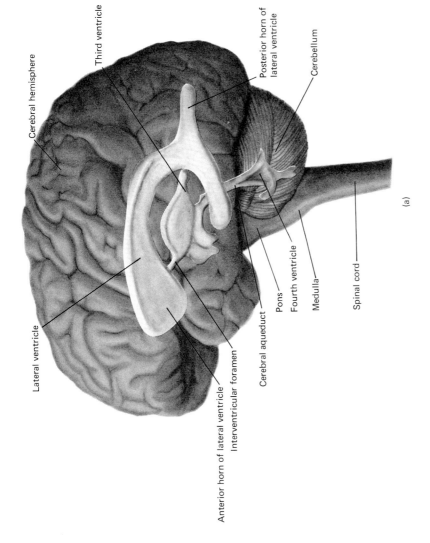

FIGURE 17-1
The functional cell unit of the nervous system, the neuron.

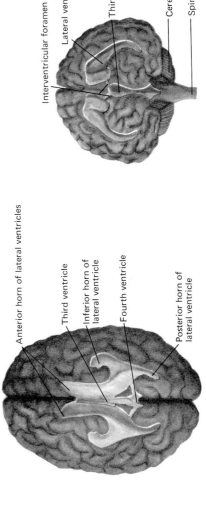

FIGURE 17-2
The ventricles: (a) sagittal view; (b) coronal view; (c) frontal view.

311

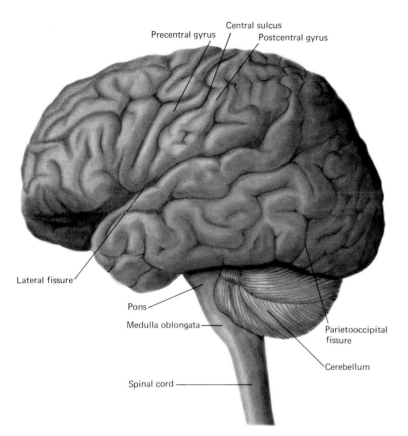

FIGURE 17-3
Major sulci and gyri of the cerebral cortex.

TABLE 17-1
Anatomical Sites of the Cerebrum and Associated Functions

ANATOMICAL SITE	FUNCTIONS
Frontal lobe	Voluntary movements Personality Some neurons of memory and speech
Parietal lobe	Conscious sensations of heat, cold, pain, touch, pressure, proprioception
Occipital lobe	Vision
Temporal lobe	Hearing Possibly smell and taste Some neurons of speech and language
Other	Reasoning, memory, emotion, foresight, intelligence, personality, interpretation of special sensations, speech mechanisms, initiations and storage of other mental activities

The major anatomical sites of the cerebrum and their known functions are listed in Table 17-1.

Deep within the cerebrum are gray matter masses known as the basal nuclei. Together with the surrounding white matter, they form the corpus striatum in each cerebral hemisphere. The basal nuclei are involved in coordination of body movements.

The cerebellum is located inferior to the occipital cerebral lobes. Like the cerebrum, it has two hemispheres connected by the vermis lobe. Gray matter makes up the outermost part of its cortex and can be found in clusters within the underlying white matter, called cerebellar nuclei. A nucleus of the nervous system is an aggregation of nerve cell bodies within the CNS. The function of the cerebellum is skeletal muscle coordination. It further controls posture and equilibrium.

The cerebellum has fiber tracts connecting it with the midbrain, pons, medulla, and spinal cord. It receives directional impulses from the cerebrum and skeletal muscles, which are then reorganized and directed as impulses to stimulate specific muscles to result in a coordinated movement or activity. Unlike the cerebrum, the cerebellar responses are purely at the unconscious level.

The brain stem is that part of the brain excluding the cerebral and cerebellar cortexes. The structures included in the brain stem are the medulla, pons, mesencephalon, diencephalon, and basal nuclei.

The medulla oblongata is anatomically a superior extension of the spinal cord from the foramen magnum (at the base of the skull). Although it is grossly similar to the spinal cord, the arrangement of gray and white matter is markedly different. Functionally, the medulla is responsible for containing the nucleic origins for four of the twelve cranial nerves: IX, glossopharyngeal; X, vagus; XI, accessory nerve; XII, hypoglossal (Figure 17-4). It further controls the vital functions of ventilation, heart rate, and vasoconstriction, as well as swallowing, coughing, vomiting, sneezing, and hiccuping. All pathways between the cord and brain must pass through the medulla.

FIGURE 17-4 (facing page)
Origins of the cranial nerves.

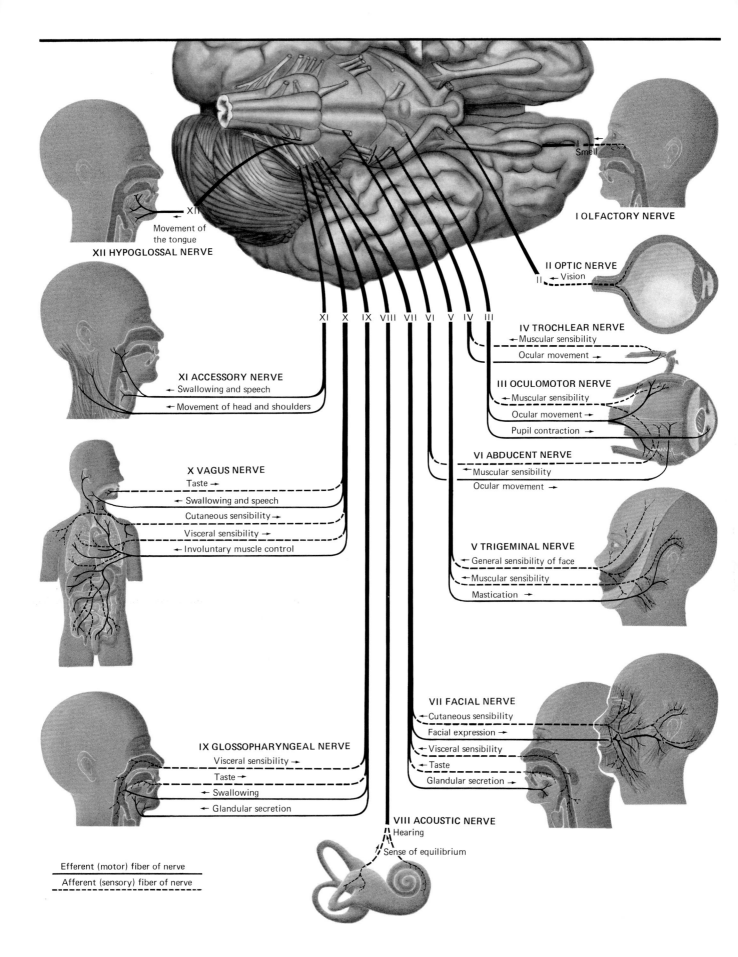

XII HYPOGLOSSAL NERVE

XII ← Movement of the tongue

I OLFACTORY NERVE

I ← Smell

XI ACCESSORY NERVE

← Swallowing and speech

← Movement of head and shoulders

II OPTIC NERVE

II ← Vision

IV TROCHLEAR NERVE

← Muscular sensibility

Ocular movement →

III OCULOMOTOR NERVE

← Muscular sensibility

Ocular movement →

Pupil contraction →

X VAGUS NERVE

Taste →

← Swallowing and speech

Cutaneous sensibility →

Visceral sensibility →

← Involuntary muscle control

VI ABDUCENT NERVE

← Muscular sensibility

Ocular movement →

V TRIGEMINAL NERVE

← General sensibility of face

← Muscular sensibility

Mastication →

VII FACIAL NERVE

← Cutaneous sensibility

Facial expression →

← Visceral sensibility

← Taste

Glandular secretion →

IX GLOSSOPHARYNGEAL NERVE

Visceral sensibility →

Taste →

← Swallowing

← Glandular secretion

VIII ACOUSTIC NERVE

Hearing

Sense of equilibrium

Efferent (motor) fiber of nerve

Afferent (sensory) fiber of nerve

XI X IX VIII VII VI V IV III

The pons is superior to the medulla. Anatomically and functionally, it connects the medulla and pons with the midbrain and joins the cerebral hemispheres. It forms the floor of the fourth ventricle. The trigeminal nerve or cranial nerve V originates from within the pons, while cranial nerves VI (abducens), VII (facial), and VIII (auditory) originate from the medulla–pons junction. Functionally, it channels some reflexes of ventilation, pupillary action, and eye movement and houses the pneumotaxic center of breathing.

The mesencephalon or midbrain is located between the forebrain (cerebrum plus diencephalon) and the hindbrain (pons and medulla). It is small in size, but contains several important connection points to allow coordination between other parts of the brain. Motor coordination is accomplished by two ventral stalks of fibers called the cerebral peduncles. On the posterior dorsal side are four posterior nuclear masses, or, collectively, quadrigeminal bodies. The two superior masses, superior colliculi, are associated with visual reflexes. The inferior colliculi deal with auditory reflexes. The colliculi are each connected individually to the thalamus by a band of fibers.

The oculomotor nerves (cranial nerves III) and the trochlear nerves (cranial nerves IV) originate between the cerebral peduncles of the midbrain and the pons. Part of the trigeminal nerve (cranial nerve) also originates in the mesencephalon.

The third ventricle (in the diencephalon) and fourth ventricle (of the hindbrain) are joined by a channel passing through the mesencephalon known as the cerebral aqueduct. The mesencephalon also contains the red nucleus, a complex integrative structure that relays impulses between the cerebrum, cerebellum, pons, and medulla.

The diencephalon consists of the thalamus, hypothalamus, and its cavity, the third ventricle. It is located between the cerebral hemispheres and is bordered inferiorly by the mesencephalon.

The thalamus is two portions of gray matter surrounding the third ventricle. It functions as an integrating center for many impulses, both motor and sensory. Many of its mediating functions are only slightly understood at this time. However, it is implicated in the control of states of wakefulness, conscious perception of sensations, and abstract feeling states.

At the inferior aspect of each thalamus is the subthalamus, which contains the nucleus and field of Forel. These structures are involved in the reception of midbrain impulses, which are then directed to the cerebral cortex. At the superior aspect of the thalamus is the epithalamus, which consists of the pineal body (involved with sexual development and behavior and secretion of melatonin), the habenular trigone (involved with the transmission of olfactory impulses), and the posterior commissure, which joins the two diencephalon halves.

The hypothalamus is inferior to the subthalamus and consists of the pituitary gland, infundibulum, the mammillary bodies, and the optic chiasm.

The pituitary gland is involved in hormonal control of growth, lactation, vasoconstriction, and metabolism. The infundibulum is the pituitary stalk. The mammillary bodies are specifically involved in directing olfactory impulses to the cerebral cortex for interpretation. The optic chiasm is the point at which the optic nerve tracts cross. Although the hypothalamus has many diverse functions, the most common function is coordination of impulses between the cerebral cortex and autonomic nervous system.

SPINAL CORD

The spinal cord provides pathways for many of the impulses traveling between the brain and the body. It is 43 cm in length or two-thirds of the length of the vertebral canal from the foramen magnum to the second lumbar vertebra. It consists of both gray matter (lying deep) and white matter. The white matter consists of pathways for impulses, whereas the gray matter consists of reflex centers.

Impulses to and from the brain via the spinal cord reach the appropriate part by means of the 31 pairs of spinal nerves that branch off the cord. Because the vertebral column grows faster than the spinal cord within it, the specific origin of each spinal nerve and the anatomical location of cord segments vary during growth periods (Figure 17-5).

PERIPHERAL NERVOUS SYSTEM

The peripheral nervous system includes the cranial nerves, spinal nerves, and autonomic nerves. The peripheral nerves have three functions,

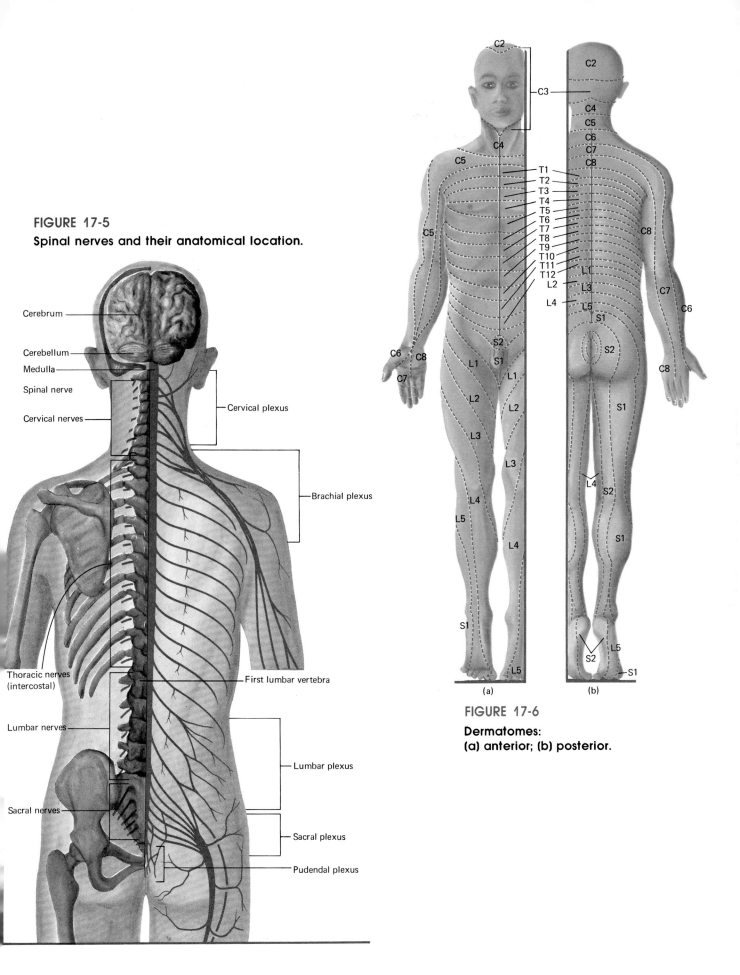

FIGURE 17-5

Spinal nerves and their anatomical location.

Cerebrum

Cerebellum

Medulla

Spinal nerve

Cervical nerves

Cervical plexus

Brachial plexus

Thoracic nerves (intercostal)

First lumbar vertebra

Lumbar nerves

Lumbar plexus

Sacral nerves

Sacral plexus

Pudendal plexus

C2
C3
C4
C5
T1
T2
T3
T4
T5
T6
T7
T8
T9
T10
T11
T12
L1
L2
L3
L4
L5
S1
S2

C6
C8
C7
L1
L2
L3
L4
L5
S1

C2
C4
C5
C6
C7
C8
L1
L3
L5
S1
S2
C8
C7
C6
S1
L4
S2
S1
L5
S1

(a)

(b)

FIGURE 17-6

Dermatomes:
(a) anterior; (b) posterior.

TABLE 17-2

Important Features of Cranial Nerves

CRANIAL NERVE	NUMBER	FUNCTIONAL CLASS	CHIEF FUNCTION
OLFACTORY	I	Sensory	Sense of smell
OPTIC	II	Sensory	Visual sense
OCULOMOTOR	III	Motor	Eye movements, dilation and constriction of pupil
TROCHLEAR	IV	Motor	Eye movements
TRIGEMINAL	V	Mixed	Movements of chewing, sensations of the head and face
ABDUCENS	VI	Motor	Lateral movement of eye
FACIAL	VII	Mixed	Movements of facial muscles, secretion of saliva, taste from anterior two-thirds of tongue
ACOUSTIC	VIII	Sensory	Hearing and equilibrium
GLOSSOPHARYNGEAL	IX	Mixed	Secretion of saliva, movements of swallowing, taste from pharynx and posterior third of tongue, reflexes of breathing, and blood pressure
VAGUS	X	Mixed	Movements and sensations of heart, digestive organs, and larynx
ACCESSORY	XI	Motor	Movements of head, shoulder, and voice-producing parts of larynx
HYPOGLOSSAL	XII	Motor	Movements of the tongue

After William F. Evans, *Anatomy and Physiology*, (2nd ed.), p. 169. Englewood Cliffs, N.J.: Prentice-Hall, Inc., 1976.

motor or efferent (toward the body), sensory or afferent (from the body), and mixed (bidirectional).

There are 12 pairs of cranial nerves. The name, number, functional class, and chief function of each cranial nerve are listed in Table 17-2.

There are 31 pairs of spinal nerves that branch off the spinal cord. In the adult, there are eight pairs of cervical spinal nerves, twelve pairs of thoracic spinal nerves, five pairs both of lumbar and sacral spinal nerves and one pair of coccygeal spinal nerves. After leaving the vertebral column, the spinal nerves branch and subbranch, forming the anterior rami and posterior rami. The anterior rami innervate the skin and muscles of the anterior and lateral trunk and upper and lower limbs. The posterior rami innervate the posterior muscles and skin of the trunk. Most of the anterior rami group together as they proceed toward related innervated sites, forming plexuses. There are five plexuses: the cervical, brachial,

lumbar, sacral, and pudendal. The rami further branch to form terminal nerves in order to accomplish innervation. The innervation of the skin from the spinal nerves is accomplished in a segmental pattern with some overlap. These segments are known as dermatomes (Figure 17-6).

Reflexes

Reflexes are involuntary responses to stimuli, many of which do not reach conscious awareness. They are predictable, but changeable, and can be facilitated or inhibited by centers in the brain. A reflex is composed of sensory perception that sends an impulse from the sensory receptor via the afferent neuron to the gray matter of the cord, and out again via an efferent neuron to the muscle or muscles for response (Figure 17-7). There are several classifications of reflexes. The major ones are described in Tables 17-6 and 17-7 with their assessment significance.

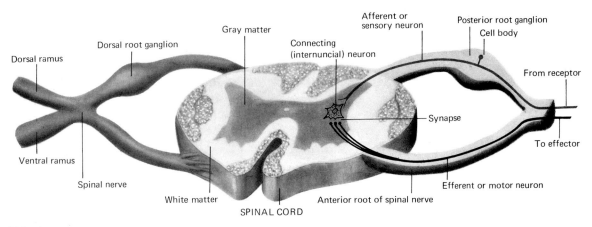

FIGURE 17-7
Reflex arch.

Autonomic Nervous System

The autonomic nervous system, an efferent nervous system also referred to as the visceral motor system, has nerve fibers that carry involuntary motor impulses to smooth muscles, cardiac muscle of the heart, and some of the exocrine and endocrine glands. All its innervations require two neuron chains. The cell body of one neuron lies within the central nervous system (primarily the spinal cord or medulla). The axon of this primary neuron synapses with the cell body and dendrite of the second neuron within a ganglion. The secondary neuron's axon carries the impulse from the ganglion to the structure of innervation. There are three types of ganglia: (1) the vertebral ganglia, which are found in two chains parallel to the spinal column; (2) the collateral ganglia, which are found in the thoracic and abdominal pelvic cavities near the aorta or its major branches; and (3) the terminal ganglia, which are located close to the structures they innervate in the abdominal and thoracic great nerve plexuses. The postganglionic fibers outnumber the preganglionic fibers about 32:1, so one primary neuron could control responses to a much greater terminal area.

The autonomic nervous system has two divisions, the sympathetic and the parasympathetic divisions. Many organs of the body are supplied by fibers of both the sympathetic and parasympathetic divisions, resulting in potentially antagonistic responses (Figure 17-8). Homeostasis is usually maintained by a balancing between these divisions.

Sympathetic The sympathetic division is referred to as the thoracolumbar division because its preganglionic cell bodies lie in the intermediolateral cell column or the horn of all thoracic and three to four lumbar segments of the spinal cord. The short preganglionic fibers leave the spinal column via the anterior roots of spinal nerves and enter the sympathetic (ganglia) trunk. This trunk contains 22 postganglionic neurons with which some of the preganglion fibers synapse. The remainder pass through the trunk and synapse in the collateral ganglia. The only exception to this system of sympathetic supply is to the adrenal gland, where no postganglionic neuron exists. Instead, the gland has cells that function as a second neuron. The primary function of the sympathetic division is fight or flight. It has a more generalized response resulting in increased blood supply to the brain, skeletal muscles, and heart, with increased central blood pressure, body temperature, alertness, and strength.

Parasympathetic The cell bodies of the parasympathetic preganglionic neurons are found in the nuclei in the medulla of cranial nerves III, VII, IX, and X and in the spinal cord segments at the second, third and fourth sacral level. The preganglionic fibers follow the cranial nerves and spinal nerves from the cord or brainstem, and extend to terminal ganglia at the surface or within the organ of innervation.

The primary function of the parasympathetic division is less generalized and has a more localized, visceral response to conserve body resources.

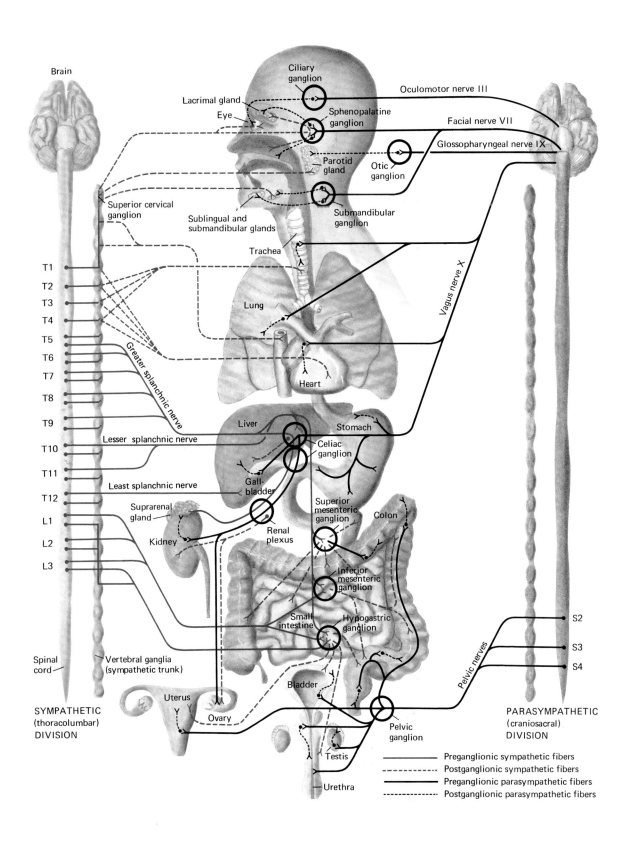

Brain

Ciliary ganglion

Oculomotor nerve III

Lacrimal gland

Sphenopalatine ganglion

Eye

Facial nerve VII

Glossopharyngeal nerve IX

Parotid gland

Otic ganglion

Superior cervical ganglion

Submandibular ganglion

Sublingual and submandibular glands

Trachea

Vagus nerve X

T1
T2
T3
T4
T5
T6
T7
T8
T9
T10
T11
T12
L1
L2
L3

Lung

Heart

Greater splanchnic nerve

Lesser splanchnic nerve

Liver

Stomach

Celiac ganglion

Least splanchnic nerve

Gall-bladder

Suprarenal gland

Superior mesenteric ganglion

Colon

Kidney

Renal plexus

Inferior mesenteric ganglion

Small intestine

Hypogastric ganglion

S2
S3
S4

Spinal cord

Vertebral ganglia (sympathetic trunk)

Bladder

Pelvic nerves

Uterus

Ovary

Pelvic ganglion

SYMPATHETIC
(thoracolumbar)
DIVISION

PARASYMPATHETIC
(craniosacral)
DIVISION

Testis

────────── Preganglionic sympathetic fibers
---------- Postganglionic sympathetic fibers
────────── Preganglionic parasympathetic fibers
---------- Postganglionic parasympathetic fibers

Urethra

FIGURE 17-8

The autonomic nervous system.

Pharmacologically, the autonomic nervous system can be divided into cholinergic and adrenergic divisions, depending upon the chemical agent that allows transmission of the impulse at the preganglionic and secondary neuron synapse and the postganglionic and visceral receptor junction. The cholinergic neurons include (1) all the preganglionic (primary) neurons, (2) the parasympathetic postganglionic (secondary) neurons, (3) sympathetic postganglionic neurons to the sweat glands, and (4) sympathetic secondary neurons that produce vasodilation of the skeletal muscle blood vessels. These cholinergic neurons release acetylcholine to transmit the impulse across the synaptic junction and cholinesterase to terminate the transmission.

The adrenergic division is confined to the other sympathetic postganglionic (secondary) neurons. These neurons release norepinephrine to transmit the impulse to their visceral effector sites (receptors). Some of these receptors are responsive to both norepinephrine and epinephrine. Norepinephrine, unlike acetylcholine, has a more generalized effect in the body and can be found in the circulating tissue along with epinephrine; both hormones are also secreted by the adrenal medulla. Receptors are further divided into two categories by their responsiveness to different types of pharmacologic agents. These two receptors are referred to as alpha and beta receptors. Stimulation of the A receptors classically results in vasoconstriction; stimulation of the B receptors causes increased cardiac output by increasing the rate and strength of myocardial contraction.

PROTECTION OF THE CENTRAL NERVOUS SYSTEM

The brain and spinal cord are protected not only by their bone casement, but also by membranes with a fluid interface to prevent shock trauma. These membranes are called the **meninges.** The dura mater is a thick fibrous membrane found outermost just beneath the epidural space and skull bone. The arachnoid mater is a more delicate membrane beneath the dura. Then there is the subarachnoid space, dividing the dura arachnoid layer from the pia mater. Cerebrospinal fluid flows within this space, providing a fluid cushion for both the brain and the spinal cord. The pia mater is the most proximal, vascular, and thin of the membranes. It approximates with the surface of the brain and houses the blood vessels that supply the brain and spinal cord.

The cerebrospinal fluid is produced by the choroid plexus in each of the four ventricles. It then circulates through these ventricles to the subarachnoid space surrounding the brain and the central canal surrounding the spinal cord. The fluid exits the ventricular system by way of openings, including the foramen of Luschka, foramen of Magendie, and cerebral aqueduct. The fluid circulates around the brain down the cord and back up in the subarachnoid space, and is reabsorbed by arachnoid villa and ultimately by the venous system. Blockage of any cerebral outlet for the fluid may lead to overaccumulation in the ventricles or subarachnoid space. If this occurs within the ventricles, it is known as internal hydrocephalus. If it occurs outside the ventricles, it is referred to as external hydrocephalus.

BLOOD SUPPLY TO THE BRAIN

The vascular supply to the brain arises from the vertebral and internal carotid arteries (Figure 17-9). The vertebral arteries are branches of the subclavian arteries, and the internal carotids branch off the common carotids. The internal carotids enter the intracranial cavity via the carotid canal and then branch into the anterior choroidal arteries, the middle cerebral arteries, and the anterior cerebral arteries. The middle cerebral artery is the main division of each internal carotid, and it supplies blood to the anterior lateral surface of the brain, including the frontal, parietal, anterior occipital, and temporal lobes of its hemisphere. It also supplies blood to the internal capsule of the brain. Occlusion results in contralateral motor and sensory impairment, with language impairment if the occlusion is on the dominant hemisphere.

The anterior cerebral arteries supply blood to the medial surface of the frontal and parietal lobes and circles around the corpus callosum. Occlusion results in weakness of the contralateral leg.

The vertebral arteries originate from the aorta and fuse at the base of the brain to form the basilar artery. The basilar artery then divides just inferior to the pons into the posterior cerebral arteries, which circulate blood to the medial and

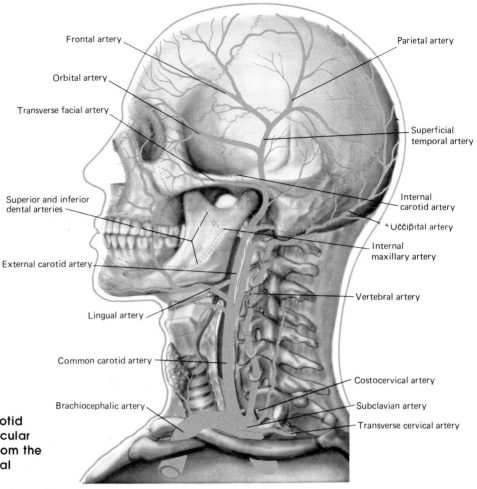

Frontal artery

Orbital artery

Transverse facial artery

Parietal artery

Superficial temporal artery

Internal carotid artery

Occipital artery

Internal maxillary artery

Superior and inferior dental arteries

External carotid artery

Vertebral artery

Lingual artery

Common carotid artery

Costocervical artery

Brachiocephalic artery

Subclavian artery

Transverse cervical artery

(a)

FIGURE 17-9

**The brain's vascular supply:
(a) origin of the internal carotid
and vertebral artery; (b) vascular
supply of the brain arising from the
internal carotid and vertebral
artery.**

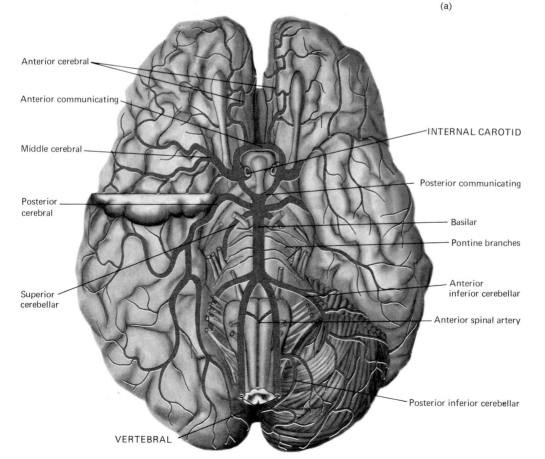

Anterior cerebral

Anterior communicating

Middle cerebral

Posterior cerebral

Superior cerebellar

INTERNAL CAROTID

Posterior communicating

Basilar

Pontine branches

Anterior inferior cerebellar

Anterior spinal artery

Posterior inferior cerebellar

VERTEBRAL

(b)

inferior aspects of the temporal lobes and the occipital lobes.

The vertebral and basilar arteries supply blood to the brain stem, cerebellum, and remaining portions of the occipital lobes. Occlusion of any of these arteries can result in cranial nerve impairments, muscle incoordination, and visual impairment.

The circle of Willis is the arterial anastomosis found at the base of the brain. The vertebral and internal carotid arteries are its primary tributaries; however, it is formed by portions of the posterior cerebral arteries and their communicating branches, the internal carotid arteries, and the anterior cerebral arteries and their communicating branch. Its primary function is to provide immediate collateral circulation to areas of the brain with decreased perfusion secondary to occlusion or rupture of other arteries.

Arterial blood supply to all areas of the brain is extensive and even brief interruption of greater than a few minutes causes irreversible damage. This is because the brain's large metabolic requirements are constant regardless of the individual's activity level. Blood flow is regulated by the cerebral arteriolar tone, which is highly sensitive to circulating levels of carbon dioxide and other metabolites.

Venous drainage of the brain is accomplished by veins that accompany the arteries. These veins then empty into sinuses: the superior sagittal, inferior sagittal, sigmoid, straight petrosal, and transverse sinuses. From these sinuses, the majority of venous blood flows into the internal jugulars, down to the brachiocephalic veins, and on to the superior vena cava.

The vertebral artery that supplies blood to the brain also supplies blood to the spinal cord by means of numerous branches called anterior and posterior spinal arteries. Venous return from the cord is accomplished through spinal veins accompanying the spinal arteries. These veins join vertebral veins, and they empty into the inferior cerebellar veins.

FUNCTIONS OF THE CENTRAL NERVOUS SYSTEM

The numerous functions of the central nervous system are summarized according to anatomical structures in Table 17-3.

The motor system functionally can be divided into the upper and lower motoneuron systems. The upper motoneuron system, known as the pyramidal tract, includes the motor cortex, corona radiata, internal capsule, motor cells of the cranial nerves III to VII and IX to XII, and the anterior horn cells of the spinal cord. The lower motoneuron system includes the motor cells of the brain stem and spinal cord and the muscles.

The upper motoneuron system controls voluntary muscle movement, and has some effect on deep tendon reflexes, muscle tonus, plantar stimulation, and abdominal reflexes in the child. Functional response to injury may cause ipsilateral, bilateral, or contralateral effects, local or generalized, depending upon the level and extent of the damage in the system. The upper motoneuron system is also involved in control of conjugate eye movement and fixation of gaze.

The lower motoneuron system primarily affects muscle tone and muscle reflexes, with the anterior horn cell of the spinal cord serving as the primary functional unit.

Sensation can be superficial or deep. Superficial sensations include pain, temperature, and light touch. These are transmitted from skin receptors to spinal nerves, and then on to a specific segment of the spinal cord depending upon the body region or dermatome from which it originated. Pain and temperature sensations are sent uninterrupted to the thalamus for immediate analysis and response. Touch sensations travel a more complicated route to the thalamus, where they are sent on to the sensory cortex.

Deep sensation, also called proprioception, originates from sensory receptors in the muscles, bones, joints, and tendons. They relate information about position and movement to the sensory cortex. They also relay information about size, shape, and texture of objects examined by touch. Finally, some of the fibers involved in deep sensation travel from the muscles and tendons to the cerebellum to provide it with information necessary to coordinate muscle movements.

Visceral sensations, including appetite, hunger, and thirst, travel along fibers originating in receptors within the visceral tissues. Appetite is a pleasurable sensation that occurs after short-term emptiness of the stomach with the anticipation of eating. Hunger is an unpleasant sensation occurring after long-term absence of food (not hours, but days) when the stomach has contracted. It is often associated with headache, weakness, irritability, and often nausea.

TABLE 17-3

Functional Anatomy of the Central Nervous System

AREA	FUNCTION	RESPONSE TO DAMAGE
CEREBRAL CORTEX ANTERIOR FRONTAL AREA	Controls personality, intellectual development	Childishness, irritability, inappropriate effect, dullness, poor judgment, loss of memory, lack of appreciation
POSTERIOR FRONTAL AREA (MOTOR CORTEX)	Voluntary motor functions: 1. Anterior portion: gross motor control 2. Posterior portion: fine motor control (contralateral innervation)	Weakness or paralysis of opposite side of the body (hemiplegia, hemiparesis)
ANTERIOR PARIETAL AREA (SENSORY CORTEX)	Receive sensory stimuli, primarily deep sensations, position in space, muscle, tendon, bone sensations (contralateral innervation)	Impaired perception of position on opposite side of body
POSTERIOR PARIETAL AND UPPER TEMPORAL AREAS	Involved in language formulation (functions only on dominant hemisphere)	Impaired language comprehension (receptive aphasia)
UPPER MEDIAL TEMPORAL AREA (AUDITORY CENTER)	Reception and interpretation of auditory stimuli	Deafness with bilateral destruction
POSTERIOR AND MEDIAL OCCIPITAL	Visual function	Complete blindness with bilateral destruction, partial blindness in both eyes with unilateral injury; injury to dominant hemisphere may affect language formulation
BRAIN STEM	Control of involuntary vital functions	Bulbar palsy, irregular, shallow and finally absent respirations, irregular, rapid pulse with decreased cardiac output, and finally cardiac arrest
	Origin of most cranial nerves	Disturbances of cranial nerve function, as outlined under the cranial nerves
CRANIAL NERVE		
I. Olfactory	Sense of smell	Loss of smell, perversion of smell
II. Optic	Vision	Ipsilateral visual impairment
III. Oculomotor	Movement of eyes, constriction of pupil and ciliary body	Ptosis, deviation of eye position and resulting double vision, fixed dilation of pupil, impaired accommodation
IV. Trochlear nerve	Eye movement	Double vision (diplopia)
V. Trigeminal	Controls muscles and sensation of mastication, facial sensation	Impaired mastication, contralateral impairment of facial sensation, paroxysmal facial pain
VI. Abducens	Movement of eyes	Absence of lateral eye movement, leading to double vision
VII. Facial	Facial expression, taste	Facial weakness or paralysis, loss of taste on anterior two-thirds of tongue
VIII. Acoustic	Sense of hearing, regulates balance	Impaired hearing, tinnitus, vertigo, nystagmus
IX. Glossopharyngeal	Taste posterior tongue, sensation of posterior tongue, throat, tonsils, movement of pharynx	No clinical manifestations (loss of sensation from mucosa of tonsils, throat and posterior tongue)
X. Vagus	Swallowing, talking, heart rate, peristalsis, secretion of some GI juices, sphincter control	Difficulty swallowing (dysphasia), difficulty talking (dysarthria), dysphonia, adverse effect on autonomic functions
XI. Spinal accessory	Elevation of shoulders and arms, lateral flexion of head	Drooping of shoulders, impaired rotation of head
XII. Hypoglossal	Movement of tongue	Atrophy and weakness of ipsilateral side of tongue

TABLE 17-3 CONTINUED

	FUNCTION	RESPONSE TO DAMAGE
CEREBELLUM	Muscle coordination, maintenance of muscle tone, establishing body equilibrium	Incoordination of movement, unsteadiness, ataxia of gait
SPINAL CORD, ANTERIOR HORN CELLS	Send motor impulse to muscle	Flaccid, weakness, and atrophy of involved muscles, decreased or absent deep reflexes
POSTERIOR HORN CELLS	Synapse for sensory impulses	Absence of sensation
PYRAMIDAL TRACT	Connects motor cortex with anterior horn cells	Muscle weakness, spasticity, hyperreflexia, positive Babinski, increased DTR's
LATERAL SPINOTHALAMIC TRACT	Conveys superficial sensations to sensory cortex	Loss of pain and temperature sensation on ipsilateral side
POSTERIOR COLUMNS	Transmit sensations from muscles, joints, and bone to sensory cortex	Decreased or loss of position sense, decrease or loss of pain in muscles and joints
AUTONOMIC NERVOUS SYSTEM: PARASYMPATHETIC	Via cranial nerve III: dilation of pupil, accommodation of eye	Fixed dilation of pupil, impaired accommodation
	Via cranial nerve VII: lacrimal and salivary gland secretion	Impaired secretion
	Via cranial nerve X: decreased heart rate, bronchial constriction, increased peristalsis, increased secretion of gastric juices	Impairment of these functions
	Muscular control of bladder, colon, and rectum	Impaired emptying
AUTONOMIC NERVOUS SYSTEM: SYMPATHETIC	Innervation of blood vessels, glands, and viscera	Impaired functions of these body parts

TABLE 17-4

Historical Information That May Possess Neurological Significance

Changes in intellectual capabilities
Mood swings
Changes in level of awareness or alertness
Changes in level of consciousness
Seizures
Headaches
Changes in visual activity
Changes or loss of hearing
Tinnitus
Vertigo
Disturbances in speech
Difficulty chewing or swallowing
Nausea and/or vomiting
Muscular weakness or wasting
Involuntary movements
Loss of sensation
Pain, tingling, prickling, or other unusual sensations
Disturbances of continence (bowel or bladder)
Sexual disturbances
Drug ingestion

Thirst, also an unpleasant sensation, occurs in increasing intensity as the body reaches a state of dehydration. The osmoreceptors of the hypothalamus respond to the increased serum osmolarity of dehydration by releasing an antidiuretic hormone, which directs the kidney to conserve water output through decreasing and concentrating urine. Thirst itself is a desire for fluid.

The sensation known as referred pain is also usually visceral in origin. It is due to the fact that many visceral organs have shared or adjacent tracts with the skin pain receptor tracts; thus, messages are often misconstrued. Similarly, phantom pain from a severed limb is transmission of sensation along the proximal unsevered segment of nerve that once extended into the limb. Usually, with time, the sensory cortex relearns the meaning of sensations from these fibers.

Finally, headache pain is one of the most common illnesses in our society. It is most frequently extracranial in origin, as the brain has little sensation to pain. It is generally a diffuse pain, often throbbing, dull, sharp, or intermittent in character that is not confined to a nerve distribution area but may be localized over the frontal, temporal, occipital, or ocular regions bilaterally or unilaterally.

Historical data play an especially important role in neurologic assessment, as problems may be difficult for the client to pinpoint, and signs and symptoms may be tangential, transient, and difficult to replicate. Table 17-4 identifies clues from the history that may have neurological significance.

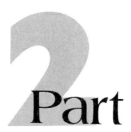

HEALTH ASSESSMENT OF THE NEUROLOGICAL SYSTEM

Part 2

A complete neurologic assessment is seldom routine, probably for several reasons. Often the examiner is uncomfortable or less familiar with the assessment; often the client is in an adverse state to perform at an optimal level; frequently, time is a limiting factor; and finally, a brief examination of key neurologic functions, along with a history, is many times a sufficient screening method to determine gross neurologic status.

Cooperation and general attitude are highly labile variables that affect the client's performance, especially in the very young. The neurologic status is frequently affected by illness of any origin. This must be considered when analyzing and interpreting the collected data. Also, it is important to realize that seldom is one finding or single examination conclusive of neurologic disease. Acceptable neurologic function varies widely among normal individuals, and neurologic abnormalities have serious social and personal ramifications. Therefore, careful consideration of all the data must be taken before conclusions are drawn and shared with the client or family.

NEUROLOGIC ASSESSMENT OF THE ADULT

There are many suggested approaches to a complete neurologic assessment of the adult or older child. The approach should be systematic and comfortable for the examiner. The following approach is by no means exhaustive but is sufficiently complete. It is unlikely, in the face of unchanged status of the client and lack of historical clues of neurologic problems, that this complete an exam would be performed on serial routine visits.

The assessment begins with general observation of the client's appearance, posture, visual activity or response, facial movements, speech, behavior, and movement. This part of the exam is usually performed by momentary, but conscious, attention of the examiner during the history-taking phase. Marked variations from the expected should be noted and used as directives throughout the remainder of the exam.

EVALUATION OF MENTAL STATUS

Observe the general appearance of the client. Grooming and personal hygiene should be consistent with the socioeconomic and intellectual status. Note the client's state of awareness and alertness as evidenced by facial expression, response to environment, and direction of conversation. Normally, the mental state of an individual varies throughout the day from keen alertness, to deep concentration, to inattentiveness and drowsiness.

Basic to assessment of mental status in a client is the determination of the client's level of consciousness. This is of greatest value in individuals who may have a primary or secondary neuropathy that could result in progressive deterioration of the sensorium level. The primary neurological cause of deterioration at this level is increased intracranial pressure due to a number of intracranial lesions, such as subdural hematomas, cerebral edema, and tumors.

The level of consciousness generally deteriorates in stages progressing from alertness to deep coma. Initially, the deterioration is characterized by a state of lethargy in which the client is drowsy and no longer alert. The level of cooperativeness then decreases, as the client is too drowsy to cooperate. The client displays disorientation; first, to time; then, to place; then, to familiar persons; and, finally, to self. Following total disorientation comes the inability to obey simple commands, which is the final stage in which personal communication is lost. The response to painful stimuli deteriorates from purposeful response, to response to painful stimuli, to purposeless response to pain, and, then, to absence of response to pain. Finally, the corneal and gag reflexes are lost.

Once the stage of sensorium deterioration is identified, the degree of unconsciousness can be classified. Coma refers to a state of insensibility which has a range of degrees. Lethargy is a light degree of coma and can be characterized by excessive drowsiness. Arousal and communication can occur. If the person is left in an undisturbed state, the person tends to rapidly drift off to sleep. Stupor is the next degree of coma. Some arousal occurs with strong stimuli (i.e., bright lights, loud noises, painful stimuli), but the ability to sustain attention and carry out simple commands is limited. In light coma, the individual responds purposefully to painful stimuli but is unable to identify and respond to other environmental factors, whereas deep coma is a state where there is no response to painful stimuli, muscle reflexes are absent, and the extremities are flaccid and motionless.

During the interviewing process, the individual's rate of speech, volume of voice, and intensity in which ideas are verbally expressed are ascertained. Also, the logical flow, organization, ability to verbalize, and ability to relate to a particular topic until discussion of it is complete are noted.

The client's beliefs about, feelings arising from, and ability to cope with factors arising in the environment are inquired into. Feelings of depression, suspicion, persecution, depersonalization, and anxiousness, as well as suicidal tendencies, delusion, illusions, and hallucinations may be ascertained during the inquiry into beliefs, feelings, and thought processes. Stability or lability of mood will be demonstrated by the client's expressive behavior, remaining appropriate to the topic of discussion or swinging from crying to laughing.

Orientation is assessed by determining the client's awareness and knowledge of time (date, month, year, time of day), place (residence, present location), and person (ability to identify significant others and self).

Memory, another asset of mental status, is assessed by ascertaining the client's ability to recall immediate and remote events. A frequently used test for immediate recall is to present the client with a series of five digits (e.g., 7, 4, 8, 1, 2), instruct him to remember them, and, in approximately 5 minutes, request the client to repeat the numerical series given earlier. Remote memory is most frequently assessed by requesting from the client information concerning birthdates and ages of children; ages of siblings; if married, the date of marriage; and dates of graduation from educational endeavors. Whatever remote events are used to determine distant recall, they must be pertinent to the client.

The ability to progress into the recall of information from the knowledge fund is assessed by requesting the individual to identify generally known information such as geographic distances or major cities; to formulate judgments as to the meanings of metaphors, such as "birds of a feather flock together"; to determine similarities and differences between objects such as radio and television; and to calculate arithmetic problems such as addition, subtraction, and multiplication. One of the most commonly used subtraction problems is to subtract sevens consecutively beginning with 100. Use of metaphors and arithmetic problems enables the examiner to assess the client's ability to deal with abstractions.

The client's language and speech are assessed. Generally, the use of language and speech is easy and free flowing, provided cultural and language barriers are not present. Slow speech, which may be articulated poorly or incompletely articulated by leaving out words, verbalization of sounds that have no meaning, repetition of what is heard without understanding its meaning, as well as inability to formulate words or failure to recognize familiar objects through the senses are deviations from normal use of language and speech.

EVALUATION OF THE CRANIAL NERVES

The first cranial nerve, the olfactory nerve, is evaluated after patency of the nares is determined. Ask the client to differentiate between several familiar aromatic substances such as coffee, peanut butter, and bananas. Do not use irritative, noxious substances such as ammonia. Test each nostril while occluding the other. Generally, females discriminate aromas more readily than males.

The second cranial nerve, the optic nerve, is assessed, if not already evaluated during the examination of the eye. Test the client's visual acuity by having him or her read newspaper print, first with one eye closed and then with the opposite eye closed. Eye glasses should be worn if required. To evaluate the client's visual fields, have the client fix on a midline point (such as the examiner's nose), then cover one eye with a card. Place your finger outside of the medial visual field and slowly bring the finger within the field. Ask the client to indicate when the finger is first seen. Repeat the test laterally, superiorly, and inferiorly, and then evaluate the opposite eye. Finally, the optic fundi are visualized.

The third (oculomotor), fourth (trochlear), and sixth (abducens) cranial nerves are evaluated together. Observe the pupils for gross abnormalities or asymmetry. Test their reactivity to light, accommodation, and note the extraocular movements or range of movement of the eyes. Abnormalities of these nerves result in ptosis, nystagmus, asymmetrical or absent reactivity of the pupils, and limited or disconjugate eye movements.

The fifth cranial nerve (trigeminal) is assessed by first palpating the strength of the temporal and masseter muscles while the client is clenching the teeth (Figure 17-10). Weakness of either of these muscles, unilateral or bilateral, is abnormal. The sensory part of the nerve is assessed first for pain sensation over the face. With the client's eyes closed, use a pin, occasionally substituting a blunt-ended object, to check the client's reliability, and touch the forehead, cheek, and chin (Figure 17-11). Ask the client to discriminate between sharp and blunt. Temperature sensation can be tested if pain sensation is absent or questionable. This is done using a cool-water-filled test tube alternating with a warm-water-filled test tube touched to the skin (Figure 17-12). The client should be able to discriminate between hot and cold. Test for light touch next by using a wisp of cotton and gently touching the forehead, cheek, and chin, having the client (eyes closed) indicate when the sensation is felt (Figure 17-13). Test the corneal reflexes using, again, a fine wisp of cotton to gently touch the cornea (approaching laterally). The normal response is blinking and usually tearing.

The seventh cranial nerve, the facial nerve, is evaluated by observing the client's facial expression. A lack of expression, a fixed expression, an unusual lack of facial wrinkles, or loss of one or both nasolabial folds, as well as asymmetry of

FIGURE 17-10
Assessment of masseter and temporal muscle strength.

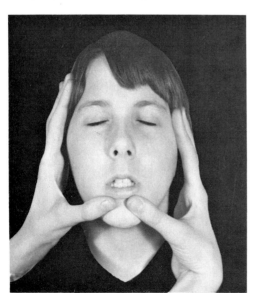

FIGURE 17-11
Assessment of pain perception through pin pricking.

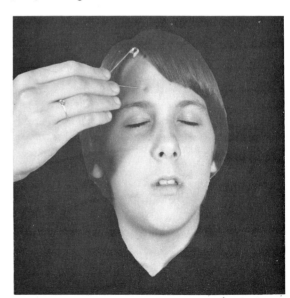

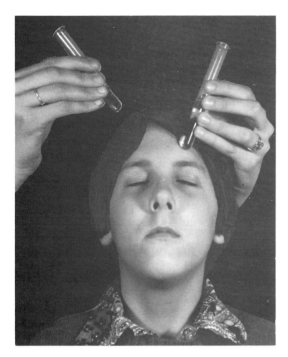

FIGURE 17-12
Assessment of temperature sensation through varied applications of heat and cold.

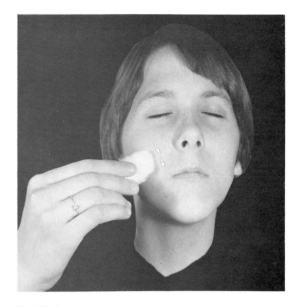

FIGURE 17-13
Assessment of light touch using a wisp of cotton.

facial movement during speaking, smiling, or laughing, may indicate damage to the lower division of this nerve. Request the client to purse the lips, puff out the cheeks, and show the teeth. Nerve damage may result in asymmetry of movement or paralysis or drooping on the ipsilateral side of the mouth. To evaluate the upper division of the nerve that controls the muscles of the forehead and eyes, have the client wrinkle the forehead and then raise the eyebrows, noting symmetry in movement. Request the client to close the eyes and keep them closed against the resistance applied when lifting on the lids (Figure 17-14). The taste sensation of the anterior two-thirds of the tongue is controlled by the sensory division of this nerve but is seldom tested routinely. When tested, four basic taste substances are used; sweet, sour, bitter, and salt. Various substances are used to elicit the taste. It is important for the examiner to ensure that the tongue is held out of the mouth while the taste of the substance, applied to the side of the tongue, is being discerned by the client.

The integrity of the eighth cranial nerve, the acoustic nerve, is assessed by evaluating the client's auditory acuity as reviewed in Chapter 5. Testing should include both air and bone conduction of sound. Hearing should be approximately equal in both ears, and bone conduction is of shorter duration than air conduction of sound. If no hearing loss is detected, assessment of vestibular function is usually deferred. However, the caloric test is easily performed if screening of vestibular function is indicated. The ear canal is irrigated with ice water, and normally nystagmus occurs within 20 seconds. Delayed or absent nystagmus occurs if vestibular function is impaired. If hearing loss is present, further evaluation is indicated by an individual with a more sophisticated diagnostic testing experience.

The ninth cranial nerve, the glossopharyngeal nerve, and tenth cranial nerve, the vagus nerve, are assessed together. First, observe the swallowing pattern and note any hoarseness upon phonation, which may indicate vagal nerve involvement. Next, ask the client to open the mouth and say "ah." Normally, the soft palate rises and the pharyngeal musculature constricts. Stimulate the lateral aspects of the pharyngeal wall using an applicatory or tongue blade. The expected response is again constriction of the pharyngeal musculature. Using the same technique, stimulate the posterior upper and lower pharynx to elicit the gag reflex. If the client is able to feel the stimuli with appropriate elevation of the palpate and constriction of the pharynx, then absence of the gag reflex is insignificant. Asymmetry in movement of the pharynx, palate, or uvula may indicate damage to either nerve.

The eleventh cranial nerve, the spinal acces-

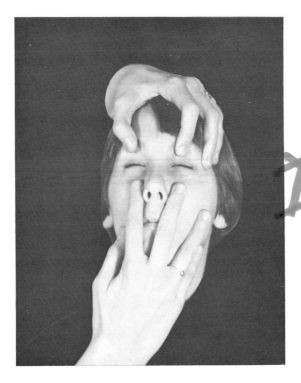

FIGURE 17-14
Assessment of eyelid strength.

FIGURE 17-15
Assessment of tongue strength.

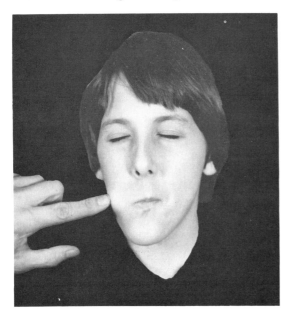

sory nerve, is assessed by evaluating the muscular strength of the trapezius muscles and the sternomastoid muscles. First, ask the client to lift the shoulder against the resistance of your hands, pressing down. Then, have the client face midline, turn the head against the resistance of your hand, first to the right, then to the left. Muscle weakness bilaterally or unilaterally is abnormal and may indicate spinal accessory nerve damage.

The twelfth cranial nerve, the hypoglossal nerve, is assessed by evaluating movement and muscle strength of the tongue. First, observe the tongue at rest and note any atrophy or fasciculation that are abnormal and indicate twelfth cranial nerve damage. Ask the client to protrude the tongue. Normally, it protrudes midline; but with unilateral paralysis, it will deviate to the affected side. The strength of the tongue can be evaluated by having the client push the tongue against the cheek while the examiner creates resistance by pushing against the outside of the same cheek (Figure 17-15). Last, have the client move the tongue in and out of the mouth and from side to side rapidly. Weakness or poor display of rapid movement of the tongue are deviations from normal.

EVALUATION OF THE MOTOR SYSTEM

The motor system is the next area evaluated in the neurologic assessment. It is generally screened for gross abnormalities. If gross abnormalities are detected during the screening or indicated in historical data collection, a more detailed examination of the motor system is undertaken.

A screening of the motor system includes evaluation of the client's station and gait through inspection. The station is evaluated by having the client stand with feet close together and with eyes opened and then closed. Involuntary swaying of the trunk with eyes closed is abnormal and is known as a positive Romberg test. Tandem standing can also be evaluated by having the client place one heel against the toes of the opposite foot leaving eyes open. Again, swaying of the trunk is abnormal. Gait is evaluated by having the client walk normally. Table 17-5 describes gait disturbances. Normal gait is reviewed in detail in Table 16-1.

The client's cerebellar or motor coordination is evaluated by asking the client to walk a straight

TABLE 17-5
Abnormal Gaits

GAIT	PATTERN OBSERVED
Hemiplegic gait	Leg is stiff and extended; movement of foot results from pelvic tilting upward on involved side; the foot is lifted and leg swung at pelvic level; arm remains flexed, adducted, and does not swing
Spastic (diplegic) gait	Short steps dragging the ball of the foot across floor; legs are extended
Steppage gait	Elevating hip and knee excessively high to lift drop foot off ground
Dystrophic gait	Legs far apart, shifting of weight from side to side like waddling; abdomen is often protruding and lordosis is common
Tabetic gait	Legs positioned far apart, lifted high, and forcibly brought down with each step, stamping heel on ground
Cerebellar gait	Staggering gait with lurching from side to side; often swaying of the trunk occurs
Parkinsonian gait	Shuffling gait with short steps; the entire trunk is flexed as are the knees, and the head is hunched forward
Dystonic gait	Jerky dancing movements that appear nondirectional
Astasia	Uncontrolled falling

line heel to toe. The expected response is that the client will have no difficulty with this maneuver.

Cerebellar integrity can also be evaluated by performing the Romberg test. This test is performed by having the client stand unsupported, feet together, with the eyes open, and then with the eyes closed. If marked swaying of the trunk occurs with the eyes open or closed, cerebellar ataxia may be present. Normally, only minimal swaying of the trunk should occur. Safety measures should be undertaken to prevent falling and injury of the client.

Next, ask the client to hop on one foot in place and then hop in place on the other foot. Note any evidence of imbalance or poor coordination. While the client is standing on one foot, have him perform a shallow knee bend with the angle of the knee at 45 degrees. Then have the client repeat this maneuver while standing on the other foot. Normally, this maneuver is performed without difficulty; however, if there is any weakness of the quadriceps, the maneuver becomes either difficult or impossible. To evaluate plantar and dorsiflexion of the ankles, ask the client to first walk on the toes and then walk on the heels.

Screening of motor function of the upper extremities is accomplished by having the client grip your hands. Subjectively evaluate the strength and symmetry of the client's grip. Have the client stand unsupported with the arms at the side, and then ask the client to raise both arms horizontal to the shoulder with the palms pronated, then supinated. Finally, ask the client to raise the arms above the head and then lower them into extension at the sides. Deviations from normal include weakness or asymmetry. A more in-depth evaluation of the motor system, including inspection and evaluation of muscle tone, muscle strength, and muscle coordination, has been reviewed in Chapter 16.

Marked abnormalities in neuromuscular function include deviations in muscular movements, deviation in muscular state or tone, and deviations in muscular coordination.

Deviations in muscular movement are evaluated first by comparative inspection of muscles and muscle groups throughout the body. Normally, the skeletal muscles are relaxed during voluntary resting of the underlying body structure. Voluntary movement creates varying strengths of contraction of those muscles required to produce the desired activity. Abnormal movements include the following:

1. Fasciculations: irregular contractions of muscle fiber bundles.

2. Myotonus: involuntary persistence of muscle contraction.
3. Choreiform movement: involuntary, intermittent, jerky movements of muscle groups, one at a time.
4. Ballism: flailing movements, usually involving limbs on one side.
5. Tremors: involuntary rhythmic movement due to alternating contractions of the flexor and extensor at a joint,
6. Dystonia: hypertonic trunk musculature resulting in slow, twisting movements of the trunk.
7. Athetosis: slow, twisting movement of the head and distal extremities.
8. Myoclonus: singular or serial, rapid, jerking movement (5 to 50 times per minute) of a muscle in the extremities, face, oral cavity, or diaphragm (hiccup).

The tone or state of the muscles is evaluated by inspection and palpation. Normally, the muscles are firm. Decreased tone is referred to as flaccidity, characterized by a soft, flabby consistency upon palpation. Chronic hypotonic muscles generally progress to atrophy or loss of bulk. Spasticity is a hypertonic state involving the flexors of the arms, adductors of the shoulders, and extensors of the legs. Rigidity is a generalized hypertonic state of the body musculature. Contractures of the muscles are shortened muscle groups that significantly limit movement.

Coordination of muscle movement is accomplished by synergistic contraction of muscle groups to produce a desired movement. Asynergy is absence of muscle coordination, and dysmetria refers to poor or suboptimal coordination. The client's coordination can be evaluated by several simple maneuvers, including the following:

1. Walking, to evaluate gait.
2. Standing, to evaluate balance.
3. Finger-to-nose maneuver with eyes closed to evaluate proprioception.
4. Performance of rapid alternating movements, such as supination and pronation of the hands.

These tests merely provide a means of screening for gross evidence of incoordination. More extensive evaluation would be necessary if deviations are present.

ASSESSMENT OF REFLEXES

There are two kinds of reflexes tested in this part of the assessment. The muscle stretch or deep tendon reflexes are elicited by sudden stretching of the muscle through percussion of the muscle tendon. The nerve conduction pathways are usually deep and segmental. The other type of reflex discussed here is the superficial reflexes that are elicited by stroking the skin. The nerve conduction pathways of these reflexes are typically more superficial and multisynaptic; however, the fundamental reflex arc is the same for both the deep reflexes and the superficial reflexes. Most of the reflexes that utilize brain stem arcs are evaluated during assessment of the cranial nerves. They include the pupillary reflex, corneal reflex, glabella tap, blink reflex, both oculo-orbicularis and audio-orbicularis reflexes, and the gag reflex.

When assessing the deep reflexes, the stimulus should be applied as a sudden brief blow over the tendon of insertion with the limb relaxed. A rubber percussion hammer is used to produce the blow. The reflex response is then evaluated in terms of speed, intensity, duration of muscle contraction, and rapidity of relaxation. The bilateral reflexes are compared for symmetry. Asymmetry of responses is much easier to observe than symmetrical deviations in response. If the reflexes are symmetrically diminished or absent, reinforcement can be used to increase reflex activity. Reinforcement involves isometric contraction of other muscles. Reinforcement of the upper extremities can be accomplished by having the client clench the teeth. Reinforcement of the lower extremities results from having the client interlock fingers and pull one hand from the other. Reflex responses can be graded from 0 to 5, as follows:

0	(0) absent
1	(+) sluggish or diminished
2	(++) active or normal
3	(+++) slightly hyperactive or increased response
4	(++++) brisk with intermittent or transient clonus
5	(+++++) very brisk wih sustained clonus

In this grading system, notation is made when reinforcement is used.

TABLE 17-6

Deep Tendon Reflexes, Methods of Assessment, and Expected Responses

REFLEX CENTER	METHOD	EXPECTED RESPONSE
PECTORALIS (C_5 to T_1)	Client's arm semiabducted, place thumb over tendon anterior axillary crease, tap the thumb (Figure 17-16)	Contraction of muscle (seen or felt)
Biceps (C_5, C_6)	Client's arm flexed and pronated, support elbow, place thumb over tendon in anticubital fossa, strike thumb (Figure 17-17)	Muscle contraction usually with flexion of the forearm
Triceps (C_7, C_8)	Client's arm flexed at elbow is supported by examiner; strike the triceps aponeurosis (do not mediate) (Figure 17-18)	Contraction ± extension of forearm
BRACHIORADIAL (C_5, C_6)	Client's forearms resting on abdomen, if lying, or lap, if sitting; the radial surface 1 to 2 in. above the wrist is tapped (do not mediate) (Figure 17-19)	Flexion and supination of forearm
FINGER FLEXOR REFLEX	Hold client's wrist relaxed and pronated; with fingers flexed and relaxed, tap a tongue blade across fingertips (Figure 17-20)	Flexion of fingers and terminal phalanx of the thumb are seen and felt
KNEE OR PATELLAR REFLEX (L_2, L_3, L_4)	Client's legs semiflexed and dangling, directly strike quadriceps tendon below patella (do not mediate) (Figure 17-21)	Contraction of muscle with extension of leg
ANKLE JERK, ACHILLES (S_1, S_2)	Client's ankle relaxed and foot extended, apply gentle pressure to ball of foot creating dorsiflexion, and strike the Achilles tendon (Figure 17-22)	Plantar flexion of foot

FIGURE 17-16

Pectoralis reflex.

FIGURE 17-17

Biceps reflex.

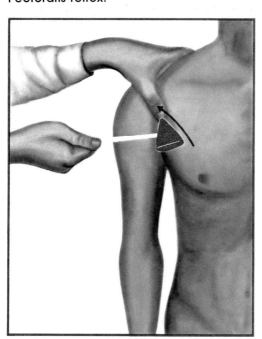

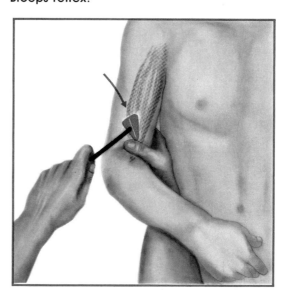

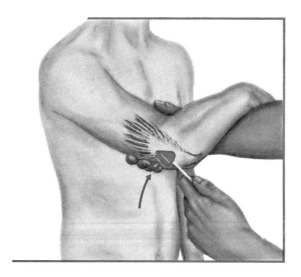

FIGURE 17-18
Triceps reflex.

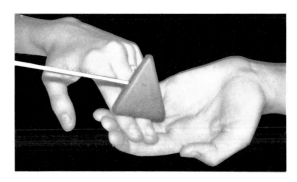

FIGURE 17-20
Finger flexor reflex.

Table 17-6 describes the major deep tendon reflexes, methods of assessment, and expected responses.

The primary superficial reflexes tested are the corneal reflex and gag reflexes (assessed during cranial nerve evaluation), the abdominal reflexes, cremasteric reflexes, anal reflex, and plantar reflexes. The abdominal, superficial reflexes should not be confused with the abdominal muscle reflexes. The latter are deep reflexes seldom tested, but elicited by tapping the muscle at its point of attachment to bone. The superficial, abdominal reflexes are elicited by stroking the skin lateral to midline with a rough-edged object (key). This can be done in the upper, middle, and lower quadrants bilaterally. The expected response is deviation of the umbilicus toward the stimulus (Figure 17-23).

The cremasteric reflex is elicited by stroking the inner aspect of the thighs (proximal to distal) of a male client, resulting in elevation of the ipsilateral testicle (Figure 17-24). The anal reflex is elicited by scratching or pricking the perianal area. The expected response is contraction of the external anal sphincter. Finally, the plantar reflex is elicited by scratching the lateral edge of the sole from heel to toe, resulting in plantar flexion of the toes (Figure 17-25).

FIGURE 17-19
Brachioradial reflex.

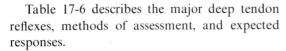

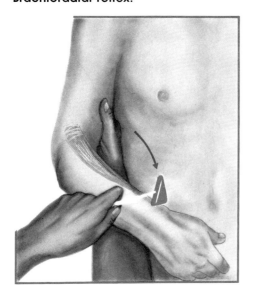

FIGURE 17-21
Knee-jerk or patellar reflex.

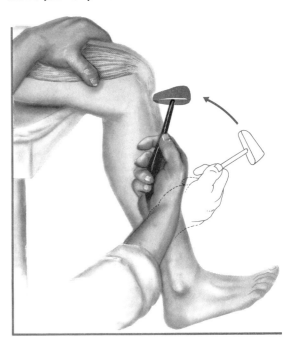

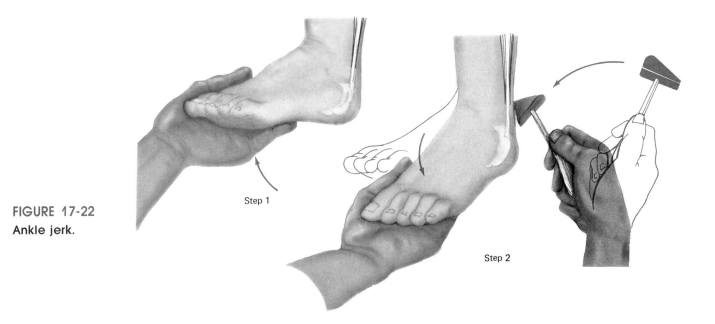

FIGURE 17-22
Ankle jerk.

Step 1

Step 2

There are several other responses that are generally tested in the assessment of reflexes, which have been referred to as pathologic reflexes. Not all these responses are reflexes, but deviations are associated with pyramidal tract disease and often seen with other hyperactive reflex responses.

Clonus is a deviation from the expected response characterized by rhythmic, alternating flexion and extension in response to muscle stretch. Oscillations may be sustained or intermittent, and may vary in rate from 50 to 5 per minute if sustained. Ankle clonus is commonly tested for by having the client relax with the

knee slightly flexed, and the foot relaxed. The foot is then dorsiflexed suddenly by the examiner's hand and held in dorsiflexion. Normally, there is no response. If clonus is present, the foot will oscillate between flexion and extension, and rhythmic clonic contractions of the quadriceps will be seen.

The Babinski phenomenon is elicited by stroking the lateral sole from heel to toe and across the ball of the foot to the medial sole with a blunt pointed object (Figure 17-26). A normal response is plantar flexion of the toes. The abnormal response (positive Babinski sign) is fanning of the toes with dorsiflexion of the great toe. Variations

FIGURE 17-23
Eliciting the abdominal reflex.

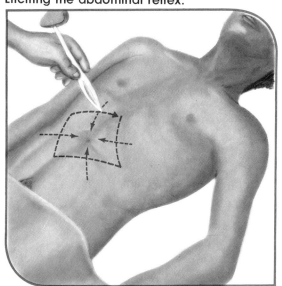

FIGURE 17-24
Eliciting the cremasteric reflex.

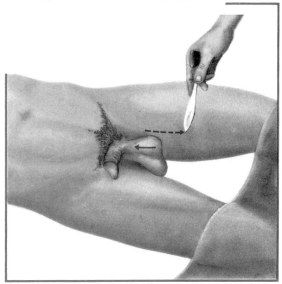

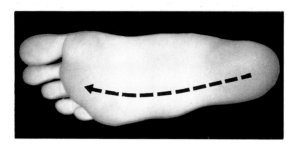

FIGURE 17-25

Eliciting the plantar reflex.

FIGURE 17-26

The Babinski reflex:
(a) negative Babinski;
(b) positive Babinski.

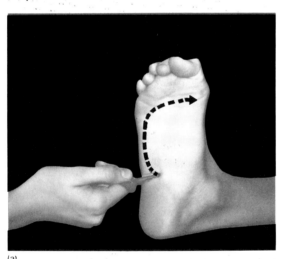

(a)

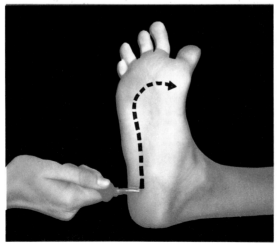

(b)

of a positive Babinski are referred to as an equivocal Babinski sign and may indicate a milder or early stage of pyramidal tract disease. An unequivocal positive Babinski sign is pathognomonic of pyramidal tract disease according to most neurologists.

Finally, Hoffmann's sign is normally an absent response to forced flexion of the distal phalanx of the middle finger. It is elicited with the wrist held horizontal, pronated, and relaxed. An abnormal response includes flexion–adduction of the fingers with opposing flexion–adduction movement of the thumb. A positive Hoffmann's sign can be seen in anxious or emotionally tense clients, but is otherwise associated with upper motor neuron lesions.

EVALUATION OF SENSATION

To obtain reliable information about the client's sensory system integrity, it is important that the client be unfatigued, cooperative, and perceptive. It is also important that the examiner be keenly skeptical of the client's reliability.

Assessment of this area includes evaluation of superficial sensation (pain, temperature, and light touch) and deep sensation (vibration sense; position sense; deep pain; discrimination; and, in the male, testicular pain). Be sure to evaluate symmetrical body parts for comparison, and if sensory loss is suspected, attempt to map out the involved area by testing from the most affected to the least affected area. The boundary of the affected area can be marked.

Begin by evaluating superficial sensation over the arms, trunk, and legs, moving in an organized, but unpatterned, manner. The client should be relaxed with eyes closed. Pain sensation is tested first using a safety pin, occasionally substituting the blunt end of the pin to test the client's reliability. Ask the client to indicate a sharp or dull sensation as it is felt. Decreased pain sensation is referred to as hypalgesia and loss of this sensation is analgesia. Paresthesia refers to an unpleasant cutaneous sensation resulting upon contact with a nonpain-producing object.

If pain sensation is intact, temperature sensation testing is often omitted. To test temperature sensation, proceed as for testing pain, using cool- and warm-water-filled test tubes. Have the client indicate cold or hot sensations as they are felt.

Light touch is evaluated using a wisp of cotton and touching each area tested above. Ask the client to indicate the sensation.

Deep sensation is evaluated first by testing vibration sense using a tuning fork (128 cycles per second) (Figure 17-27). Begin by familiarizing the client with the sensation over the sternum where it is seldom lost. Vibration is tested over bony prominences. Losses commonly occur distal to proximal; so test distal areas first and, if losses are evident, proceed proximally. Vibratory sense is commonly disturbed in the lower extremities before the upper extremities are involved; so in screening for vibration sense, always test the feet. This test is of less value in the elderly as vibration sense normally reduces with age.

Position sense is usually tested in a finger and the great toe bilaterally. Grasp the distal phalanx of the digit on its lateral surfaces between the thumb and index finger and move it up then down gently (Figure 17-28). Ask the client to indicate the position of the digit. If position sense is impaired, continue the testing at the next proximal joint.

Deep pain is evaluated by first applying painful pressure on the calf muscle with the thumb. Have the client indicate when the pain is felt and note the degree of pressure needed to elicit pain. Normally, deep pressure is required. Pinch the Achilles tendon between the thumb knuckle and index finger until the client indicates pain. Usually slight pressure will be painful.

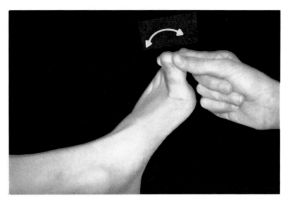

FIGURE 17-28
Assessment of position sense.

Cortical sensory function is tested by evaluating sensory discrimination. Stereognosis consists of the ability to identify familiar objects placed in the hand while the eyes are closed. Sufficient time should be given to the client to examine the object. Familiar objects used may include coins, keys, marbles, and paper clips. Graphesthesia, the recognition of figures (numbers) drawn on the hand, is tested with the client's eyes closed (Figure 17-29). The hand is opened, palmar surface facing up, and the examiner draws out the symbol on the entire palmar surface. Normally, these symbols are recognized easily if drawn in a manner familiar to the client.

Finally, testicular pain is evaluated in males by gently squeezing the testicle between the thumb and index finger. Usually, pain is elicited by slight pressure.

FIGURE 17-27
Assessment of vibratory sensation.

FIGURE 17-29
Assessment of graphesthesia.

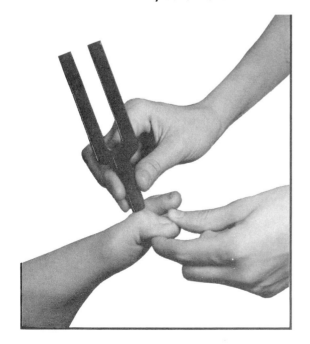

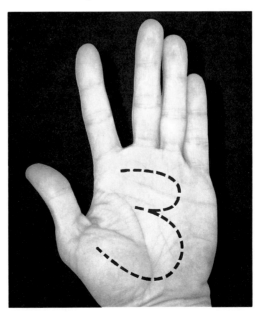

NEUROLOGIC ASSESSMENT OF THE INFANT AND CHILD

Maturation of the nervous system occurs well beyond birth, so assessment of the neurological integrity of the infant or young child must be modified accordingly. Much of this immaturity is due to incomplete myelination of nerves and nerve tracts. The major myelination process occurs during the first few years, as evidenced by the significant developmental accomplishments; however, neurological refinement continues well into adulthood.

The neurologic assessment of the infant and young child differs for three primary reasons. First, the neuromuscular and cortical immaturity of the child varies from the expected findings of the exam in many areas and requires modified modalities to elicit valid testing. Second, the physical endurance of the child (especially the infant) seldom permits extensive neurologic testing with reliable results. Finally, the variability in the child's ability to cooperate or willingness to cooperate requires modification of most testing modalities, as well as the interpretation of findings.

FIGURE 17-30

Normal and abnormal positions assumed by the infant: (a) normal flexion; (b) scissoring of lower extremities; (c) frog-leg positioning of the premature.

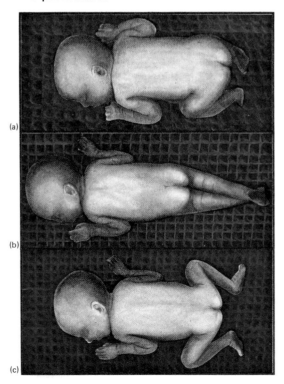

Neuromuscular development is most dramatic during the first years of life. Although this developmental process occurs at an uneven pace throughout the body and at varied rates in different individuals, it possesses certain common characteristics. One of these characteristics is that development and control progress in a cephalo-caudal direction from proximal to distal. Motor skill also progresses from diffuse, uncontrolled movement to specific, controlled movements.

Probably the most significant modification in evaluation of neurologic function must be made in assessment of the infant. As the child progresses into the toddler preschool age, modifications in testing are lessened; and by school age, few changes need be made in the assessment process. The importance of recognizing the child's maturational stage of development should always be reflected in interpretation of findings.

In the newborn, special consideration should be made for the time of day with regard to feeding and sleep schedules. It is best to evaluate the infant about 1 to 2 hours after a feeding and during a waking state. Allowances are made for prematurity until about 1 to 2 years of age. Also, it is important to make all the observations indicated before stimulating the infant, and to remember that a single deviation is of limited significance unless recurrent, asymmetric, or functionally handicapping.

To begin, observe the infant's level of alertness and response to stimuli. Subcortical functions predominate in the newborn, but by 6 weeks, early cerebral function becomes evident, and the infant should be aware and responsive to various environmental stimuli. Marked irritability, extended posturing, high-pitched cry, or unresponsiveness are abnormal at any age. The normal posture of the newborn is one of flexion in the supine and prone position with tight fisting of the hands until about 2 months. Obligate scissoring of the lower extremities is a sign of spasticity and frog-leg position is indicative of hypotonia in the term infant (Figure 17-30(a), (b), and (c)). The premature, however, has decreased tone, and normally assumes a more extended position of the extremities.

Evaluation of head size and shape as well as inspection of the head for signs of trauma and transillumination are especially important in the newborn. This is covered in more detail in Chapter 4.

TABLE 17-7
Primitive Reflexes of Infancy

REFLEX	METHOD: EXPECTED RESPONSE	ONSET/DISAPPEARANCE	SIGNIFICANCE
BLINK	Flash bright light in face: Blink (Figure 17-31)	Birth/Persists	Absence may indicate blindness
PUPILLARY	Bright light in eye: Pupillary constriction (Figure 17-32)	Birth*/Persists	Absence or asymmetry
COCHLEOPALPEBRAL	Loud noise: Blink ± startle	Birth*/6 to 9 months	Most consistent auditory response
SUCKING	Insert fingertip or nipple in mouth: Sucking (Figure 17-33)	Birth*/Variable	Absence indicates CNS depression or immaturity
ROOTING	Stroke each corner of mouth, middle upper lip, and middle lower lip: Head and mouth move toward stimulus (Figure 17-34)	Birth*/3 to 4 months	Absence: CNS depression, immaturity Persistence: prolonged immaturity of neuro-organization
PALMAR GRASP	Press on palm with finger: Tight grasp of finger (Figure 17-35)	Birth*/5 to 6 months	Persistence: spasticity Weak: CNS depression Absent: paralysis
PLANTAR GRASP	Press on ball of foot: Plantar flexion of toes (Figure 17-36)	Birth*/8 to 12 months	Absent: spinal cord or root damage
CROSSED EXTENSION	In supine position, hold one leg in extension and prick sole with pin: Extension and adduction of opposite leg (Figure 17-37)	Birth*/1 to 2 months	Absent: cord or nerve damage Persistence: pyramidal tract lesions
TONIC NECK	Active or passive turning of head in supine position: Extension of limbs on opposite side (Figure 17-38)	±Birth (2 to 3 months/6 to 7 months	Persistence: lack of motor organization
MORO	Sudden disalignment of head from spine in retroflexion: Abduction, extension and supination of arms, extension of third and fourth fingers, flexion of thumb and index finger bilaterally; extension of legs and cry may also result (Figure 17-39)	Birth*/4 to 6 months	Absent: CNS depression Asymmetry: paralysis Persistence: CNS damage
STEPPING	Held erect, feet on surface, tilt forward and lateral: Walking movements (Figure 17-40)	Birth/3 to 4 months	Persistence or recurrence: cord injury
PLACING	Held erect, touch dorsal surface of foot: Flexion of ipsilateral leg at knee and hip (Figure 17-41)	Birth/1 year	Absent: neuromuscular degeneration, cord injuries
LANDAU	Hold infant over one hand, prone, and tuck chin to chest: Flexion of legs (Figure 17-42)	3 months/12 to 24 months	Absent: spinal cord labyrinthine damage
PARACHUTE	Suspend infant prone position above surface and thrust infant suddenly down: Extension of arms, fingers, and legs toward surface (Figure 17-43)	7 to 12 months/Persists	Asymmetry: Neuro or muscular disorder unilaterally

*Indicates preterm appearance.

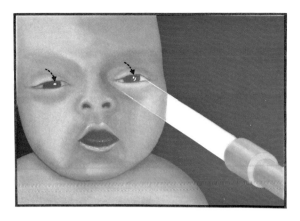

FIGURE 17-31
Blink reflex.

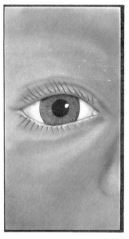
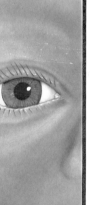

FIGURE 17-32
Pupillary reflex.

FIGURE 17-33
Sucking reflex.

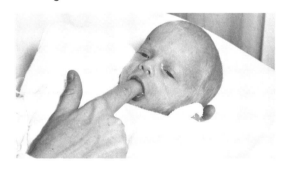

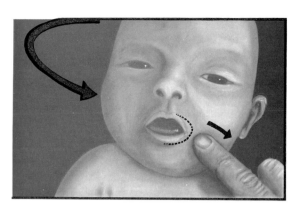

FIGURE 17-34
Rooting.

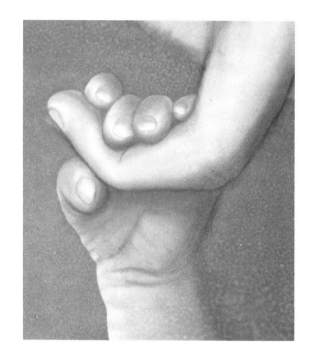

FIGURE 17-35
Palmar grasp.

FIGURE 17-36
Plantar grasp.

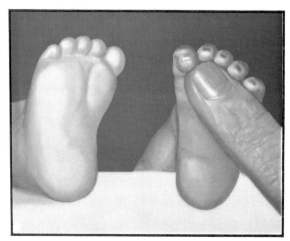

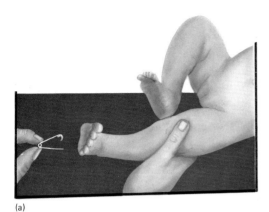

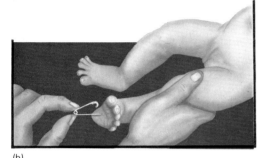

FIGURE 17-37
Crossed-extensor reflex.

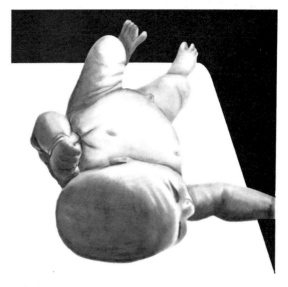

FIGURE 17-38
Tonic neck.

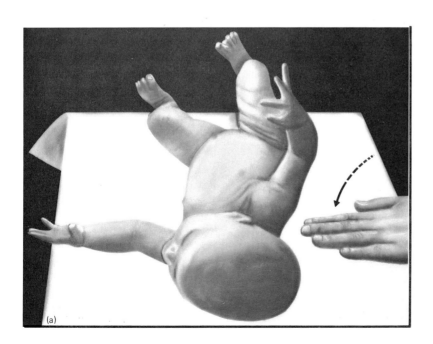

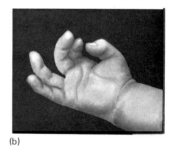

FIGURE 17-39
Moro reflex: (a) elicited by striking the table; (b) characteristic "C" formation of fingers.

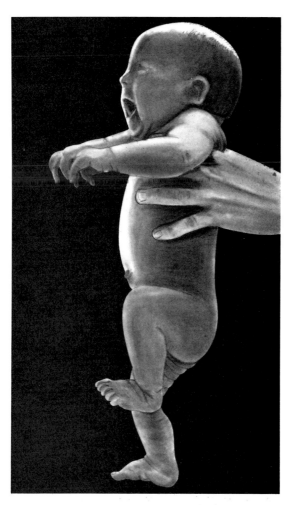

FIGURE 17-40
Stepping reflex.

FIGURE 17-42
Landau reflex.

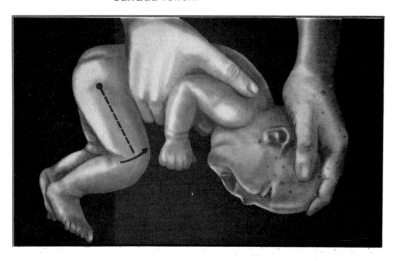

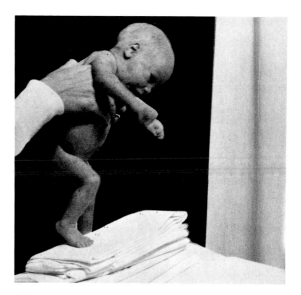

FIGURE 17-41
Placing reflex.

Sensory testing of the newborn, infant, and child is similar to the adult with modification for level of cooperativeness. Normally, in the infant, response to superficial sensory stimuli is often decreased because of increased thresholds. Pain sensation can be evaluated using a safety pin to stimulate several areas. As with the adult, asymmetry of response is abnormal. Normally, the infant will cry and withdraw the extremity. Light touch can be tested by gentle touching, which elicits either a change in activity or a change in facial expression.

The deep sensory responses to vibratory and position stimuli are not tested until about 3 years when the child will best cooperate if it is presented as a game.

Assessing the cranial nerve function in the newborn is limited. The olfactory nerve is seldom tested reliably before school age. Cranial nerves III, IV, and VI can be tested in the newborn by moving a light or bright-colored object from the periphery to midline. Until $1\frac{1}{2}$ months, the infant's response is periodic and difficult to sustain. After that time, the infant should be able to follow the light. A funduscopic exam is usually referred to the expert examiner if visual acuity is questionable. The doll's eye maneuver can be employed to test conjugate movement of the eyes. The infant is held face up with examiner and moved in circular rotation, first to one side and then the other. Normally, the eyes look toward the direction of movement and, when movement stops, they look to the opposite direction. Sustained disconjugate eye movement and jerky movements may be abnormal. Pupillary reactivity can also be tested as in the adult, with similar expected findings.

Evaluation of cranial nerves V, VII, IX, X, and XI is done in the newborn with little modification. Hearing and vestibular functions of cranial nerve VIII are difficult to evaluate in the newborn or infant. Reliable response to sound is not expected much before 8 months. Vestibular function is evaluated in the newborn by the doll's eye maneuver or caloric test. The nerve XII function can be tested by occluding the infant's nares. Normally, the infant opens the mouth and protrudes the tongue out and up. Lateral deviation of the tongue is abnormal.

The reflex responses to muscle stretch in the newborn are often equivocal because of immature corticospinal nerve pathways. Therefore, increased or decreased (and even absent) reflex responses are not necessarily significant unless persistence of the deviation or asymmetry is noted. The triceps reflex is absent until 6 months, and the Babinski may be equivocal until 2 years. Unsustained ankle clonus (up to 12 beats) is not uncommon in infants until 5 or 6 months and, occasionally, at times of exhaustion or irritability; several (three to five beats) of ankle clonus may be seen until about 12 months.

The primitive reflexes of the newborn and infant are listed in Table 17-7. Although some of these responses persist as voluntary activity during infancy and later, they are uniquely involuntary during the specified time of infancy. Early absence of some of these reflexes and persistence of others may be neurologically significant.

Motor function of the infant includes observation of muscular movement, noting evidence of asymmetry, palpation of muscle size, testing of muscle strength and tone, and range of motion in extremities. Head control is tested by pulling the infant by the hand from supine to sitting position and then lowering the infant down again. Head lag is not abnormal in premature infants, but term infants should be able to right the head momentarily at a 45 degree angle from the surface. Early hand preference before 15 months is abnormal and may indicate spasticity or weakness of the unpreferred extremity. Neuromuscular function is a helpful indicator of gestational age in the newborn. A commonly used tool for

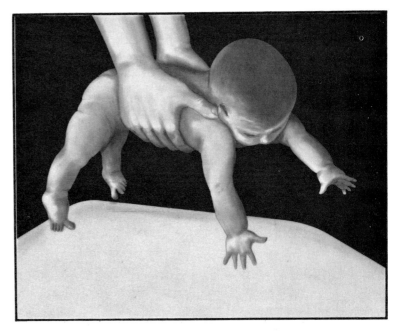

FIGURE 17-43
Parachute reflex.

determining gestational age involving both physical characteristics and neuromuscular function is the Clinical Estimation of Gestational Age with Confirmatory Neurologic Examination (Figure 17-44).

Neurologic assessment of the infant beyond the neonatal period is similar to that in the newborn. Expectations should be appropriate for age with correction for prematurity. The Denver Developmental Screening tool is usually used initially at 4 months, then repeated at 8 to 10 months. The neurologic assessment of the toddler varies little from that in the preschool child with modification for developmental maturation and cooperativeness.

FIGURE 17-44 (pages 342–343)
Clinical estimation of gestational age, an approximation based on published data, including neuromuscular assessment:
(a) examination first hours; (b) confirmatory neurologic examination to be done after 24 hours. Reproduced with permission from C. H. Kempe, H. K. Silver, and D. O'Brien (eds.), Current Pediatric Diagnosis and Treatment, 5th ed., Lange Medical Publications, 1978.

FIGURE 17-44(a)

PATIENT'S NAME _____

◁ Examination First Hours

CLINICAL ESTIMATION
OF GESTATIONAL AGE
An Approximation Based on Published Data*

WEEKS GESTATION

PHYSICAL FINDINGS		20–48 (by week)
VERNIX		APPEARS (20) · COVERS BODY, THICK LAYER · ON BACK, SCALP, IN CREASES (38) · SCANT, IN CREASES (40–41) · NO VERNIX (44–48)
BREAST TISSUE AND AREOLA		AREOLA & NIPPLE BARELY VISIBLE, NO PALPABLE BREAST TISSUE · AREOLA RAISED (34–35) · 1–2 MM NODULE (36–37) · 3–5 MM (38) · 5–6 MM (39) · 7–10 MM (40–42) · ?12 MM (45–48)
EAR – FORM		FLAT, SHAPELESS · BEGINNING INCURVING SUPERIOR (34–35) · INCURVING UPPER 2/3 PINNAE (36–37) · WELL-DEFINED INCURVING TO LOBE (40–48)
EAR – CARTILAGE		PINNA SOFT, STAYS FOLDED · CARTILAGE SCANT RETURNS SLOWLY FROM FOLDING (33–34) · THIN CARTILAGE SPRINGS BACK FROM FOLDING (36–37) · PINNA FIRM, REMAINS ERECT FROM HEAD (40–48)
SOLE CREASES		SMOOTH SOLES c̄ CREASES · 1–2 ANTERIOR CREASES (32–33) · 2–3 ANTERIOR CREASES (35) · CREASES ANTERIOR 2/3 SOLE (36–37) · CREASES INVOLVING HEEL (38–39) · DEEPER CREASES OVER ENTIRE SOLE (44–48)
SKIN – THICKNESS & APPEARANCE		THIN, TRANSLUCENT SKIN, PLETHORIC, VENULES OVER ABDOMEN; EDEMA · SMOOTH THICKER NO EDEMA (34) · PINK (36) · FEW VESSELS (38–39) · SOME DESQUAMATION PALE PINK (40–41) · THICK, PALE, DESQUAMATION OVER ENTIRE BODY (44–48)
SKIN – NAIL PLATES		AP-PEAR (21) · NAILS TO FINGER TIPS (33) · NAILS EXTEND WELL BEYOND FINGER TIPS (44–48)
HAIR		APPEARS ON HEAD (22) · EYE BROWS & LASHES · FINE, WOOLLY, BUNCHES OUT FROM HEAD · SILKY, SINGLE STRANDS LAYS FLAT (38–39) · RECEDING HAIRLINE OR LOSS OF BABY HAIR SHORT, FINE UNDERNEATH (44–48)
LANUGO		AP-PEARS (22) · COVERS ENTIRE BODY · VANISHES FROM FACE (33) · PRESENT ON SHOULDERS (38–39) · NO LANUGO (44–48)
GENITALIA – TESTES		TESTES PALPABLE IN INGUINAL CANAL · IN UPPER SCROTUM (36–37) · IN LOWER SCROTUM (44–48)
GENITALIA – SCROTUM		FEW RUGAE · RUGAE, ANTERIOR PORTION (38–39) · RUGAE COVER (40–41) · PENDULOUS (44–48)
GENITALIA – LABIA & CLITORIS		PROMINENT CLITORIS, LABIA MAJORA SMALL WIDELY SEPARATED · LABIA MAJORA LARGER NEARLY COVERED CLITORIS (36–37) · LABIA MINORA & CLITORIS COVERED (44–48)
SKULL FIRMNESS		BONES ARE SOFT · SOFT TO 1" FROM ANTERIOR FONTANELLE (30) · SPONGY AT EDGES OF FONTANELLE CENTER FIRM (36) · BONES HARD SUTURES EASILY DISPLACED (38–39) · BONES HARD, CANNOT BE DISPLACED (44–48)
POSTURE – RESTING		HYPOTONIC LATERAL DECUBITUS · HYPOTONIC (28) · BEGINNING FLEXION THIGH (30) · STRONGER HIP FLEXION (32–33) · FROG-LIKE (34) · FLEXION ALL LIMBS (36) · HYPERTONIC (39–40) · VERY HYPERTONIC (44–48)
RECOIL – LEG		NO RECOIL · PARTIAL RECOIL (34–35) · PROMPT RECOIL (41–48)
ARM		NO RECOIL · BEGIN FLEXION NO RECOIL (34) · PROMPT RECOIL MAY BE INHIBITED (36) · PROMPT RECOIL AFTER 30" INHIBITION (41) · PROMPT RECOIL AFTER 30" INHIBITION (43–48)

| 20 | 21 | 22 | 23 | 24 | 25 | 26 | 27 | 28 | 29 | 30 | 31 | 32 | 33 | 34 | 35 | 36 | 37 | 38 | 39 | 40 | 41 | 42 | 43 | 44 | 45 | 46 | 47 | 48 |

FIGURE 17 (cont.)

Confirmatory Neurologic Examination to be Done After 24 Hours

WEEKS GESTATION: 20 – 48

Category	Finding	Milestones (by weeks gestation)
TONE	HEEL TO EAR	NO RESISTANCE (20–24) → SOME RESISTANCE (~30) → IMPOSSIBLE (34+)
	SCARF SIGN	NO RESISTANCE (23–26) → ELBOW PASSES MIDLINE (~31) → ELBOW AT MIDLINE (~36) → ELBOW DOES NOT REACH MIDLINE (41+)
	NECK FLEXORS (HEAD LAG)	ABSENT (~31) → HEAD IN PLANE OF BODY (~38) → HOLDS HEAD (~44)
	NECK EXTENSORS	HEAD BEGINS TO RIGHT ITSELF FROM FLEXED POSITION (~32) → GOOD RIGHTING CANNOT HOLD IT (~36) → HOLDS HEAD FEW SECONDS (~38) → KEEPS HEAD IN LINE $\bar{c}$ TRUNK >40" (~40) → TURNS HEAD FROM SIDE TO SIDE (~44)
	BODY EXTENSORS	STRAIGHTENING OF LEGS (~33) → STRAIGHTENING OF TRUNK (~36) → STRAIGHTENING OF HEAD & TRUNK TOGETHER (~39)
	VERTICAL POSITIONS	WHEN HELD UNDER ARMS, BODY SLIPS THROUGH HANDS (28–30) → ARMS HOLD BABY LEGS EXTENDED (~34) → LEGS FLEXED GOOD SUPPORT $\bar{c}$ ARMS (~37)
	HORIZONTAL POSITIONS	HYPOTONIC ARMS & LEGS STRAIGHT (~28) → ARMS AND LEGS FLEXED (~36) → HEAD & BACK EVEN FLEXED EXTREMITIES (~38) → HEAD ABOVE BACK (~43)
FLEXION ANGLES	POPLITEAL	NO RESISTANCE (23–26) → 150° (~28) → 110° (~32) → 100° (~34) → 90° (~38) → 80° (~40)
	ANKLE	90° (~29) → 45° (~32) → 20° (~36) → 0° (41+) · A PRE-TERM WHO HAS REACHED 40 WEEKS STILL HAS A 40° ANGLE
	WRIST (SQUARE WINDOW)	90° (~29) → 60° (~32) → 45° (~36) → 30° (~38) → 0° (41+)
REFLEXES	SUCKING	WEAK NOT SYNCHRONIZED $\bar{c}$ SWALLOWING (~26) → STRONGER SYNCHRONIZED (~32) → PERFECT (~35) → PERFECT HAND TO MOUTH (~38) → PERFECT (~44)
	ROOTING	LONG LATENCY PERIOD SLOW, IMPERFECT (~30) → HAND TO MOUTH (~32) → BRISK, COMPLETE, DURABLE (~37) → COMPLETE (~45)
	GRASP	FINGER GRASP IS GOOD STRENGTH IS POOR (~28) → STRONGER (~34) → CAN LIFT BABY OFF BED INVOLVES ARMS (~39) → HANDS OPEN (~46)
	MORO	BARELY APPARENT / WEAK NOT ELICITED EVERY TIME (24–26) → STRONGER (~33) → COMPLETE $\bar{c}$ ARM EXTENSION OPEN FINGERS, CRY (~34) → ARM ADDUCTION ADDED (~39) → ?BEGINS TO LOSE MORO (~47)
	CROSSED EXTENSION	FLEXION & EXTENSION IN A RANDOM, PURPOSELESS PATTERN (~26) → EXTENSION BUT NO ADDUCTION (~32) → STILL INCOMPLETE (~36) → EXTENSION ADDUCTION FANNING OF TOES (~40) → COMPLETE (~45)
	AUTOMATIC WALK	MINIMAL (~31) → BEGINS TIPTOEING GOOD SUPPORT ON SOLE (~33) → FAST TIPTOEING (~37) → HEEL-TOE PROGRESSION WHOLE SOLE OF FOOT (~40) → A PRE-TERM WHO HAS REACHED 40 WEEKS WALKS ON TOES (~43) → ?BEGINS TO LOSE AUTOMATIC WALK (~47)
	PUPILLARY REFLEX	ABSENT (20–29) → APPEARS (~30) → PRESENT (31+)
	GLABELLAR TAP	ABSENT (20–33) → APPEARS (~34) → PRESENT (35+)
	TONIC NECK REFLEX	ABSENT (20–34) → APPEARS (~35) → PRESENT (36+)
	NECK-RIGHTING	ABSENT (20–36) → APPEARS (~37) → PRESENT AFTER 37 WEEKS (38+)

Week scale: 20 21 22 23 24 25 26 27 28 29 30 31 32 33 34 35 36 37 38 39 40 41 42 43 44 45 46 47 48

The neurologic assessment of the preschooler is much the same as evaluation in the adult. Cerebral function has matured greatly since birth. Recent and remote memory can be tested, as well as immediate recall using up to three digits.

All cranial nerves are tested, as in the adult, except the olfactory nerve, which is difficult to evaluate reliably before school age. Reflexes are evaluated as in the adult.

Evaluation of motor function is usually best received by the child if it is presented as a game. Muscle strength can be tested by assisting the child in a wheelbarrow maneuver to assess arm strength; observing the child get up from the floor to assess unilateral or bilateral weakness; and, finally, climbing stairs. Muscular size and tone are evaluated. Coordination is evaluated as in the adult, but adult coordination is not expected prior to 8 years.

Finally, sensory responses are tested. Vibratory and position sense can now be tested, and stereognosis and graphesthesia are evaluated.

The neurological assessment of the infant or young child is performed most efficiently if integrated throughout the entire assessment. Neurologic function and evaluation of this function is dependent upon developmental maturation. Likewise, developmental maturation is dependent upon intact neurologic function. Therefore, any complete assessment during infancy and childhood should include neurologic evaluation and also developmental screening.

Developmental Assessment

Developmental assessment has classically been an integrated part of the neurological assessment in the medical model. This approach is justified during the first 12 to 18 months of life when the child's neuromuscular development is most dramatic. During this period of time, neuromuscular deficits are likely to present as developmental delays. Shortly after the first year of life, however, the neuromuscular development becomes less dramatic, and psychosocial development is more impressive. Therefore, after 12 to 18 months, it is more appropriate that development be assessed as an area or system separate from neurological assessment. Data collected from developmental assessment, as well as the data collected from the rest of the physical examination, remain important supplements to the neurological assessment.

Routine developmental screening is an important part of pediatric health assessment. It requires the use of a tool to aid the examiner in observation and description of the child's developmental progress at various ages, and enables the examiner to determine whether the child's present development falls within the normal range of expectations for his or her age. It is important that the developmental screening tool to be used facilitate the examiner's assessment of each individual area of development, that is, gross motor, fine motor, language, self-help, and personal–social: that it outline both the course and sequence of normal development with a range of normal; and that it enable the examiner to follow the child's rate of development in terms of developmental milestones. One of the most widely used developmental screening tests is the Denver Developmental Screening Test. This tool can be used for children of 1 month to 6 years of age; however, it is most reliable for children 1 to 4 years of age. The Denver Developmental Screening Test correlates age and expected performance with regard to the areas of gross motor, fine motor, language, and social developmental milestones. It is not a diagnostic test; however, properly performed and interpreted, it will indicate possible development delays in specific functional areas (Figure 17-45).

FIGURE 17-45 (pages 345–346)
Denver Developmental Screening Test:
(a) scoring form; (b) instructions for scoring and testing. Copyright © 1969 by William K. Frankenburg, M.D., and Josiah B. Dodds, University of Colorado Medical Center. Reproduced with permission.

FIGURE 17-46 (pages 347–349)
Minnesota Child Development Inventory profile for: (a) a male; (b) a female. Scoring instructions are found in (c). Copyright © 1974, 1972 by Harold R. Ireton and Edward J. Thwing. Reproduced with permission.

FIGURE 17-45(a)

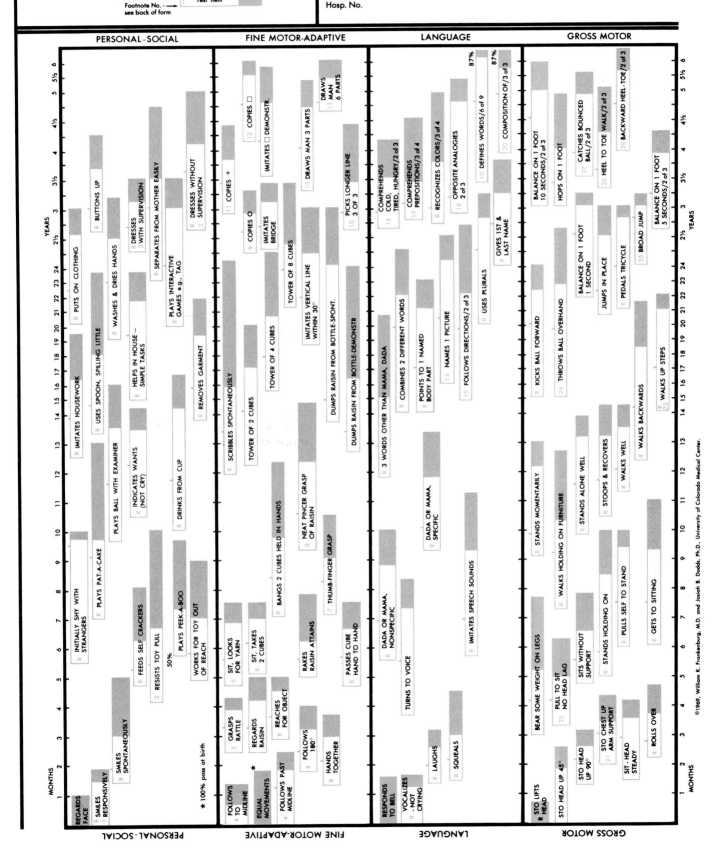

DENVER DEVELOPMENTAL SCREENING TEST

STO.= STOMACH
SIT = SITTING

PERCENT OF CHILDREN PASSING

Date
Name
Birthdate
Hosp. No.

©1969, William K. Frankenburg, M.D. and Josiah B. Dodds, Ph.D., University of Colorado Medical Center.

FIGURE 17-45(b)

1. Try to get child to smile by smiling, talking or waving to him. Do not touch him.
2. When child is playing with toy, pull it away from him. Pass if he resists.
3. Child does not have to be able to tie shoes or button in the back.
4. Move yarn slowly in an arc from one side to the other, about 6" above child's face. Pass if eyes follow 90° to midline. (Past midline; 180°)
5. Pass if child grasps rattle when it is touched to the backs or tips of fingers.
6. Pass if child continues to look where yarn disappeared or tries to see where it went. Yarn should be dropped quickly from sight from tester's hand without arm movement.
7. Pass if child picks up raisin with any part of thumb and a finger.
8. Pass if child picks up raisin with the ends of thumb and index finger using an over hand approach.

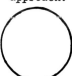   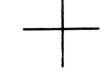

9. Pass any enclosed form. Fail continuous round motions.
10. Which line is longer? (Not bigger.) Turn paper upside down and repeat. (3/3 or 5/6)
11. Pass any crossing lines.
12. Have child copy first. If failed, demonstrate

When giving items 9, 11 and 12, do not name the forms. Do not demonstrate 9 and 11.

13. When scoring, each pair (2 arms, 2 legs, etc.) counts as one part.
14. Point to picture and have child name it. (No credit is given for sounds only.)

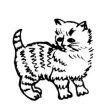 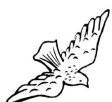 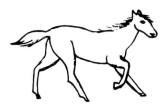 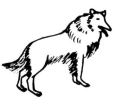 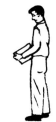

15. Tell child to: Give block to Mommie; put block on table; put block on floor. Pass 2 of 3. (Do not help child by pointing, moving head or eyes.)
16. Ask child: What do you do when you are cold? ..hungry? ..tired? Pass 2 of 3.
17. Tell child to: Put block on table; under table; in front of chair, behind chair. Pass 3 of 4. (Do not help child by pointing, moving head or eyes.)
18. Ask child: If fire is hot, ice is ?; Mother is a woman, Dad is a ?; a horse is big, a mouse is ?. Pass 2 of 3.
19. Ask child: What is a ball? ..lake? ..desk? ..house? ..banana? ..curtain? ..ceiling? ..hedge? ..pavement? Pass if defined in terms of use, shape, what it is made of or general category (such as banana is fruit, not just yellow). Pass 6 of 9.
20. Ask child: What is a spoon made of? ..a shoe made of? ..a door made of? (No other objects may be substituted.) Pass 3 of 3.
21. When placed on stomach, child lifts chest off table with support of forearms and/or hands.
22. When child is on back, grasp his hands and pull him to sitting. Pass if head does not hang back.
23. Child may use wall or rail only, not person. May not crawl.
24. Child must throw ball overhand 3 feet to within arm's reach of tester.
25. Child must perform standing broad jump over width of test sheet. (8-1/2 inches)
26. Tell child to walk forward, 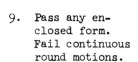 heel within 1 inch of toe. Tester may demonstrate. Child must walk 4 consecutive steps, 2 out of 3 trials.
27. Bounce ball to child who should stand 3 feet away from tester. Child must catch ball with hands, not arms, 2 out of 3 trials.
28. Tell child to walk backward, 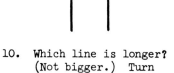 toe within 1 inch of heel. Tester may demonstrate. Child must walk 4 consecutive steps, 2 out of 3 trials.

DATE AND BEHAVIORAL OBSERVATIONS (how child feels at time of test, relation to tester, attention span, verbal behavior, self-confidence, etc,):

FIGURE 17-46(a)

Minnesota Child Development Inventory Profile

Harold R. Ireton and Edward J. Thwing

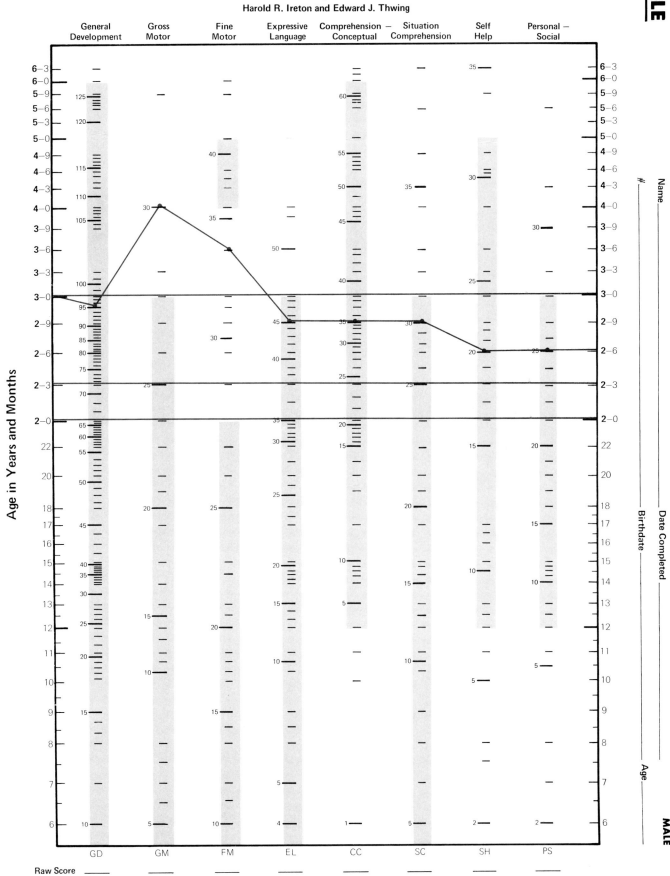

FIGURE 17-46(b)

Minnesota Child Development Inventory Profile

Harold R. Ireton and Edward J. Thwing

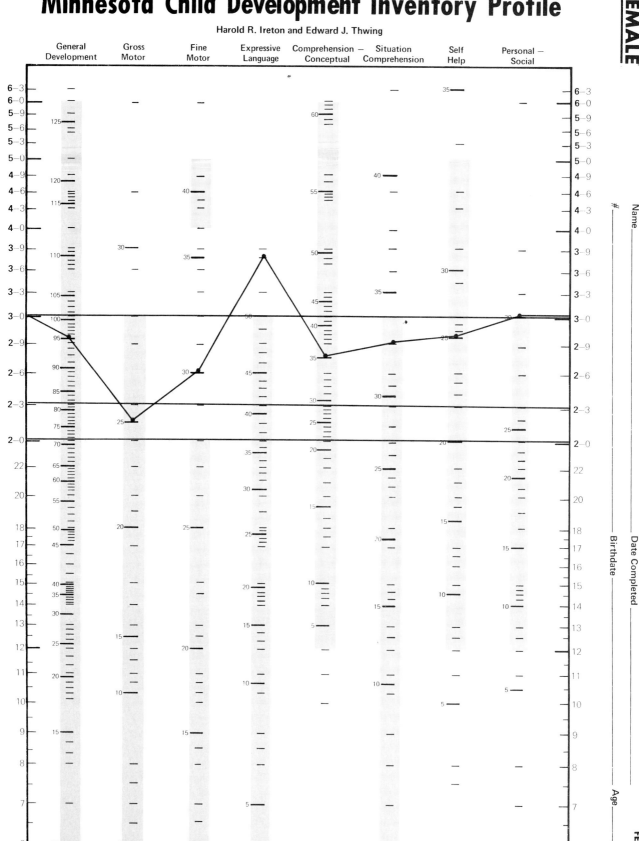

Raw Score

FIGURE 17-46(c)

MINNESOTA CHILD DEVELOPMENT INVENTORY PROFILE*

Instructions

1. Select a profile form for the appropriate sex. Sex is indicated on the right margin.

2. Record the child's name, identification number, the date the Inventory was completed, and the child's birthdate on the right margin of the profile form.

3. Calculate the child's age by subtracting his birthdate from the date the Inventory was completed. See example below:

```
          AGE CALCULATION

                  Year     Month    Day

Date Completed    1971      7  6     8  38

Birthdate         1968      5        14

Age               3         1        24
```

This child has passed the age of 3 years, 1 month, but is not yet 3 years, 2 months. His age is recorded as 3-1. Drop the days *after* calculating the age, not before.

For children under age two, the age is recorded in months. For example, a child whose age is calculated as 1 year, 7 months, is recorded as 19 months. Record the child's age in the lower right corner of the profile form.

4. Determine the score for each scale according to the instructions on the scoring templates. Record the scores in the appropriate spaces at the foot of the scales on the profile form.

5. Plot the score for each scale as a point at the corresponding number on the scale. If a score exceeds the highest number on the scale, plot the score at the highest number on the scale. Connect the points with lines to obtain the Minnesota Child Development Inventory Profile.

6. Draw a line across the profile at the age interval within which the child's age falls. For example, a child age 3-1 would fall within the 3-0 interval which represents children age 3-0 through 3-2, so a line would be drawn across the profile at 3-0.

7. The table to the right (Percent Below Age Guide) lists, for each age, the age intervals which are 20% below age and 30% below age. From the table, determine the 20% and 30% below-age intervals for the child. Draw a green line across the profile at the age interval which is 20% below the child's age, and a red line across the profile at the age interval which is 30% below the child's age. For children younger than 2-3, these below age lines may fall mid-way between age intervals.

*Age norms by sex are based upon 796 white suburban children.

```
          AGE CALCULATION

                  Year     Month    Day

Date Completed  _____     _____    _____

Birthdate       _____     _____    _____

Age             _____     _____    _____
```

PERCENT BELOW AGE GUIDE

Age	20% below age	30% below age
9	7.0	6.5
10	8.0	7.0
11	9.0	7.5
12	9.5	8.5
13	10.5	9.0
14	11.0	10.0
15	12.0	10.5
16	13.0	11.0
17	13.5	12.0
18, 19	14.5	12.5
20, 21	16.0	14.0
22, 23	17.5	15.5
2-0/2-2	20.0	17.5
2-3/2-5	22.0	18.0
2-6/2-8	2-0	20.0
2-9/2-11	2-3	22.0
3-0/3-2	2-3	2-0
3-3/3-5	2-6	2-3
3-6/3-8	2-9	2-6
3-9/3-11	3-0	2-6
4-0/4-2	3-3	2-9
4-3/4-5	3-3	3-0
4-6/4-8	3-6	3-0
4-9/4-11	3-9	3-3
5-0/5-2	4-0	3-6
5-3/5-5	4-3	3-6
5-6/5-8	4-3	3-9
5-9/5-11	4-6	4-0
6-0/6-2	4-9	4-3
6-3/6-5	5-0	4-3

TABLE 17-8
Summary of Milestones in Infant and Child Development*

	REFLEX FUNCTIONS AND INTEGRATED MOTOR ACTIVITIES	ADAPTIVE AND SOCIAL BEHAVIOR
Newborn period	Strong sucking, rooting, swallowing, and Moro reflexes. Infantile grasping, hands and feet. Tonic neck reflexes variable. Plantars flexor. Knee jerks, biceps reflexes present, other tendon reflexes variable, abdominal reflexes difficult to elicit. Flexion postures predominate. Extension and flexion movement of limbs. Briefly extends neck in prone position. Reflex walking.	
6 weeks	Tonic neck reflexes prominent. Tendon reflexes usually present. Unsustained ankle clonus not unusual. Plantars usually extensor. Asymmetrical postures usual. Extends and turns neck in prone position. Marked head lag when pulled to sit. Reflex walking usually lost unless facilitated by practice.	Smiles in response to play.
12 weeks (3 mo)	Incomplete tonic neck reflexes. Infantile grasp and sucking reflexes variable and modified by volition. Slight head lag when pulled to sit. Head bobs in sitting position. Briefly holds object placed in hand. Better organized movement of individual extremities. Holds head above plane of body for long periods in prone position.	Ready smile and makes pleasant sounds when talked to.
16 weeks (4 mo)	Hand grasp, sucking, and tonic neck reflexes subservient to volition and evident only when drowsy. Minimal head lag, holds head well and looks about when held in sitting position. Makes swimming movements when in prone position. Holds and shakes rattle, but cannot retrieve it if dropped. Moro response absent or nearly so. Symmetrical attitudes of extremities predominate and precede two-hand reach (20 weeks).	Laughs aloud. Shows pleasure when played with and at sight of food and friendly faces.
20 weeks (5 mo)	Extends knees when soles of feet contact surface if held in standing position (positive supporting reaction). Some movements of progression. No head lag on pull to sit, maintains head posture when body pulled or pushed by examiner. Grasps objects with both hands. Holds on to bottle.	Primitive articulated sounds ga-goo. Regards self in mirror and smiles. Pulls cloth from over face in play.
24 weeks (6 mo)	Beginning to grasp with one hand rather than with both hands. Sits with support. Supports upper parts of body on hands in prone position. Rolls from prone to supine. Grasps own feet and takes object with whole hand.	Range of sounds greater. Vocalizes spontaneously in social play. Tries to recover lost object. Extends arms in anticipation of being lifted. Expresses displeasure clearly.
28 weeks (7 mo)	Sits with hands for support (tripod). Stands with support. Rolls supine to prone. Transfers object from hand to hand. Bangs object on table.	A, ba, da, ga sounds usually heard. Repeats sounds in imitative way. Refuses food or things he does not want. Feeds self a cracker. Responds to name. Mimics.
32 weeks (8 mo)	Sits briefly without support. Supports weight and may stand holding on. Mounting of objects prominent.	Uses da-da, ba-ba sounds. Imitates sounds readily. Responds to "No."

TABLE 17-8 CONTINUED

AGE	REFLEX FUNCTIONS AND INTEGRATED MOTOR ACTIVITIES	ADAPTIVE AND SOCIAL BEHAVIOR
36 to 40 weeks (9 to 10 mo)	Sits well and pulls self to sitting position. Crawls using arms; grasps small object between thumb and forefinger. Beginning to release objects. Stands holding on. Sits well.	Nursery tricks, e.g., waves bye-bye and plays patty-cake on request. Seeks attention.
44 to 48 weeks (10 to 11 mo)	Creeps well. Usually puts object into and removes it from container. Walks holding on.	Usually one or two words with meaning. Shakes head for "No." Responds to questions such as, "Where is daddy?" Releases object for examination on request. Plays peek-a-boo.
52 weeks (1 year)	Plantar reflexes flexor in 50% of children. Abdominal reflexes elicited easily. Cruises and walks, one hand held. Dexterous in manipulating small objects. Throws objects. Less mouthing of objects.	Two to four words with meaning. Assists in dressing. Often shy. May kiss on request. Understands the names of several objects in environment.
15 months	Walks by self, toddles. Falls easily. Can feed self clumsily if allowed. Scribbles with crayon.	Several intelligible words. Often babbles in communicating. Imitates family in play, may build tower of two to four blocks. Requests things by pointing.
18 months (1 1/2 years)	Walks up and down stairs holding on. May pull toy and carry objects. Seats self in chair. Throws ball. Removes shoes, socks, and unzips clothing. Uses spoon well.	Many intelligible words. Well-developed jargon language. Points to two to three parts of body, common objects, pictures in books. Answers question: "Where is the . . . ?" Carries out simple commands, e.g., "Bring the ball."
24 months (2 years)	Plantar reflexes flexor in 100% of normal children. Walks up and down stairs by self (two feet per step). Bends over and picks up objects without falling. Runs, kicks ball, turns knob, washes hands, puts on shoes, socks, and pants.	Makes two- to three-word sentences. Uses I, me, and you. Asks for things by name. Imitates circle. Points to four or five parts of body. Organized play (e.g., puts doll to bed). Turns single pages of book. Builds tower of six to seven blocks. Toilet training often completed.
30 months (2 1/2 years)	Jumps both feet. Walks on tiptoes when requested.	Communicates well with simple sentences, asks questions. Knows full name. Helps put away toys. Holds pencil in hand. Builds tower of eight blocks. Can complete three-piece form board. Understands one to three colors. Tends to own toilet needs.
36 months (3 years)	Can stand on one foot. Rides tricycle. Dresses self except for buttons. Confuses feet.	Constantly talking, asking "Why?" Uses pronouns accurately. Recites nursery rhymes. Copies circle. Often can identify five colors. Obeys commands, recognizing three prepositions. Dresses and undresses doll. Plays with others. Tells sex.
48 to 54 months (4 to 4 1/2 years)	Walks one foot to a step on stairs. Hops and skips on one foot. Throws ball overhand. Laces shoes.	Articulation no longer infantile. Tells fanciful stories. Copies cross and square. Counts three to four objects and answers "How many?" Builds block building. Cooperates in play; boastful and critical.

*Modified with permission from Farmer, T. W., *Pediatric Neurology* 2nd ed., New York: Harper and Row.

TABLE 17-9
Developmental Map for the First Five Years

AGE	GROSS MOTOR	FINE MOTOR	LANGUAGE	SELF-HELP	SOCIAL
3 months	Lifts head and chest when prone	Reaches for objects overhead	Coos, laughs, squeals		Smiles, laughs
6 months	Sits without support	Picks up objects	Vocal play, wide range of sounds	Feeds self cracker	Reaches for familiar person
9 months	Crawls	Picks up small objects, e.g., raisin; thumb and finger grasp	Repetitive sounds like "baba, mama, dada"; understands "no-no"	Chews food	Plays pat-a-cake
1 yr	Walks alone (12 to 15 months)	Pencil, makes marks	Words or word-sounds (beyond "mama, dada"); comes when called	Drinks from cup	Gives affection
1 1/2 yr	Runs stiff-legged	Builds block tower, 4 cubes	3 plus intelligible words; follows simple instructions	Eats with spoon	Asks for help in doing things
2 yr	Walks up and down stairs alone	Imitates vertical line	2 to 3 work phrases; understandable half the time; names at least three body parts when asked	Washes and dries hands	Imitates household tasks
3 yr	Goes up and down stairs, one foot per tread	Copies (picture of) circle	Phrases of 4 or more words; understandable three-quarters of the time; understands simple concepts like "cold, tired, hungry"	Toilet trained	Understands sharing and taking turns
4 yr	Broad jumps or skips	Cross (+) copies	Talks in sentences; completely understandable (some articulation errors); follows short series of simple instructions: first . . . , then . . . , then . . .	Dresses self, except tying	Plays cooperatively following simple game rules
5 yr	Good balance and coordination in active play (vs. "clumsy")	Copies square, with good corners	Defines concrete words in practical terms, i.e., ball . . . "to play with"	Takes a bath without help	

With permission from Harold Ireton, Ph.D., Department of Family Practice. University of Minnesota.

TABLE 17-10
Developmental Screening

PRESENT STATUS	GROSS MOTOR	FINE MOTOR	LANGUAGE	SELF-HELP	SOCIAL
Parental report					
Clinical observation					
Screening tests					
Minnesota Child Development Inventory					
HISTORY					
Developmental					

	LABOR	DELIVERY	NEONATAL STATUS		
PREGNANCY				HEALTH HISTORY	

With permission from Harold Ireton, Ph.D., Department of Family Practice, University of Minnesota.

Another tool useful for developmental screening, which requires little professional time to administer, is the Minnesota Child Development Inventory (MCDI). This tool is a standardized questionnaire based on developmental skills achieved by children 1 to 6½ years of age as reported by the parent. The developmental areas assessed by the tool include gross motor, fine motor, expressive language, comprehension–conceptual, situation comprehension, self-help, personal social, and, finally, general development, which is an overall index of development. After compiling the parent's responses on the questionnaire, each area is evaluated separately, and the child's score is plotted on a profile for his or her sex. This profile then allows comparison of the child's developmental stage with that of children of the same age and other ages. The child's development in each area is considered normal if it falls at or above the developmental expectations of children 30 percent younger. Scores falling below the 30 percent level indicate developmental delay in that area. Figure 17-46(a), (b), and (c) are examples of the MCDI profile for both a male and a female with the directions for scoring.

There are many other tools available to assess development in the preschool-age child, including Draw a Man Test, Vineland Social Maturity Scale, Gesell's Scales, and the Vane Kindergarten Test. Whatever assessment tool is used, it is helpful if the examiner identifies areas to be assessed and sources for data collection in each area.

There are also numerous tables and developmental maps available that can serve as references for surveying major areas of development and specific behaviors or developmental skills expected at each age level. It is important to choose a developmental map that looks at all the areas of development. Table 17-8 is an example of a very detailed developmental map of neuromuscular development. Table 17-9 is a developmental map that is less detailed in each area; however, it covers a wide range of areas. Often it is helpful to refer to two such references for a more holistic approach to a developmental survey. Table 17-10 provides a format for developmental screening and data recording.

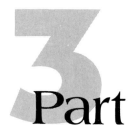

Part 3

STUDY GUIDE QUESTIONS

In the following client situations, identify and describe the subjective and objective data to be collected, the specific tools and procedures to be utilized in the collection of those data, and the rationale for the nursing assessment.

1. Alfred Meels, 36 years old, is hospitalized as a result of trauma to the head. You are to assess his level of consciousness.
2. Janice Milfred, a 24-year-old female, enters the clinic with numbness progressing from her feet to her thighs. Your responsibility is to perform an initial neurological screening examination.
3. During a home visit to Mr. and Mrs. Miltown, Mrs. Miltown states her 70-year-old husband has been having "black-out spells" over the last 2 weeks.
4. Mrs. Loretta Mitus brings her 6-week-old infant daughter in for a 6-week well-baby check. You are to assess her neurological status.
5. Jimmy, age 3, is brought to the clinic for a nursery school examination. You are to perform a developmental assessment.
6. Mrs. Mildred Smith brings her 12-year-old son, Ralph, to clinic for a routine physical. Mrs. Smith's primary complaint is that Ralph is clumsy.

SAMPLE FORMAT TO BE USED IN RESPONDING TO THE STUDY GUIDE QUESTIONS

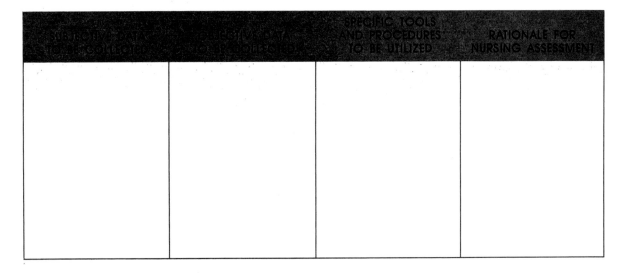

SUBJECTIVE DATA TO BE COLLECTED	OBJECTIVE DATA TO BE RECORDED	SPECIFIC TOOLS AND PROCEDURES TO BE UTILIZED	RATIONALE FOR NURSING ASSESSMENT

BIBLIOGRAPHY

ALPERS, BERNARD J., and ELIOTT L. MONCALL, *Essentials of the Neurological Examination.* Philadelphia: F. A. Davis Co., 1971.

BAKER, A. B., *An Outline of Applied Neurology.* Dubuque, Iowa: Kendall/Hunt Publishing Company, 1970.

BATES, BARBARA, *A Guide to Physical Examination,* pp. 263–293. Philadelphia: J. B. Lippincott Co., 1974.

CARTER, SIDNEY, and ARNOLD P. GOLD, *Neurology of Infancy and Childhood.* New York: Appleton-Century-Crofts, 1974.

CHUSID, JOSEPH G., *Correlative Neuroanatomy and Functional Neurology* (14th ed.). Los Altos, Calif.: Lange Medical Publications, 1970.

DEMYER, WILLIAM, *Technique of the Neurologic Examination* (2nd ed.). New York: McGraw-Hill Book Company, 1974.

DYKEN, PAUL R., "Neurologic Examination of the Neonate," *G.P.,* 39, no. 3, March 1969, pp. 108–115.

EVANS, WILLIAM F., *Anatomy and Physiology* (2nd ed.), pp. 146–205. Englewood Cliffs, N.J.: Prentice-Hall, Inc., 1976.

FARMER, THOMAS W., *Pediatric Neurology* (2nd ed.), pp. 1–43. New York: Harper & Row, Inc., 1975.

HOGAN, GWENDOLYN R., and NELL J. RYAN, "Neurological Evaluation of the Newborn," *Clinics in Perinatology,* 4, no. 1, March 1977, pp. 31–42.

HOLLINSHEAD, W. HENRY, *Textbook of Anatomy* (2nd ed.), pp. 37–70. New York: Harper & Row, Inc., 1967.

IRETON, HAROLD, and EDWARD THWING, "Appraising the Development of a Preschool Child by Means of a Standardized Report Prepared by the Mother: The Minnesota Child Development Inventory," *Clinical Pediatrics,* 15, no. 10, October 1976, pp. 875–882.

LEZAK, MURIEL D., *Neuropsychological Assessment.* New York: Oxford University Press, 1976.

NOBACK, CHARLES R., *The Human Nervous System.* New York: McGraw-Hill Book Company, 1967.

SALIBI, BAHIJ S., "The State of Consciousness—from Alertness to Deep Coma." Unpublished work. St. Mary's Junior College, Minneapolis, Minn., n.d.

STEEGMANN, A. THEODORE, *Examination of the Nervous System* (3rd ed.). Chicago: Year Book Medical Publishers, Inc., 1970.

VAN ALLEN, M. W., *Pictorial Manual of Neurological Test.* Chicago: Year Book Medical Publishers, Inc., 1969.

WELLS, CHARLES E., "Neurologic Evaluation in General Practice: Part I," *World-Wide Abstracts of General Medicine,* 9, no. 1, January 1966, pp. 8–14.

———, "Neurologic Evaluations in General Practice: Part II," *World-Wide Abstracts of General Medicine,* 9, no. 2, February 1966, pp. 8–18.

SECTION 4

Appendix
Tables

CLINICAL
ASSESSMENT
GUIDES
FOR VARIOUS
AGE GROUPS

TABLE I

Clinical Assessment Guide for Various Age Groups: The Integument

INTEGUMENT	NEWBORN/INFANCY	TODDLER/PRESCHOOL	SCHOOL AGE/PREPUBESCENCE	ADOLESCENCE/ADULTHOOD	ELDERLY	DEVIATIONS FROM NORMAL
EPIDERMIS/DERMIS	Premature skin color ruddy and translucent. Skin color in Caucasion newborn is uniform and pink. Hands and feet may present physiological cyanosis Skin color in the black newborn is pink with pigmented areas visible in deep crevices and creases. Pigmentation becomes established in first year 36 to 48 hours postbirth, a yellowish-orange or yellowish-green (jaundice) develops from head to toe with maximal intensity in 3 to 6 days and remission in 7 to 10 days	Skin color variable, dependent upon genetic background and exposure to sun	Skin color variable, dependent upon genetic background and exposure to sun	Skin color variable, dependent upon genetic background and exposure to sun Localized, increased pigmentation of areola and genitalia following biological maturity Hyperpigmentation of forehead, bridge of nose, and cheeks forming a masklike design during pregnancy or while on birth-control pills may occur (cholasma)	Skin color variable, dependent upon genetic background and exposure to sun Skin color may be faded, slightly yellowish Uneven skin color with exposure to sun or tanning	Bronze Hyperpigmentation Hypopigmentation Bluish color Bluish gray Purplish Erthema Albinism Localized yellowish-white or silverish discolorations Rapid development of jaundice in first 24 hours of life Prolonged jaundice in newborn
	VARIATIONS OF NORMAL Flat, pink, red or purplish vascular nevi (capillary hemangioma) frequently in nuchal area Nonblanching, bright red, raised vascular nevi, which gradually enlarge (strawberry marks)	VARIATIONS OF NORMAL Flat, pink, red or purplish vascular nevi (capillary hemangioma) frequently in nuchal area Nonblanching, bright red, raised vascular nevi that no longer increase in size and may regress in size (strawberry marks)	VARIATIONS OF NORMAL Flat, pink, red or purplish vascular nevi (capillary hemangioma) frequently in nuchal area Small, nonblanching, bright red, raised vascular nevi, which may disappear by age 7 with residual of a brownish pigmented or puckered atrophic area (strawberry marks)	VARIATIONS OF NORMAL Flat, pink, red or purplish vascular nevi (capillary hemangioma) frequently in nuchal area Small, nonblanching, red, raised vascular nevi or residual of a brownish pigmented or puckered atrophic area (strawberry marks)	VARIATIONS OF NORMAL Flat, pink, red or purplish, vascular nevi (capillary hemangioma) frequently in nuchal area Small, nonblanching, red, raised vascular nevi or residual of a brownish pigmented or puckered atrophic area (strawberry marks)	

TABLE I CONTINUED

EPIDERMIS/DERMIS (cont.)					
Dark blue or localized purple discolorations generally in lower lumbar region, buttock, or scrotal regions (Mongolian spots)	Dark blue or localized purple discolorations generally in lower lumbar region, buttock, or scrotal regions (Mongolian spots) May disappear spontaneously by 4 years of age	Dark blue or localized purple discolorations generally in lower lumbar region, buttock, or scrotal regions (Mongolian spots)	Faded blue or purplish discolorations generally located in lower lumbar region, buttock, or scrotal regions (Mongolian spots)	Multiple light-brown, nonraised, localized pigmentations (cafe au lait)
A single, light-brown, nonraised, localized pigmentation (cafe au lait)	A single, light-brown, nonraised, localized pigmentation (cafe au lait)	A single, light-brown, nonraised, localized pigmentation (cafe au lait)	A single, light-brown, nonraised, localized pigmentation (cafe au lait)	
Moles that are flat or raised, localized, light to dark brown in pigmentation	Moles that are flat or raised, localized, light to dark brown in pigmentation	Moles that are flat or raised, localized, light to dark brown in pigmentation	Moles that are flat or raised, localized, light to dark brown in pigmentation	
Freckles: flat, light brown areas that increase in color intensity with sun exposure and fade with nonexposure to sun	Freckles: flat, light brown areas that increase in color intensity with sun exposure and fade with nonexposure to sun	Freckles: flat, light brown areas that increase in color intensity with sun exposure and fade with nonexposure to sun	Freckles: flat, light brown areas that increase in color intensity with sun exposure and fade with nonexposure to sun	
		Lentigo: small, flat, light to dark brown pigmented area may be present	Lentigo: small, flat, light to dark brown pigmented area may be present	
Yellowish-orange deposits in forehead, nasolabial folds, palms of hands, and soles of feet (carotinemia)				

				SURFACE OF THE INTEGUMENT

Telangiectasis: bright red stellate or linear-shaped dilation of small vessels that fade when pressure is applied. In darkly pigmented individuals, they appear reddish brown

Telangiectasis: bright red stellate or linear-shaped dilation of small vessels that fade when pressure is applied. In darkly pigmented individuals, they appear reddish brown

Telangiectasis: bright red stellate or linear-shaped dilation of small vessels that fade when pressure is applied. In darkly pigmented individuals, they appear reddish brown

bright red stellate or linear-shaped dilation of small vessels that fade when pressure is applied. In darkly pigmented individuals, they appear reddish brown

Senile angioma: slightly raised, red in color, and composed of blood vessels. Usually formed during middle age

Venous stars: bluish in color, radiating from a central point, forming a stellate or flaring pattern

Senile angioma: slightly raised, red in color, and composed of blood vessels

Venous stars: bluish in color, radiating from a central point, forming a stellate or flaring pattern

Spider angioma: deep red in color, resembles shape of spider and fades when pressure is applied

Smooth and taut in full term
Wrinkled and loose in premature
Smoothness may be interrupted by vernix caseosa, milia, especially the nose, chin and cheeks as small, white papules and erythema toxicum, a macropapular lesion with erythematous border

Smooth and elastic

Smooth and elastic

Smooth and elastic

Smooth. Loss of tissue and elastic tissue may give rise to loose, wrinkled skin, especially in eyelids, neck, axillae, trunk, and body creases, overgrowths of normal skin forming stalk and head

Raised lesions
Indurations
Scaling
Exanthems
Localized hypertrophy
Chafing
Primary lesions
Secondary lesions
Skin tags
Orange-peel effect
Domed, tense, round or oval cyst filled with whitish-yellow substance
Follicular orifices filled with white or yellowish-white substances
Follicular orifices filled with black substances

TABLE I CONTINUED

INTEGUMENT	NEWBORN/INFANCY	TODDLER/ PRESCHOOL	SCHOOL AGE/ PREPUBESCENCE	ADOLESCENCE/ ADULTHOOD	ELDERLY	DEVIATIONS FROM NORMAL
SUBCUTANEOUS TISSUE	In premature, little or no subcutaneous tissue. In full-term infant, elastic and resilient	Elastic and resilient	Elastic and resilient	Elastic and resilient	Elastic and resilient. Atrophy of subcutaneous tissue occurs gradually	Dehydration. Tenting of skin. Overhydration. Edema. Excessive subcutaneous fat in all age ranges. Atrophy
HAIR: FUZZ	Lanugo: a fine, downy hair, most prominent on back and shoulders in premature. In full-term, universal distribution of variable amounts of hair, which is fine, light in color, and possesses a short hair shaft	Universal distribution of variable amounts of hair which is fine, light in color, and possesses a short hair shaft	Universal distribution of variable amounts of hair, which is fine, light in color, and possesses a short hair shaft	Universal distribution of variable amounts of hair, which is fine, light in color, and possesses a short hair shaft	Universal distribution of variable amounts of hair, which is fine, light in color, and possesses a short hair shaft	
HAIR: TERMINAL	Present on scalp. Color and amount varies. Fine to coarse texture. May have an uneven distribution	Present on scalp. Color and amount varies. Fine to coarse texture. Even distribution	Present on scalp. Color and amount varies. Fine to coarse texture. Even distribution	Present on scalp, axilla, pubic area, and legs in males and females. Universal distribution especially noted in males. In adolescent males, some scalp hair line recession occurs. Adult male may present male pattern of baldness. Color and amount of hair varies. Fine to coarse texture. Even distribution	Present on scalp, axilla pubic area, and legs in males and females. Universal distribution especially noted in males. Generalized thinning and graying of hair. Males may present male pattern of baldness. Color and amount of hair varies. Fine to coarse texture. Even distribution	Abrupt patchy loss of hair. Total loss of scalp hair with the exception of balding. Total loss of all body hair. Hirsutism. Brittle hair shafts. Development of prominent, terminal body hairs prior to pubertal changes

					Deviations
Thin	Thin	Thin	Thin	Thin	Atrophy Hard Brittle Soft
Firm	Firm	Firm	Firm	Firm	
Convex	Convex	Convex	Convex	Convex	Concave
Nail plate is clear with grayish-white free edge that protrudes straight out from end of finger. Frequently, the lunula is visible	Nail plate is clear with grayish-white free edge that protrudes straight out from end of finger. Frequently, the lunula is visible	Nail plate is clear with grayish-white free edge that protrudes straight out from end of finger. Frequently, the lunula is visible	Nail plate is clear with grayish-white free edge that protrudes straight out from end of finger. Frequently, the lunula is visible	Nail plate is clear with grayish-white free edge that protrudes straight out from end of finger. Frequently, the lunula is visible	Longitudinal pigmented line Yellowish coloration Brownish coloration Slate blue Transverse white striations Free edge curved upward or downward
Nail bed pinkish in color. May present physiological cyanosis in the immediate newborn period or with cold stress	Nail bed pinkish in color. May present physiological cyanosis with cold stress	Nail bed pinkish in color. May present physiological cyanosis with cold stress	Nail bed pinkish in color. May present physiological cyanosis with cold stress	Nail bed pinkish in color. May present physiological cyanosis with cold stress	Cyanosis Transient flushing or redness Ecchymosis
Approximate angle of 160°	Approximate angle of 160°	Approximate angle of 160°	Approximate angle of 160°	Approximate angle of 160°	Increase in angle (180°)
LATERAL AND POSTERIOR NAIL FOLDS Smooth, firm, and nontender	Smooth, firm, and nontender	Smooth, firm, and nontender	Smooth, firm, and nontender	Smooth, firm, and nontender	Hangnails Skin tags Tense Swollen Tender

TABLE II

Clinical Assessment Guide for Various Age Groups: The Head

HEAD	NEWBORN/INFANCY	TODDLER PRESCHOOL	SCHOOL AGE PREADOLESCENCE	ADOLESCENCE ADULTHOOD	ELDERLY	DEVIATIONS FROM NORMAL
SKULL	Sutures palpable as splits or ridges	Sutures palpable as breaks in bone continuity	Sutures palpable as breaks in bone continuity	Sutures palpable as breaks in bone continuity	Sutures palpable as breaks in bone continuity	Premature ossification of sutures. Postmature (delayed) ossification of sutures
	Skull surface smooth	Skull surface smooth	Skull surface smooth	Skull surface smooth	Skull surface smooth	Cephalohematoma Caput succedaneum Irregularity of surface
	Anterior fontanel open, ranging from 1 by 1 to 6 by 6 cm	Anterior fontanel closed by 18 months	Anterior fontanel closed	Anterior fontanel closed	Anterior fontanel closed	Premature closure with cessation of head growth. Delayed or late closure.
	Posterior fontanel open, 0.5 to 1 cm in diameter, closes between 6 and 9 months of age	Posterior fontanel closed	Posterior fontanel closed	Posterior fontanel closed	Posterior fontanel closed	Premature closure with cessation of head growth. Delayed or late closure
	Fontanels flat and soft	Open fontanels flat and soft	Fontanels closed	Fontanels closed	Fontanels closed	Bulging Sunken Tense Marked pulsation
	Frontal region yields illumination ring of 2 cm or less	Not assessed	Not assessed	Not assessed	Not assessed	Illumination ring greater than 2 cm Asymmetrical illumination
	Posterior occipital region yields a light ring of 1 cm or less	Not assessed	Not assessed	Not assessed	Not assessed	Asymmetrical illumination
	Lateral head transilluminates a ring smaller than the frontal region	Not assessed	Not assessed	Not assessed	Not assessed	Asymmetrical illumination
	Percussion yields "crackpot" sound with open fontanel	Percussion yields a resonant sound following closure of fontanel	Percussion yields a resonant sound	Percussion yields a resonant sound	Percussion yields a resonant sound	Nonresonant sound Crackpot sound following closure of

					Abnormal Findings
Symmetrical shape, unless molded from birth process for first week of life or positional compression	Symmetrical shape Normocephalic	Symmetrical shape Normocephalic	Symmetrical shape Normocephalic	Symmetrical shape Normocephalic	Oxycephaly Scaphocephaly Trigonocephaly Plagiocephaly
Mean head circumference in newborn is 34 cm (female), 34.5 to 35 cm (male), and in infants is 36 to 45.5 cm (female), 37 to 47 cm (male)	Mean head circumference in toddler is 45.5 to 49 cm (female), 47 to 50 cm (male), and in preschooler is 49 to 50.5 cm (female), 50 to 51 cm (male)	Mean head circumference in school age is 50.5 to 52 cm (female), 51 to 53 cm (male), and in prepubescence is 52 to 53 cm (female), 53 to 54 cm male	Mean head circumference of biologically mature is 55 cm (female), 56 cm (male)	Mean head circumference of elderly is 55 cm (female), 56 cm (male)	Microcephaly Macrocephaly
FACE Symmetrical shape	Symmetrical shape	Symmetrical shape	Symmetrical shape	Symmetrical shape	Asymmetrical shape Masked facies Ptosis
SCALP Smooth, slightly oily	Smooth, slightly oily	Smooth, slightly oily	Smooth, slightly oily	Smooth, dry or oily	Rough Scaly Dry Cradle cap Dandruff Seborrhea Lacerations Inflammation
HAIR Even distribution except in occipital region	Even distribution	Even distribution	Even distribution of hair. Males may demonstrate thinning and baldness	Even distribution of hair. Thinning may be present in both male and female	Asymmetrical distribution of hair. In male, loss of hair prior to adulthood. In female, patchy thinning or balding
Grows toward face and neck except for cowlicks	Grows toward face and neck except for cowlicks	Grows toward face and neck except for cowlicks	Grows toward face and neck except for cowlicks	Grows toward face and neck except for cowlicks	Growth toward occiput of head

TABLE III
Clinical Assessment Guide for Various Age Groups: The Ear

EAR	NEWBORN/INFANCY	TODDLER/PRESCHOOL	SCHOOL AGE/PREPUBESCENCE	ADOLESCENCE/ADULTHOOD	ELDERLY	DEVIATIONS FROM NORMAL
AURICLE	Pink, creases of auricles in black newborn may present pigmentation	Pink to dark brown, dependent upon genetic characteristics	Pink to dark brown, dependent upon genetic characteristics	Pink to dark brown, dependent upon genetic characteristics	Pink to dark brown, dependent upon genetic characteristics. May present a faded appearance or yellowing	Cyanotic Erythematous Pallied Irregular color Pale
	Bilaterally, superior portion of helix crosses a line from the lateral angle of the eye to the occipital protuberance	Bilaterally, superior portion of helix crosses a line from the lateral angle of the eye to the occipital protuberance	Bilaterally, superior portion of helix crosses a line from the lateral angle of the eye to the occipital protuberance	Bilaterally, superior portion of helix crosses a line from the lateral angle of the eye to the occipital protuberance	Bilaterally, superior portion of helix crosses a line from the lateral angle of the eye to the occipital protuberance	Helix lower than imaginary line from lateral angle of eye to the occipital protuberance
	Almost vertical with and not greater than a 10° lateral posterior angle	Almost vertical with and not greater than a 10° lateral posterior angle	Almost vertical with and not greater than a 10° lateral posterior angle	Almost vertical with and not greater than a 10° lateral posterior angle	Almost vertical with and not greater than a 10° lateral posterior angle	Protrusion from head at a right angle (lop ear)
	Elastic, firm texture unless premature	Elastic, firm texture	Elastic, firm texture	Elastic, firm texture	Elastic, firm texture	Rigid
	Symmetrical curvature May possess Darwinian tubercle	Symmetrical curvature May possess Darwinian tubercle	Symmetrical curvature May possess Darwinian tubercle	Symmetrical curvature May possess Darwinian tubercle	Symmetrical curvature May possess Darwinian tubercle	Pointed pinna: satyr ear Curling pinna: scroll ear Asymmetrical without familial characteristics
	Large to small in size dependent on genetic composition	Large to small in size dependent on genetic composition	Large to small in size dependent on genetic composition	Large to small in size dependent on genetic composition	Large to small in size dependent on genetic composition	Large without familial characteristics (macrotia) Small (microtia) Absence: Aztec ear
	Lobule present	Lobule present	Lobule present	Lobule present	Lobule present. May appear large	
EAR CANAL	Patent	Patent	Patent	Patent	Patent	Atresia Foreign object obstruction
	Wet or dry wax present	Wet or dry wax present	Wet or dry wax may be present	Wet or dry wax may be present	Wet or dry wax may be present	Polyp Wax occlusion or

	Smooth, pink	Smooth, pink In blacks, meatus highly pigmented	Smooth, pink In blacks, meatus highly pigmented	Smooth, pink In blacks, meatus highly pigmented	In blacks, meatus highly pigmented	Erythematous Scaly
		Hair follicles present	Hair follicles present	Hair follicles present	Hair follicles present	
TYMPANIC MEMBRANE	Transparent, glistening, pearly-gray	Transparent, glistening, pearly-gray	Transparent, glistening, pearly-gray	Transparent, glistening, pearly-gray	Transparent, glistening, pearly-gray	Partial or complete loss of transparency / Erythematous / Bluish / Purplish / Black / Absence of color / Dull appearance
	Smooth	Smooth	Smooth	Smooth	Smooth	Perforation / Scarring / Plaque formation / Absence of malleus
	Malleus extends from superior hemisphere as a dense whitish object	Malleus extends from superior hemisphere as a dense whitish object	Malleus extends from superior hemisphere as a dense whitish object	Malleus extends from superior hemisphere as a dense whitish object	Malleus extends from superior hemisphere as a dense whitish object	
	Umbo presents as an area of concavity	Umbo presents as an area of concavity	Umbo presents as an area of concavity	Umbo presents as an area of concavity	Umbo presents as an area of concavity	Umbo presents convexity / Absence of umbo
	Light reflex in anterior inferior quadrant	Light reflex in anterior inferior quadrant	Light reflex in anterior inferior quadrant	Light reflex in anterior inferior quadrant	Light reflex in anterior inferior quadrant	Light reflex absent or diminished
	Newborn: light reflex diffuse over membrane with minimal point directed toward the umbo	Diffusely conical in shape with point directed toward the umbo	Diffusely conical in shape with point directed toward the umbo	Diffusely conical in shape with point directed toward the umbo	Diffusely conical in shape with point directed toward the umbo	
	At approximately 3 months assumes cone shape, although diffuse					
	Vascular structures present smooth course	Vascular structures present smooth course	Vascular structures present smooth course	Vascular structures present smooth course	Vascular structures present smooth course	Distended / Tortuous / Numerous vessels apparent
	Vary in number, visible	Vary in number, visible	Vary in number, visible	Vary in number, visible	Vary in number, visible	
	Vibratory to air current	Vibratory to air current	Vibratory to air current	Vibratory to air current	Vibratory to air current	Minimal to absent vibrability
HEARING	Newborn: blink in response to sudden noise stimuli	If cooperative, hears whispered word at 15 ft	Hears whispered word at 15 ft	Hears whispered word at 15 ft	Hears whispered word at 15 ft	Failure to respond to sudden noise / Intermittent failure to respond to sudden loud noise

367

TABLE III CONTINUED

EAR	NEWBORN/INFANCY	TODDLER/PRESCHOOL	SCHOOL-AGE/PREPUBESCENCE	ADOLESCENCE/ADULTHOOD	ELDERLY	DEVIATIONS FROM NORMAL
HEARING (cont.)	14 days old: "jump" or body jerk to sudden noise stimuli	If cooperative, hears spoken word at 20 ft	Hears spoken word at 20 ft	Hears spoken word at 20 ft	Hears spoken word at 20 ft	Prysbycusis
	2 to 3 months: temporary cessation of body activity to sudden noise stimuli	If cooperative, watch tick heard equal to examiner's hearing distance	Watch tick heard equal to examiner's hearing distance	Watch tick heard equal to examiner's hearing distance	Watch tick heard equal to examiner's hearing distance	Failure to turn in direction of sudden loud noise
	3 to 4 months: Eyes and head turn in direction sound originated from					Cessation of attempts to vocalize
	6 months to 1 year: continued development of vocalized sounds					No response to name or simple direction
	React to verbalizations of name and simple directions (e.g., no)	If cooperative at age 3, can identify equal intensity of sound bilaterally with Weber test	Equal intensity of sound bilaterally with Weber test	Equal intensity of sound bilaterally with Weber test	Equal intensity of sound bilaterally with Weber test	Lateralization of sound. Conductive loss, sound readily perceived in ear with loss while in sensorineural loss. Sound heard best in intact ear
		If cooperative at age 3, air to bone conduction of sound ratio 2:1 in Rinne test	Air conduction to bone conduction of sound ratio 2:1 in Rinne test	Air conduction to bone conduction of sound ratio 2:1 in Rinne test	Air conduction to bone conduction of sound ratio 2:1 in Rinne test	Bone conduction of sound longer than air conduction due to conduction loss
			Cessation of bone-conducted sound simultaneously for examiner and client (Schwabach test)	Cessation of bone-conducted sound simultaneously for examiner and client (Schwabach test)		Sound duration shorter than examiners. May indicate sensorineural loss
			Sounds transmitted from vertex of skull with ear occluded are heard by occluded ear	Sounds transmitted from vertex of skull with ear occluded are heard by occluded ear	Sounds transmitted from vertex of skull with ear occluded are heard by occluded ear	Sound duration longer than examiners may indicate conductive loss

TABLE IV
Clinical Assessment Guide for Various Age Groups: The Eye

EYE	NEWBORN/INFANCY	TODDLER/PRESCHOOL	SCHOOL AGE/PREPUBESCENCE	ADOLESCENCE/ADULTHOOD	ELDERLY	DEVIATIONS FROM NORMAL
VISUAL PERCEPTION	3 to 7 months: 20/200 10 to 12 months: 20/200 Fascinated by bright colors between 1 and 3 months of age At 4 1/2 to 7 months has preference for reds and yellows Second month: stares at bright objects and able to fixate gaze Third month: follows objects If removed from sight suddenly, acts as if object is gone. Eyes converge on object as it approaches nose Fourth month: recognizes significant others	18 months to 2 years: 20/40 2 to 3 years: 20/30 (Snellen illiterate chart) Development of color recognition is occurring	20/20 (Snellen alphabet chart) with corrective lenses if worn By 5 years, color recognition established By 6 years, may be able to differentiate color shading	20/20 (Snellen alphabet chart) with corrective lenses if worn Discriminates between colors and shading	20/20 (Snellen alphabet chart) with corrective lenses if worn Differentiates between colors. Ability to discriminate in shadings of color may be decreased	Inability to accommodate: presbyopia Sensitivity to glare: photophobia Loss of peripheral field vision Loss of central vision Myopia (near-sighted) Hyperopia (far-sighted) Sudden loss of vision Blurred vision Diplopia Distortion of shape of object focused on Color blindness Inability to discriminate shadings of color

369

TABLE IV CONTINUED

EYE	NEWBORN/INFANCY	TODDLER/PRESCHOOL	SCHOOL AGE/PREPUBESCENCE	ADOLESCENCE/ADULTHOOD	ELDERLY	DEVIATIONS FROM NORMAL
VISUAL PERCEPTION (cont.)	Blinks to sudden bright light stimulus Protective blink to threatening stimulus at approximately 7 to 8 weeks of age	Blinks to sudden bright light stimulus Blinks in response to threatening stimuli	Blinks to sudden bright light stimulus Blinks in response to threatening stimuli	Blinks to sudden bright light stimulus Blinks in response to threatening stimuli	Blinks to sudden bright light stimulus Blinks in response to threatening stimuli	Failure to blink with a sudden bright light stimulus Absence of blink to threatening stimuli
BINOCULAR VISION	Epicanthal folds can give false appearance of cross eyes Bilaterally, eye globes directed in same plane. At 6 weeks, conjugate positioning and movement Cover test not performed	Epicanthal folds can give false appearance of cross eyes Bilaterally, eye globes directed in same plane and position Cover test yields object-fixed focus	Bilaterally, eye globes directed in same plane and position Cover test yields object-fixed focus	Bilaterally, eye globes directed in same plane and position Cover test yields object-fixed focus	Bilaterally eye globes directed in same plane and position Cover test yields object-fixed focus	Asymmetry of eye globe direction and position Wandering of eye or drifting with refocus once cover removed from eye
VISUAL FIELDS	Not assessed due to inability to cooperate with examiner	Confrontation With one eye covered, should visualize objects 60° nasalward 50° upward 90° temporally 70° downward	Confrontation With one eye covered, should visualize objects 60° nasalward 50° upward 90° temporally 70° downward	Confrontation With one eye covered, should visualize objects 60° nasalward 50° upward 90° temporally 70° downward	Confrontation With one eye covered, should visualize objects 60° nasalward 50° upward 90° temporally 70° downward	Unilateral or bilateral visualization of confronting object in degrees less than those stipulated
EXTRAOCULAR MUSCLES	Conjugate movement with slow moving objects at approximately 6 weeks old	Conjugate movement in same direction	Conjugate movement in same direction	Conjugate movement in same direction	Conjugate movement in same direction	Disconjugate movement Diplopia

					Abnormal Findings
Globe movement	Globe movement in:	Globe movement in:	Globe movement in:	Globe movement in:	failure of globe to move in any one or more of the specified directions. Limited movement of the globe in any one of the specified directions.
Globe movement in: 1. superior temporal plane 2. midline temporal plane 3. inferior temporal plane 4. superior nasal plane 5. midline nasal plane 6. inferior nasal plane	1. superior temporal plane 2. midline temporal plane 3. inferior temporal plane 4. superior nasal plane 5. midline nasal plane 6. inferior nasal plane	1. superior temporal plane 2. midline temporal plane 3. inferior temporal plane 4. superior nasal plane 5. midline nasal plane 6. inferior nasal plane	1. superior temporal plane 2. midline temporal plane 3. inferior temporal plane 4. superior nasal plane 5. midline nasal plane 6. inferior nasal plane	1. superior temporal plane 2. midline temporal plane 3. inferior temporal plane 4. superior nasal plane 5. midline nasal plane 6. inferior nasal plane	Pathologic nystagmus Pendular nystagmus Oscillating nystagmus Vertical nystagmus Rotary nystagmus Spontaneous nystagmus
Limited horizontal nystagmus from rotational eye movement up to 1 month					
May present end point nystagmus in extremes of gazing position	May present end point nystagmus in extremes of gazing position	May present end point nystagmus in extremes of gazing position	May present end point nystagmus in extremes of gazing position	May present end point nystagmus in extremes of gazing position	
Third month: eyes converge on object as it approaches nose					
UPPER EYELID	Thin, smooth, and resilient	Thin, smooth, and resilient	Thin, smooth, and resilient	Thin and smooth. Atrophy of elastic and fibrous tissue. May have elongation of skinfold and baggy-appearing lid	Localized swelling stye, chalazion Thickening of skin Generalized swelling Tenseness Senile keratotic growths Lipomas Warts
Thin, smooth, and resilient					
Color of lid resembles surrounding skin	Color of lid resembles surrounding skin	Color of lid resembles surrounding skin	Color of lid resembles surrounding skin	Color of lid resembles surrounding skin or may have increased pigmentation	Increased pigmentation during pregnancy Bluish in color Red Pallid Ecchymotic Increased pigmentation before completion of adulthood Hypopigmentation Yellow stiff plaques

TABLE IV CONTINUED

EYE	NEWBORN/INFANCY	TODDLER/PRESCHOOL	SCHOOL AGE/PREPUBESCENCE	ADOLESCENCE/ADULTHOOD	OLDER ADULT	DEVIATIONS FROM NORMAL
UPPER EYELID (cont.)	Covers the eye to the limbus	Covers the eye to the limbus	Covers the eye to the limbus	Covers the eye to the limbus	Covers the eye to the limbus	White scleral strip showing between lid and limbus (retraction) Lid lag with movements of the globe Spasm Ptosis Increased or decreased width of palpebral fissure Ectropion Squinting
	Lid margins contain dark hairs that curve outward	Lid margins contain dark hairs that curve outward	Lid margins contain dark hairs that curve outward	Lid margins contain dark hairs that curve outward	Lid margins contain dark hairs that curve outward	Entropion Absence of hairs Marked long lashes, especially newborn and infant Dry or oily crust or scales at hair base Eyelash root on posterior border of eyelid Whitening of lash color
	Lid covers eye globe totally when closed	Lid covers eye globe totally when closed	Lid covers eye globe totally when closed	Lid covers eye globe totally when closed	Lid covers eye globe totally when closed	Failure to cover eye globe when closed
LOWER EYELID	Smooth and resilient	Smooth and resilient	Smooth and resilient	Smooth and resilient	Smooth Atrophy of elastic and fibrous tissue May appear boggy	Localized swelling Thickening of skin Generalized swelling Tenseness Senile keratotic growths Whitish-gray, raised lymph glands on internal surface
	Color of lid resembles surrounding skin	Color of lid resembles surrounding skin	Color of lid resembles surrounding skin	Color of lid resembles surrounding skin	Color of lid resembles surrounding skin or may have increased pigmentation	Bluish in color Ecchymotic Red Pallid Increased pigmentation before completion of adulthood

						Deviations from Normal
	Small white scleral strip between lower lid and limbus	Small white scleral strip between lower lid and limbus	Small white scleral strip between lower lid and limbus	Small white scleral strip between lower lid and limbus	Small white scleral strip between lower lid and limbus	...palpebral fissure; Squinting
	Lid margins contain dark hairs that curve outward	Lid margins contain dark hairs that curve outward	Lid margins contain dark hairs that curve outward	Lid margins contain dark hairs that curve outward	Lid margins contain dark hairs that curve outward	Ectropion; Entropion
PALPEBRAL CONJUNCTIVA	Transparent, presenting pink color of underlying structures	Transparent, presenting pink color of underlying structures	Transparent, presenting pink color of underlying structures	Transparent, presenting pink color of underlying structures	Transparent, presenting pink color of underlying structures	Erythematous; Cyanotic
	Meibomian glands visible as yellowish striations	Meibomian glands visible as yellowish striations	Meibomian glands visible as yellowish striations	Meibomian glands visible as yellowish striations	Meibomian glands visible as yellowish striations	Marked enlargement of striations; Distention of meibomian gland (cyst)
	Smooth	Smooth	Smooth	Smooth	Smooth	Bulges
	Fine, nonprominent vessels	Fine, nonprominent vessels	Fine, nonprominent vessels	Fine, nonprominent vessels	Fine, nonprominent vessels	Dilated, prominent vessels
BULBAR CONJUNCTIVA	Transparent, presenting opaque white color of sclera	Transparent, presenting opaque white color of sclera	Transparent, presenting opaque white color of sclera	Transparent, presenting opaque white color of sclera	Transparent, presenting opaque white color of sclera	Extravasation of blood; Intense blueness; Raised yellow plaque; Pterygium
	Episcleral vessels visible	Episcleral vessels visible	Episcleral vessels visible	Episcleral vessels visible	Episcleral vessels visible	Dilated, tortuous
	Superficial vessels visible in periphery	Superficial vessels visible in periphery	Superficial vessels visible in periphery	Superficial vessels visible in periphery	Superficial vessels visible in periphery	Dilated
LACRIMAL APPARATUS	Begin to function in 2 to 4 weeks; Respond to emotion in 4 to 12 weeks				Decreased amount of tearing may occur	Stenotic; Obstructed; Lacrimation; Epiphoria; Congenital alacrima; Erythema
	Patent	Patent	Patent	Patent	Patent	
	Deep pink in color	Deep pink in color	Deep pink in color	Deep pink in color	Deep pink in color	

373

TABLE IV CONTINUED

EYE	NEWBORN/INFANCY	TODDLER/PRESCHOOL	SCHOOL AGE/PREPUBESCENCE	ADOLESCENCE/ADULTHOOD	ELDERLY	DEVIATIONS FROM NORMAL
SCLERA	At birth, sclera may have bluish coloration, which dissipates and a glistening opaque white color develops	Glistening Opaque White May have spots of melanin	Glistening Opaque White May have spots of melanin	Glistening Opaque White May have spots of melanin	Glistening Opaque White to whitish yellow May have spots of melanin	Jaundice, evenly distributed Blue Lackluster appearance Dry appearance Yellowish collection of fatty tissue Sensation of foreign body Red
IRIS	Color of iris established in 26 to 28 wk Round, uniform in color	Uniform color, symmetrically round	Uniform color, symmetrically round	Uniform color, symmetrically round	Uniform color, symmetrically round Color of iris fades	Heterochromia Irregular color intensity Asymmetrical Coloboma Cleft in iris
CORNEA	May be hazy for short period of time after birth, then clear and transparent	Clear Transparent	Clear Transparent	Clear Transparent	Clear Transparent	Grayish white ring around cornea Red or green ring encircling cornea Pigmented areas Scars Visible vascularization Redness encircling cornea (limbal flush) Erosions Cloudy Opacities Dull Grayish infiltration into cornea
	Dome shaped Smooth	Dome shaped Smooth	Dome shaped Smooth	Dome shaped Smooth	Dome shaped Smooth	Irregular surface Edematous Grayish-white elevated lesions near limbus Ulcerations Pits

							Abnormal Findings
	Moist	Moist			Moist	Moist	Unilateral or bilateral absence of blink with corneal stimulation
	Corneal reflex in response to touch (cranial nerve V)	Corneal reflex in response to touch (cranial nerve V)	Corneal reflex in response to touch (cranial nerve V)	Corneal reflex in response to touch (cranial nerve V)	Corneal reflex in response to touch (cranial nerve V)	Corneal reflex in response to touch (cranial nerve V)	
	Symmetrical corneal light reflex	Symmetrical corneal light reflex	Symmetrical corneal light reflex	Symmetrical corneal light reflex	Symmetrical corneal light reflex	Symmetrical corneal light reflex	Asymmetrical corneal light reflex
PUPIL	Round Equal in size	Round Equal in size	Round Equal in size	Round Equal in size	Round Equal in size	Round Equal in size Smaller than in adulthood	Mydriatic Miosis Anisocoria Irregularity of pupil
	Constriction to direct light	Constriction to direct light	Constriction to direct light	Constriction to direct light	Constriction to direct light	Constriction to direct light	Absence Sluggish
	Consensual constriction to light	Consensual constriction to light	Consensual constriction to light	Consensual constriction to light	Consensual constriction to light	Consensual constriction to light	Absence Sluggish Dilation of the pupil
	Bilateral symmetry in response to light	Bilateral symmetry in response to light	Bilateral symmetry in response to light	Bilateral symmetry in response to light	Bilateral symmetry in response to light	Bilateral symmetry in response to light	Asymmetrical response
	Accommodation, begins to develop at 2 to 10 weeks	18 months to 2 years becomes well developed and accommodates to near and distant objects promptly	Accommodates to near and distant objects promptly	Accommodates to near and distant objects promptly	Accommodates to near and distant objects promptly	Accommodates to near and distant objects promptly	Unilateral or bilateral failure to accommodate Sluggish accommodation
LENS	Clear and transparent	Clear and transparent	Clear and transparent	Clear and transparent	Clear and transparent	Clear and transparent	Subluxation Dislocation Milky color Stellate opacities Black reflection on light of ophthalmoscopic exam
STRUCTURAL PARALLELISM	Symmetrical light reflex in center of pupil	Symmetrical light reflex in center of pupil	Symmetrical light reflex in center of pupil	Symmetrical light reflex in center of pupil	Symmetrical light reflex in center of pupil	Symmetrical light reflex in center of pupil	Exophthalmos Enophthalmos Asymmetrical light reflex on pupils
LENS, CORNEA, PUPIL	Round, full, red, reflex with funduscopic exam	Round, full, red, reflex with funduscopic exam	Round, full, red, reflex with funduscopic exam	Round, full, red, reflex with funduscopic exam	Round, full, red, reflex with funduscopic exam	Round, full, red, reflex with funduscopic exam	Opacities Shadows Irregularly shaped red reflex White reflex

TABLE IV CONTINUED

EYE	NEWBORN/INFANCY	TODDLER/PRESCHOOL	SCHOOL AGE/PREPUBESCENCE	ADOLESCENCE/ADULTHOOD	ELDERLY	DEVIATIONS FROM NORMAL
OPTIC DISC	Round or oval in shape	Round or oval in shape	Round or oval in shape	Round or oval in shape	Round or oval in shape	Coloboma; large inferior elongation of the disc Vertically oval shape
	Superior, inferior, and temporal margins clearly defined. Nasal margin may be less well defined. Margins may be blurred near large vessels	Superior, inferior, and temporal margins clearly defined. Nasal margin may be less well defined. Margins may be blurred near large vessels	Superior, inferior, and temporal margins clearly defined. Nasal margin may be less well defined. Margins may be blurred near large vessels	Superior, inferior, and temporal margins clearly defined. Nasal margin may be less well defined. Margins may be blurred near large vessels	Superior, inferior, and temporal margins clearly defined. Nasal margin may be less well defined. Margins may be blurred near large vessels	Blurred margins Elevated Disc margins interrupted Partial occlusion of disc to examiner's vision Excavation of disc margin
	Glistening, creamy pink or grayish in color	Glistening, creamy-pink color	Glistening, creamy-pink color	Glistening, creamy-pink color	Glistening, creamy-pink color	Diffuse or localized pallor Extreme whiteness Erythema Grayness
	Minimal numbers of small-caliber vessels confined to the disc present smooth pathways	Minimal numbers of small-caliber vessels confined to the disc present smooth pathways	Minimal numbers of small-caliber vessels confined to the disc present smooth pathways	Minimal numbers of small-caliber vessels confined to the disc present smooth pathways	Minimal numbers of small-caliber vessels confined to the disc present smooth pathways	Dilated Tortuous Numerous vessels
	Large vessels emerge from disc in a smooth symmetric pattern	Large vessels emerge from disc in a smooth symmetric pattern	Large vessels emerge from disc in a smooth symmetric pattern	Large vessels emerge from disc in a smooth symmetric pattern	Large vessels emerge from disc in a smooth symmetric pattern	Vessels pushed to nasal side Dilated Tortuous Sharply bent vessels as they emerge from disc
	White scleral ring (crescent) may partially or totally encompass disc	White scleral ring (crescent) may partially or totally encompass disc	White scleral ring (crescent) may partially or totally encompass disc	White scleral ring (crescent) may partially or totally encompass disc		
	Grayish-black segmented rings or crescents may be present, especially on temporal side of disc	Grayish-black segmented rings or crescents may be present, especially on temporal side of disc	Grayish-black segmented rings or crescents may be present, especially on temporal side of disc	Grayish-black segmented rings or crescents may be present, especially on temporal side of disc	Grayish-black segmented rings or crescents may be present, especially on temporal side of disc	Grayish-black area penetrating disc area

PHYSIOLOGIC CUP	Whitish-gray depression centrally located or just temporal to center of disc. Does not extend to disc edge	Whitish-gray depression centrally located or just temporal to center of disc. Does not extend to disc edge	Whitish-gray depression centrally located or just temporal to center of disc. Does not extend to disc edge	Whitish-gray depression centrally located or just temporal to center of disc. Does not extend to disc edge	Whitish-gray depression centrally located or just temporal to center of disc. Does not extend to disc edge	...of disc
	Blood vessels converge to cup	Blood vessels converge to cup	Blood vessels converge to cup	Blood vessels converge to cup	Blood vessels converge to cup	Absence of vessels
	Size and shape vary	Size and shape vary	Size and shape vary	Size and shape vary	Size and shape vary	
	Generally pale					
RETINA	Color varies with racial characteristics from light reddish-orange to a deep brownish color as growth occurs	Color varies with racial characteristics from light reddish-orange to a deep brownish color	Color varies with racial characteristics from light reddish-orange to a deep brownish color	Color varies with racial characteristics from light reddish-orange to a deep brownish color	Color varies with racial characteristics from light reddish-orange to a deep brownish color	Grayish white exudate patches
						Fuzzy-bordered or well-demarcated dull-gray or white patches
						Black patches
						Red hemorrhages of varied shapes and diameters
	Uniform in color	Uniform in color	Uniform in color	Uniform in color	Uniform in color	Bilaterally symmetrical round gray or yellow spots (drusen)
	Smooth surface	Smooth surface	Smooth surface	Smooth surface	Smooth surface	Ulcerated
						Bulging
						Smooth surface
RETINAL ARTERIES	Bright red in color, vessel wall not visible	Bright red in color, vessel wall not visible	Bright red in color, vessel wall not visible	Bright red in color, vessel wall not visible	Bright red in color, vessel wall not visible	Orange
						Copper
						Reddish-gray
						Dull gray
						Bluish
	Longitudinal light reflex, centrally located, and one-quarter the width of the artery	Longitudinal light reflex, centrally located, and one-quarter the width of the artery	Longitudinal light reflex, centrally located, and one-quarter the width of the artery	Longitudinal light reflex, centrally located, and one-quarter the width of the artery	Longitudinal light reflex, centrally located, and one-quarter the width of the artery	Gray lines on either side of the artery
						Occlusion of visualization due to overlaying hemorrhage
						Light reflex one-third to one-half the width of the vessel
						Absence of light reflex

377

TABLE IV CONTINUED

	NEWBORN/INFANCY	TODDLER/PRESCHOOL	SCHOOL AGE/PREPUBESCENCE	ADOLESCENCE/ADULTHOOD	ELDERLY	DEVIATIONS FROM NORMAL
RETINAL ARTERIES (cont.)	Arteries two-thirds the diameter of veins	Arteries two-thirds the diameter of veins	Arteries two-thirds the diameter of veins	Arteries two-thirds the diameter of veins	Arteries two-thirds the diameter of veins	Arteries equal in size to veins; Arteries significantly less than two-thirds the diameter of veins; Constriction of arterials
	Smooth and regular margins with caliber of vessels decreasing toward periphery	Smooth and regular margins with caliber of vessels decreasing toward periphery	Smooth and regular margins with caliber of vessels decreasing toward periphery	Smooth and regular margins with caliber of vessels decreasing toward periphery	Smooth and regular margins with caliber of vessels decreasing toward periphery	Irregular margins; Bulging of margins; Distention of a segment; Bending or segmental enlargement
	Orderly pattern of branching	Orderly pattern of branching	Orderly pattern of branching	Orderly pattern of branching	Orderly pattern of branching	No visible pattern of branching; Tortuous course; Numerous small vessels closely packed together
RETINAL VEINS	Dark red or bluish red in color, occasionally may have a minor, centrally located light reflex	Dark red or bluish red in color, occasionally may have a minor, centrally located light reflex	Dark red or bluish red in color, occasionally may have a minor, centrally located light reflex	Dark red or bluish red in color, occasionally may have a minor, centrally located light reflex	Dark red or bluish red in color, occasionally may have a minor, centrally located light reflex	Brownish; Inability to visualize vein due to overlaying hemorrhage
	One-third wider than artery	One-third wider than artery	One-third wider than artery	One-third wider than artery	One-third wider than artery	Engorgement; Distention
	Smooth and regular margins	Smooth and regular margins	Smooth and regular margins	Smooth and regular margins	Smooth and regular margins	Tortuosity
	Arterial venous crossings relaxed and smooth with an angle of less than 90°	Arterial venous crossings relaxed and smooth with an angle of less than 90°	Arterial venous crossings relaxed and smooth with an angle of less than 90°	Arterial venous crossings relaxed and smooth with an angle of less than 90°	Arterial venous crossings relaxed and smooth with an angle of less than 90	Concealment of vein below artery; Deflection of vein
	Slight pulsation of veins near optic disc	Slight pulsation of veins near optic disc	Slight pulsation of veins near optic disc	Slight pulsation of veins near optic disc	Slight pulsation of veins near optic	90° or greater angle

					Dilation at end of venous segment
Caliber of vein decreases in size toward periphery	Caliber of vein decreases in size toward periphery	Caliber of vein decreases in size toward periphery	Caliber of vein decreases in size toward periphery	Caliber of vein decreases in size toward periphery	Neovascularizations
Avascular Reddish in color	Avascular Reddish in color	Avascular Reddish in color	Avascular Reddish in color	Avascular Reddish in color	Pigmentation irregularities, deep red spots, yellow waxy patches
MACULA					
Avascular Reddish in color	Avascular Reddish in color	Avascular Reddish in color	Avascular Reddish in color	Avascular Reddish in color	Pigmentation Occlusion of visibility
Becomes distinguishable between 3 and 5 months					
Centrally located is a bright, miniature yellow depression, the fovea centralis	Centrally located is a bright, miniature yellow depression, the fovea centralis	Centrally located is a bright, miniature yellow depression, the fovea centralis	Centrally located is a bright, miniature yellow depression, the fovea centralis	Centrally located is a bright, miniature yellow depression, the fovea centralis Frequently absent over age 50	

TABLE V
Clinical Assessment Guide for Various Age Groups: The Nose

NOSE	NEWBORN INFANT	TODDLER PRESCHOOL	SCHOOL AGE ADOLESCENT	ADOLESCENT ADULT	DEVIATIONS FROM NORMAL
EXTERNAL NASAL STRUCTURE	Broad	Breadth decreases as face lengthens	Breadth decreases as face lengthens	Triangular in shape with base of triangle proximal to face	Triangular in shape with increase in length	Swelling
	Minimal if any movement during respiration	Minimal if any movement during respiration	Minimal if any movement during respiration	Minimal if any movement during respiration	Minimal if any movement during respiration	Displacement
						Nasal flaring
						Fracture
						Saddle nose
						Crepitation
NARES	Patent	Patent	Patent	Patent	Patent	Excessive secretions from nares
	Nares chamber small	Nares chamber increased in size, but remains small	Nares chamber medium in size	Nares chamber large in size	Nares chamber large in size	Choanal atresia
						Stenosis
						Obstruction: unilateral, bilateral
						Polyp
						Foreign body
VESTIBULE	Smooth, pink, hairless	Smooth, pink, hairless	Smooth, pink, hair follicles present	Smooth, pink, amount of hair increases with age	Smooth, pink, amount of hair increases with age	Swelling
						Inflammation of hair follicles
						Presence of crusty purulent discharge
						Fissure
						Furunculosis
MUCOSA	Pink, moist	Pink, moist	Pink, moist	Pink, moist	Pink, moist	Shiny gray color
						Extreme pallor
						Erythema, dry
NASAL SEPTUM	Straight	Straight	Straight	Straight or slight lateral deviation	Straight or slight lateral deviation	Gross lateral deviation
	Intact	Intact	Intact	Intact	Intact	Sharp angles
						Spurs
						Perforations
						Ulcerations
						Crusting
						Abscess
						Absence of whole or part of septum

KIESSELBACH'S PLEXUS	Not assessed	If assessed, smooth and nontortuous	If assessed, smooth and nontortuous	Smooth Nontortuous	smooth nontortuous	...Epistaxis
INFERIOR TURBONATE	Not assessed	Pink Firm Small	Pink Firm Small	Pink Firm Size varying bilaterally	Pink Firm Size varying bilaterally	Engorgement Boggy Dusky red or bluish Polyps
FRONTAL AND MAXILLARY SINUSES	Not assessed	Not assessed / Full cavity transilluminates / Nontender to direct pressure	Resonant and nontender with percussion / Full cavity transilluminates / Nontender to direct pressure	Resonant and nontender with percussion / Full cavity transilluminates / Nontender to direct pressure	Resonant and nontender with percussion / Full cavity transilluminates / Nontender to direct pressure	Inflammation Tumor: dull or flat sound to percussion Tenderness to percussion / Absence of transillumination / Pain elicited with direct pressure

TABLE VI
Clinical Assessment Guide for Various Age Groups: The Mouth and Oropharynx

						Deviations from Normal
LIPS	Pinkish red in color. May have bluish hue if cold	Pinkish red in color. May have bluish hue if cold	Pinkish red in color. May have bluish hue if cold	Pinkish red in color. May have bluish hue if cold	Pale pinkish red in color. May have bluish hue if cold	Red / Cherry red / Cyanotic / Pallid
	Smooth, may develop callous during newborn period	Smooth	Smooth	Smooth	Smooth	Cracking / Peeling of skin / Ulcerations / Vesicles / Fissures / Crusting
MUCOUS MEMBRANE	Pinkish red / Blacks may have bluish coloration	Pinkish red / Blacks may have bluish coloration	Pinkish red / Blacks may have bluish coloration	Pinkish red / Blacks may have bluish coloration	Pink to pale pink / Blacks may have bluish coloration	Erythematous / Pallid / Increased pigmentation / Cyanotic
	Smooth / Moist	Smooth, may have scars along occlusal line / Moist	Smooth, may have scars along occlusal line / Moist	Smooth, may have scars along occlusal line / Moist	Smooth, may have scars along occlusal line / Moist	Dry / Irregular surface / Ulcerations / Denuded / Abraded areas / Vesicles / Xanthomas / Plaque buildup of various colors / Erythematous / Stenson's duct
GUMS	Pink	Pink / Bluish with brown pigmented areas in blacks	Pink / Bluish with brown pigmented areas in blacks	Pink / Bluish with brown pigmented areas in blacks	Pink / Bluish with brown pigmented areas in blacks	Erythematous / Cyanotic / Pallid / Black or silver streaks
	Smooth / May appear irregular with tooth buds, and beginning eruption of deciduous teeth	Smooth / Irregular with continued eruption of deciduous teeth	Smooth / Irregular with loss of deciduous teeth and eruption of permanent teeth	Smooth / Atrophic if endentulous	Smooth / Atrophic if endentulous	Atrophy / Hypertrophy / Lesions
	Closely approximated around erupting teeth	Closely approximated to deciduous teeth	Closely approximated to deciduous teeth	Closely approximated to deciduous teeth	Closely approximated to deciduous teeth	Retraction of tooth edge / Recession of gum between teeth

						Abnormal Findings
	Firm	Firm	Firm	Firm	Firm	Hard; Boggy; Tender; Bleeding
TEETH	Toothbuds may be visible in newborn; Deciduous tooth eruption at approximately 6 months	Toddler: deciduous teeth complete eruption process; Preschool: may begin to lose deciduous teeth; Adult teeth may begin eruption; Spacing of teeth variable	Deciduous teeth being lost and replaced by adult or permanent teeth; Spacing of teeth variable	Adult or permanent teeth generally completed eruption process; May have had "wisdom" teeth extracted; May have dentures or edentulous	May have dentures or edentulous	Cavities; Missing members; Eruption of deciduous teeth shortly after birth; Failure of tooth eruption
	Ivory color	Ivory color	Ivory color	Ivory color; Yellowed from smoking	Ivory color; Yellowed from smoking	Stained black; Bluish discoloration
	Surface smooth; Contact edge often serrated	Surface smooth; Contact edge smooth with wear; Serrated edge of newly erupted teeth	Surface smooth; Contact edge smooth with wear; Serrated edge of newly erupted teeth	Surface smooth; Contact edge smooth with wear; Serrated edge of newly erupted teeth	Surface smooth; Contact edge smooth with wear	Notching; Pitting; Chipped or cracked; Aplasia or hypoplasia of enamel and dentin
TONGUE	Pink color	Dull red color; Thin, removable whitish coating	Dull red color; Thin, removable whitish coating	Dull red color; Thin, removable whitish coating	Dull red color; Thin, removable whitish coating	Bright red; Grayish plaques; Adherent white curds; Beefy; Boggy; Ulcerations; Craters; Plaques
	Smooth and firm	Smooth and firm	Smooth and firm	Smooth and firm	Smooth and firm	
	Smooth coordinated movement	Smooth coordinated movement	Smooth coordinated movement	Smooth coordinated movement	Smooth coordinated movement	Bulky movement; Restricted movement; Slowed movement; Rhythmic protrusions from mouth; Asymmetrical movement
	Fits floor of mouth	Fits floor of mouth	Fits floor of mouth	Fits floor of mouth	Fits floor of mouth	Protrudes from oral cavity; Occludes airway
HARD PALATE	Pale pink color, almost whitish	Pale pink color	Pale pink color	Pale pink color	Pale pink color	Hyperemic; Pallid; Cyanotic

383

TABLE VI CONTINUED

HARD PALATE (cont.)	Irregular surface with transverse rugae May present midline protuberance	Irregular surface with transverse rugae May present midline protuberance	Irregular surface with transverse rugae May present midline protuberance	Irregular surface with transverse rugae May present midline protuberance	Irregular surface with transverse rugae May present midline protuberance	Irregular surface with transverse rugae May present midline protuberance	Smooth Bulging Cleft Marked groove or arch
SOFT PALATE	Pink Palate rises in midline on phonation	Pink Palate rises in midline on phonation	Pink Palate rises in midline on phonation	Pink Palate rises in midline on phonation	Pink Palate rises in midline on phonation	Pink Palate rises in midline on phonation	Red Pallid White patches Unilateral or bilateral sagging upon phonation Cleft or absence of palate
UVULA	Pink Single structure hanging in midline Rises in midline on phonation	Pink Single structure hanging in midline Rises in midline on phonation	Pink Single structure hanging in midline Rises in midline on phonation	Pink Single structure hanging in midline Rises in midline on phonation	Pink Single structure hanging in midline Rises in midline on phonation	Pink Single structure hanging in midline Rises in midline on phonation	Pallid Erythematous White patchy exudate Bifid Absent Misplaced Lateral deviation upon phonation
TONSILS	Pink Small in size Smooth	Pink Increasing in size Smooth Crypts may be noted	Pink Increasing in size Smooth Crypts may be noted	Pink Increasing in size Smooth Crypts may be noted	Pink Begin to atrophy Smooth Crypts may be noted	Pink Atrophic Smooth Crypts may be noted	Absent Red White patchy exudate Increase in size during adulthood and elderly phases of life Edematous Ulcerated areas Plaquelike buildup vesicles Irregular surface
GAG REFLEX	Present Strong	Present Strong	Present Strong	Present Strong	Present Strong	Present Strong but may be slightly diminished	Diminished Absent
VOCAL CORDS	Variable range and intensity of vocalization upon phonation	Variable range and intensity of vocalization upon phonation	Variable range and intensity of vocalization upon phonation	Variable range and intensity of vocalization upon phonation	Variable range and intensity of vocalization upon phonation	Variable range and intensity of vocalization upon phonation	Hypophonation Aphonation Paralytic aphonation

TABLE VII

Clinical Assessment Guide for Various Age Groups: The Neck

NECK	NEWBORN/INFANCY	TODDLER/PRESCHOOL	SCHOOL-AGE/PREPUBESCENCE	ADOLESCENCE/ADULTHOOD	ELDERLY	DEVIATIONS FROM NORMAL
CERVICAL CONTOUR	Bilateral symmetry of angles	Bilateral symmetry of angles	Bilateral symmetry of angles	Bilateral symmetry of angles	Bilateral symmetry of angles	Asymmetry of angles Hypertrophy of thyroid tissue Atrophy of muscle structures
	Neck appears short, multiple skin folds	Neck may or may not appear short, multiple skin folds disappear unless obese	Longitudinal growth of neck evident. Neck folds present if obese	Neck assumes adult proportions. In male, larynx may be prominent. Skin folds if obese	Neck shortens Skin folds if obese	Brevicollis
SUPRASTERNAL NOTCH	Occasional visible pulsation associated with elongated aorta	Occasional visible pulsation associated with elongated aorta	Occasional visible pulsation associated with elongated aorta	Occasional visible pulsation associated with elongated aorta	Occasional visible pulsation associated with elongated aorta	Continuous marked pulsations occur simultaneously with carotid artery pulsation
	No movement with respiration	No movement with respiration	No movement with respiration	No movement with respiration	No movement with respiration	Bulging Retraction
JUGULAR VEINS	Visible only with marked hyperextension of neck	Visible only with marked hyperextension of neck	Visible in supine position	Veins distended in supine position Veins collapse at 30 to 45° angle	Veins distended in supine position Veins collapse at 30 to 45° angle	Cervical venous distention 4 cm above angle of Louis line Sustained rise in level of venous distention with compression of abdomen in region of liver Venous distention remaining when client semiflexed above 45° angle
	High-pitched continuous sound may be present	High-pitched continuous sound may be present	High-pitched continuous sound may be present	High-pitched continuous sound may be present	High-pitched continuous sound may be present	Continuation of high-pitched sound with compression of jugular bulb

TABLE VII CONTINUED

	Newborn/Infant	Toddler/Preschool	School Age	Adult	Elderly	Deviations or Abnormalities
CAROTID ARTERIES	Newborn: rate 120 to 140 regular rhythm quality; rapid crescendo with slower decrescendo of impulse Infant: rate 80 to 140 regular rhythm quality; rapid crescendo with slower decrescendo of impulse Bilateral equality Distant S_1 and S_2 sounds on auscultation	Toddler: rate 80 to 130 regular rhythm quality; rapid crescendo with slower decrescendo of impulse Preschool: rate 70 to 115 regular rhythm quality; rapid crescendo with slower decrescendo of impulse Bilateral equality Distant S_1 and S_2 sounds on auscultation	Rate 60 to 110 regular rhythm quality; rapid crescendo with slower decrescendo of impulse Bilateral equality Distant S_1 and S_2 sounds on auscultation	Rate 60 to 100 regular rhythm quality; rapid crescendo with slower decrescendo of impulse Bilateral equality Distant S_1 and S_2 sounds on auscultation	Rate 60 to 100 regular rhythm quality; rapid crescendo with slower decrescendo of impulse Bilateral equality Distant S_1 and S_2 sounds on auscultation	Rates above or below identified ranges of normal Slow rise and fall of pulsation Rapid decrescendo of pulsation Waxing and waning Inequality of pulsation Bruits
LYMPH GLANDS	Not palpable	Occasional shotty node frequently located in submental or submandibular area	Occasional shotty node frequently located in submental or submandibular area	Occasional shotty node frequently located in submental or submandibular area	Occasional shotty node frequently located in submental or submandibular area	Swollen Hard Tender Matted Adherent to skin or underlying structures Nonmobile
RANGE OF MOTION	Flexion 45° Hyperextension 45° Right and left lateral rotation 45° Right and left lateral bending 45°	Flexion 45° Hyperextension 45° Right and left lateral rotation 45° Right and left lateral bending 45°	Flexion 45° Hyperextension 45° Right and left lateral rotation 45° Right and left lateral bending 45°	Flexion 45° Hyperextension 45° Right and left lateral rotation 45° Right and left lateral bending 45°	Flexion 45° Hyperextension 45° Right and left lateral rotation 45° Right and left lateral bending 45°	Limited range of motion Torticollis Splinting with ROM Asymmetrical movement
THYROID	Midline	Midline	Midline Symmetrical Lobe size and contour	Midline Smooth, firm Symmetrical Lobe size and contour	Midline Smooth, firm Symmetrical Lobe size and contour	Positive Kocker's test Enlargement Displacement from midline

386

TABLE VIII
Clinical Assessment Guide for Various Age Groups: The Chest and Pulmonary System

CHEST AND PULMONARY	NEWBORN/INFANCY	TODDLER/PRESCHOOL	SCHOOL AGE/PREADOLESCENCE	ADOLESCENCE/ADULTHOOD	ELDERLY	DEVIATIONS FROM NORMAL
CHEST WALL	Rounded, barrel-like	Lateral chest becomes broader than anterior-posterior diameter	Lateral chest broader than anterior-posterior diameter	Lateral chest broader than anterior-posterior diameter; Anterior-posterior to lateral ratio of 1:2 or 5:7	Increase in anterior-posterior diameter; Barrel chest	Pectus excavatum; Pectus carinatum; Barrel chest; Kyphosis; Scoliosis
	Symmetrical	Symmetrical	Symmetrical	Symmetrical	Symmetrical	Asymmetry
SKIN	Smooth	Smooth	Smooth	Smooth	Smooth	Rough, dry, scaly; Lesions; Rash
	Color reflects genetic makeup; Pink in newborn with increased pigmentation in races characterized by such	Color reflects genetic makeup; Pink to dark brown	Color reflects genetic makeup; Pink to dark brown	Color reflects genetic makeup; Pink to dark brown	Color reflects genetic makeup, may appear faded with a slightly yellowish hue	Cyanotic; Pallid; Striated; Prominent; Tortuous blue venous tracts; Increase or loss of pigmentation; Erythema; Petechia
	Resilient, elastic	Resilient, elastic	Resilient, elastic	Resilient, elastic	Resilient, some loss of elasticity	Tenting; Rigidity; Edema
	Fine hairs	Fine hair, varying amount	Fine hair, varying amount	Fine hair in male; Varying amount of dark coarse terminal hair; In female, may have coarse hairs around nipples	Fine hair, varying amount; Graying and softening of terminal hairs	Hirsutism; Folliculitis; Appearance of coarse dark terminal hairs prior to 10 years of age; Parasitic infestation
MUSCLE STRUCTURE	Firm	Firm	Firm	Firm	Firm	Spasticity; Flaccidity
	Symmetrical in shape	Symmetrical in shape	Symmetrical in shape	Symmetrical in shape	Symmetrical in shape	Asymmetry of shape
	Smooth	Smooth	Smooth	Smooth and may be fibrous in athletic	Smooth	Nodular; Tender

TABLE VIII CONTINUED

CHEST AND PULMONARY	NEWBORN-INFANT	TODDLER OR PRESCHOOL	SCHOOL-AGE OR PREADOLESCENCE	ADOLESCENCE-ADULTHOOD	DEVIATIONS FROM NORMAL
CHEST MOVEMENT RESPIRATORY CYCLE	Symmetrical on inspiration and expiration	Symmetrical on inspiration and expiration	Symmetrical on inspiration and expiration	Symmetrical on inspiration and expiration	Asymmetrical intercostal retraction or bulging Suprasternal notch retraction
	Abdominal respirations	Abdominal respirations	Abdominal or thoracic respirations	Abdominal or thoracic respirations	Thoracic respirations prior to age 7 Immediate change from abdominal to thoracic or thoracic to abdominal respirations
	Inspiration to expiration ratio of 1:3	Inspiration to expiration ratio of 1:3	Inspiration to expiration ratio of 2:3	Inspiration to expiration ratio of 2:3	Ratios above or below normal ratios for age
	Inspiration active	Inspiration active	Inspiration active	Inspiration active	Cessation of active inspiration
	Expiration passive	Expiration passive	Expiration passive	Expiration passive	Obligatory active expiration
	Regular rhythm rate of 30 to 60	Regular rhythm rate of 15 to 25	Regular rhythm rate of 15 to 25	Regular rhythm rate of 10 to 25	Regular rhythm rate of 15 to 25	Tachypnea Bradypnea Apnea Hyperpnea Cheyne–Stokes Dyspnea Apneusis
	Symmetrical movement Seldom assessed by palpation	If cooperative, symmetrical divergence of thumbs on inspiration with palpation at apex, mid-thoracic, and base of thoracic cage	Symmetrical divergence of thumbs on inspiration with palpation at apex, mid-thoracic, and base of thoracic cage	Symmetrical divergence of thumbs on inspiration with palpation at apex, mid-thoracic, and base of thoracic cage	Symmetrical divergence of thumbs on inspiration with palpation at apex, mid-thoracic, and base of thoracic cage	Asymmetrical divergence of thumbs on inspiration with palpation at apex, mid-thoracic, and base of thoracic cage

THORACIC VIBRATIONS	Not assessed	If cooperative, palpable vocal fremitus throughout chest Generally not assessed	Palpable vocal fremitus remains intense, bilaterally equal with beginning differentiation between regions near origin of sound Decreased intensity toward periphery	...ble vocal fremitus is equal, greatest intensity near origin of sound Decreased intensity toward periphery	Palpable vocal fremitus is equal, greatest intensity near origin of sound Decreased intensity toward periphery Palpable vibrations have decreased intensity compared to adulthood	... of vibrations: lung consolidation Decreased vibrations Absence of vibrations: pleural effusion
THORACIC SOUNDS	Percussion yields resonance over lung fields Dullness over heart, sternum, liver	Percussion yields resonance over lung fields Dullness over heart, sternum, liver	Percussion yields resonance over lung fields Dullness over heart, sternum, liver	Percussion yields resonance over lung fields Dullness over heart, sternum, liver	Percussion yields resonance over lung fields Dullness over heart, sternum, liver	Hyper-resonant: emphysema Flat or dull sounds in lung fields
LUNG SOUNDS	Tubular or bronchial vesicular throughout lung fields	Tubular sounds persist during early toddler, progressing to more differentiation of sounds in preschooler	Tracheal in region of trachea / Inspiration and expiration equal in duration / Loud, tubular, harsh, high pitch / Bronchial in region of the manubrium / Tubular, harsh, high pitch / Bronchovesicular upper third of sternum and interscapular space	Tracheal in region of trachea / Inspiration and expiration equal in duration / Loud, tubular, harsh, high pitch / Bronchial in region of the manubrium / Tubular, harsh, high pitch / Bronchovesicular upper third of sternum and interscapular space	Tracheal in region of trachea / Inspiration and expiration equal in duration / Loud, tubular, harsh, high pitch / Bronchial in region of the manubrium / Tubular, harsh, high pitch / Bronchovesicular upper third of sternum and interscapular space	Fine, medium, or coarse rales / Rhonchi; sibilant or sonorous / Wheezes / Pleural friction rub / Stridor / Expiratory grunt / Delayed or decreased air entry

TABLE VIII CONTINUED

CHEST AND PULMONARY	NEWBORN/INFANCY	TODDLER/PRESCHOOL	SCHOOL AGE/PREPUBESCENCE	ADOLESCENCE/ADULTHOOD	ELDERLY	DEVIATIONS FROM NORMAL
LUNG SOUNDS (cont.)			Medium to high pitch, moderate amplitude, blowing muffled characteristic	Medium to high pitch, moderate amplitude, blowing muffled characteristic	Medium to high pitch, moderate amplitude, blowing muffled characteristic	
			Vesicular, periphery of lung fields	Vesicular, periphery of lung fields	Vesicular, periphery of lung fields	
			Medium to low pitch	Medium to low pitch	Medium to low pitch	
			Low amplitude	Low amplitude	Low amplitude	
			Breezy, swishing, rustling	Breezy, swishing, rustling	Breezy, swishing, rustling	
	Bilateral symmetry of air entry	Bilateral symmetry of air entry	Bilateral symmetry of air entry	Bilateral symmetry of air entry	Bilateral symmetry of air entry	Asymmetry of air entry in bilateral comparison
VOICE SOUNDS	Not assessed	If cooperative, resonant syllables or nonresonant sound highly intense to auscultation	Resonant syllables or nonresonant sound intense in early school age Decrease in intensity toward prepubescence, yielding muffled sounds at auscultation	Resonant syllables are muffled to auscultation	Resonant syllables are muffled to auscultation	Bronchophony (clear auscultation of resonant sound verbalized) Egophony (clear auscultation of nonresonant sound verbalized) Whispered pectoriloquy

390

TABLE IX

Clinical Assessment Guide for Various Age Groups: The Heart

HEART	NEWBORN/INFANCY	TODDLER/PRESCHOOL	SCHOOL AGE/PREPUBESCENCE	ADOLESCENCE/ADULTHOOD	ELDERLY	DEVIATIONS FROM NORMAL
BLOOD PRESSURE	Newborn: $\frac{80 \pm 16}{46 \pm 16}$ 6 months to 1 year: $\frac{89 \pm 29}{60 \pm 10}$	1 year: $\frac{96 \pm 30}{66 \pm 25}$ 2 years: $\frac{99 \pm 25}{64 \pm 25}$ 3 years: $\frac{100 \pm 25}{67 \pm 23}$ 4 years: $\frac{99 \pm 20}{65 \pm 20}$	5 to 6 years: $\frac{94 \pm 14}{55 \pm 9}$ 6 to 7 years: $\frac{100 \pm 15}{56 \pm 8}$ 7 to 8 years: $\frac{102 \pm 15}{56 \pm 8}$ 8 to 9 years: $\frac{105 \pm 16}{57 \pm 9}$ 9 to 10 years: $\frac{107 \pm 16}{57 \pm 9}$ 10 to 11 years: $\frac{111 \pm 17}{58 \pm 10}$	11 to 12 years: $\frac{113 \pm 18}{59 \pm 10}$ 12 to 13 years: $\frac{115 \pm 19}{59 \pm 10}$ 13 to 14 years: $\frac{118 \pm 19}{60 \pm 10}$ Although there is no established normal blood pressure for the adult, acceptable measures are: Young Adult to 45 years: $\frac{110 \text{ to } 140}{65 \text{ to } 90}$ 45 to 65 years: $\frac{140 \text{ to } 160}{80 \pm 10}$	Although there is no established normal blood pressure for the adult, a generally accepted measure of the systolic pressure for age is 100 mm of Hg plus the client's age in years. A generally accepted normotensive pressure is $\frac{150 \pm 10}{80 \pm 10}$	Repeated systolic measurements exceeding 100 mm of Hg plus client's age Repeated diastolic measurements exceeding: 80 mm of Hg in 5-yr old 85 mm of Hg in 12-yr old 90 mm of Hg in adults
	Infant less than 1 year, arm pressure commonly greater than leg pressure	Difference of 10+ or −5 mm of Hg between brachial and popliteal artery systolic pressure	Difference of 10+ or −5 mm of Hg between brachial and popliteal artery systolic pressure	Difference of 10+ or −5 mm of Hg between brachial and popliteal artery systolic pressure	Difference of 10+ or −5 mm of Hg between brachial and popliteal artery systolic pressure	Gradient difference greater than 40 mm of Hg Newborn to early infancy: gradient difference greater than 20 mm of Hg
		Diastolic pressure is equal between brachial and popliteal artery	Generally, diastolic pressure is equal between brachial and popliteal artery	Generally, diastolic pressure is equal between brachial and popliteal artery	Generally, diastolic pressure is equal between brachial and popliteal artery	Marked inequality of diastolic pressure between brachial and popliteal artery
	Pressure between right and left brachial artery is + or −5 mm of Hg	Pressure between right and left brachial artery is + or −5 mm of Hg	Pressure between right and left brachial artery is + or −5 mm of Hg	Pressure between right and left brachial artery is + or −5 mm of Hg	Pressure between right and left brachial artery is + or −5 mm of Hg	Pressure difference greater than 15 mm of Hg
	Systolic pressure change of 10 to 15 mm of Hg decrease from lying to standing blood pressure. Diastolic difference of + or −5 mm of Hg	Systolic pressure change of 10 to 15 mm of Hg decrease from lying to standing blood pressure. Diastolic difference of + or −5 mm of Hg	Systolic pressure change of 10 to 15 mm of Hg decrease from lying to standing blood pressure. Diastolic difference of + or −5 mm of Hg	Systolic pressure change of 10 to 15 mm of Hg decrease from lying to standing blood pressure. Diastolic difference of + or −5 mm of Hg	Systolic pressure change of 10 to 15 mm of Hg decrease from lying to standing blood pressure. Diastolic difference of + or −5 mm of Hg	Systolic pressure change greater than 15 mm of Hg; diastolic pressure difference greater than 5 mm of Hg

TABLE IX CONTINUED

HEART	NEWBORN/INFANCY	TODDLER/PRESCHOOL	SCHOOL AGE/PREPUBESCENCE	ADOLESCENCE/ADULTHOOD	ELDERLY	DEVIATIONS FROM NORMAL
PULSE	Newborn: 120 to 140 beats per minute Infancy: 80 to 140 beats per minute	Toddler: 80 to 130 beats per minute Preschool: 70 to 115 beats per minute	School age: 60 to 110 beats per minute Prepubescence: 60 to 100 beats per minute	60 to 100 beats per minute	60 to 00 beats per minute	Newborn: rate above 180 or below 90 beats per minute Infancy: rate above 160 or below 80 beats per minute Toddler: rate above 140 or below 80 beats per minute Preschool: rate above 125 or below 70 beats per minute School age: rate above 120 or below 60 beats per minute Prepubescence through elderly: rate above 110 or below 60 beats per minute
	Regular rhythm	Regular rhythm	Regular rhythm	Regular rhythm	Regular rhythm	Regular irregular rhythm Irregular irregular rhythm
	Consistent intensity in the rise and fall of pulsation	Consistent intensity in the rise and fall of pulsation	Consistent intensity in the rise and fall of pulsation	Consistent intensity in the rise and fall of pulsation	Consistent intensity in the rise and fall of pulsation	Diminished Bounding Waxing and waning Weak pulse alternations
MOVEMENT OF THORACIC STRUCTURE	Point of maximal impulse presents as a localized, quick, forward projection located above and lateral to the anatomical apex of the heart, to the left of the midsternal line	Point of maximal impulse presents as a localized, quick, forward projection located above and lateral to the anatomical apex of the heart, at or to the left of the midsternal line	Point of maximal impulse presents as a localized, quick, forward projection located above and lateral to the anatomical apex of the heart approximately 8 cm to left of the midsternal line	Point of maximal impulse presents as a localized, quick, forward projection located above and lateral to the anatomical apex of the heart approximately 8 cm to left of the midsternal line. The PMI may not be visible after age 20 and not palpable after age 30	Point of maximal impulse not visible or palpable	Diffuse PMI movement Sustained forward PMI movement PMI displacement to the right, left, upward, or downward

	Precordial regions quiescent when palpated	Precordial regions quiescent when palpated	Precordial regions quiescent when palpated	Precordial regions quiescent when palpated	Precordial regions quiescent when palpated	Thrust Heaves Lifts Bulges Retractions
AUSCULTATED CARDIAC SOUNDS	S_1 and S_2 readily transmitted throughout the chest. In the aortic and pulmonic auscultatory sites, S_2 is prominent and S_1 is less pronounced	S_2 and S_2 readily transmitted throughout the chest in the toddler. In the aortic and pulmonic auscultatory sites, S_2 is prominent and S_1 is less pronounced	In the aortic and pulmonic auscultatory sites, S_2 is prominent and S_1 is less pronounced. S_1 and S_2 may be distant when obese or barrel chested	In the aortic and pulmonic auscultatory sites, S_2 is prominent and S_1 is less pronounced. S_1 and S_2 may be distant when obese, extremely muscular, or barrel chested	In the aortic and pulmonic auscultatory sites, S_2 is prominent and S_1 is less pronounced. S_1 and S_2 may be distant when obese, extremely muscular, or barrel chested	Increased or decreased intensity of S_1; Increased or decreased intensity of S_2; Decreased intensity of S_1 and S_2
	S_1 and S_2 may be physiologically split in the aortic and pulmonic auscultatory sites	S_1 and S_2 may be physiologically split in the aortic and pulmonic auscultatory sites	S_1 and S_2 may be physiologically split in the aortic and pulmonic auscultatory sites	S_1 and S_2 may be physiologically split in the aortic and pulmonic auscultatory sites	S_1 and S_2 may be physiologically split in the aortic and pulmonic auscultatory sites	Widely split S_2 during expiration; Narrowing of a widely split S_2 during inspiration; Widely split S_2 that remains widely split during inspiration and expiration
	Aortic component of S_2 is louder than the pulmonic component when auscultated in the second ICS to the left or right of the sternum	Aortic component of S_2 is louder than the pulmonic component when auscultated in the second ICS to the left or right of the sternum	Aortic component of S_2 is louder than the pulmonic component when auscultated in the second ICS to the left or right of the sternum	Aortic component of S_2 is louder than the pulmonic component when auscultated in the second ICS to the left or right of the sternum	Aortic component of S_2 is louder than the pulmonic component when auscultated in the second ICS to the left or right of the sternum plus increased sound intensity difference between components	Aortic component softer than pulmonic component of S_2
	In the tricuspid and mitral auscultatory sites, S_1 is prominent and S_2 is less pronounced	In the tricuspid and mitral auscultatory sites, S_1 is prominent and S_2 is less pronounced	In the tricuspid and mitral auscultatory sites, S_1 is prominent and S_2 is less pronounced	In the tricuspid and mitral auscultatory sites, S_1 is prominent and S_2 is less pronounced	In the tricuspid and mitral auscultatory sites, S_1 is prominent and S_2 is less pronounced	Increased or decreased intensity of S_1; Increased or decreased intensity of S_2
	S_1 may be physiologically split in the mitral and tricuspid auscultatory sites	S_1 may be physiologically split in the mitral and tricuspid auscultatory sites	S_1 may be physiologically split in the mitral and tricuspid auscultatory sites	S_1 may be physiologically split in the mitral and tricuspid auscultatory sites	S_1 may be physiologically split in the mitral and tricuspid auscultatory sites	Widely split S_1

TABLE IX CONTINUED

HEART	NEWBORN/INFANCY	TODDLER/PRESCHOOL	SCHOOL AGE/PREPUBESCENCE	ADOLESCENCE/ADULTHOOD	ELDERLY	DEVIATIONS FROM NORMAL
AUSCULTATED CARDIAC SOUNDS (cont.)	A physiologic S_3 may be auscultated. Generally, it disappears in a sitting position. Infrequently, a physiologic S_4 may be heard	A physiologic S_3 may be auscultated. Generally, it disappears in a sitting position. Infrequently, a physiologic S_4 may be heard during toddlerhood	A physiologic S_3 may be auscultated. Generally, it disappears in a sitting position	A physiologic S_3 may be auscultated until the approximate age of 20. The physiologic S_3 generally it disappears in the sitting position	S_3 should not be heard	S_3 subsequent to the age of 20 S_4 subsequent to toddlerhood Pathological gallops
	Systole and diastole quiescent or systole may contain a soft, low-pitched, blowing, innocent murmur, which usually decreases in intensity or disappears during expiration	Systole and diastole quiescent or systole may contain a soft, low-pitched, blowing, innocent murmur, which usually decreases in intensity or disappears during expiration	Systole and diastole quiescent or systole may contain a soft, low-pitched, blowing, innocent murmur, which usually decreases in intensity or disappears during expiration	Systole and diastole quiescent or systole may contain a soft, low-pitched, blowing, innocent murmur, which usually decreases in intensity or disappears during expiration	Systole and diastole quiescent or systole may contain a soft, low-pitched, blowing, innocent murmur, which usually decreases in intensity or disappears during expiration	Clicks Snaps Pathological murmurs
				In pregnancy, a mammary souffle may be present		

TABLE X

Clinical Assessment Guide for Various Age Groups: The Breast

BREAST	NEWBORN/INFANCY	TODDLER/PRESCHOOL	SCHOOL AGE/PREPUBESCENCE	ADOLESCENCE/ADULTHOOD	ELDERLY	DEVIATIONS FROM NORMAL
SKIN	Color varies with genetic characteristics	Color varies with genetic characteristics	Color varies with genetic characteristics	Color varies with genetic characteristics / Linear bluish vascular coloration / Red, pale white on silvery striae	May present a faded, slightly yellowish-orange coloration / Pale white or silvery striations may be present	Unilateral bluish vascular coloration / Unilateral striae / Erythema / Petechai
	Smooth	Smooth	Smooth	Smooth	Smooth	Lesions / Indrawn / Puckered / Dimpling / Orange-peel effect / Tense
	Resilient	Resilient	Resilient	Resilient	Resilient	Tense / Nonelastic
BREAST TISSUE	2 mm or less at 36 weeks gestation or less / 4 mm at 37 to 38 weeks gestation / 7 mm or more at 39 weeks gestation	Minimal or no change in amount of breast tissue	Minimal change in amount of breast tissue in school age / Prepubescence: initial prominence as fat is layered in tissue with elevation of the papilla	Puberty: glandular tissue development with fat deposits results in breast size resembling adult / Average adult breast is 150 to 200 g	May have atrophy of glandular and fatty breast tissue	Extremely large breast / Discomfort from large breast / Unilateral increase in size / Failure to develop breast tissue after 16 years of age / Precocious development prior to 10 years of age
	May be swollen due to maternal hormone influence, which subsides in 2 to 4 weeks / Flat and even with tissue structures of the chest	Little or no change in shape and contour	Little or no change in shape and contour in school age / Prepubescence: initial prominence as fat is deposited with elevation of the papilla	Progresses to conical shape in postpubertal female / Bilaterally symmetrical	May have loss of structural support with sagging, pendulous breast / May have atrophy of tissue with subsequent loss of breast tissue, resulting in "flat chest" appearance / Bilaterally symmetrical	Asymmetrical shape / Puckering / Dimpling / Unilateral development
				In male adolescent, swelling of breast tissue may occur with subsequent subsiding / Male breast tissue remains rudimentary		Conical shape unilaterally or bilaterally / Gynecomastia

TABLE X CONTINUED

BREAST	NEWBORN/INFANCY	TODDLER/PRESCHOOL	SCHOOL AGE/PREPUBESCENCE	ADOLESCENCE/ADULTHOOD	ELDERLY	DEVIATIONS FROM NORMAL
BREAST TISSUE (cont.)	Rudiments of glandular tissue	Rudiments of glandular tissue	Rudiments of glandular tissue	Glandular	Glandular or nodular	Nodules or tumors that are poorly defined Unilateral nodules, especially upper outer quadrant Cystic
AREOLA	Located centrally on breast tissue	Located centrally on breast tissue	Located centrally on breast tissue	Located centrally on breast; hair follicle at periphery 1 to 2 1/2 cm in diameter	Located centrally on breast tissue Hair follicle may be present at periphery Terminal ducts readily palpable due to fibrosis and calcification	Asymmetrical shape other than circular Retraction Bulging
	Pale pink to deep brown pigmentation with a smooth surface	Pale pink to deep brown pigmentation with a smooth surface	Pale pink to deep brown pigmentation with a smooth surface	Pale pink to deep brown pigmentation with a smooth surface Irregular due to papilla	Pale pink to deep brown pigmentation with a smooth surface Irregular due to papilla	Erythematous Hyperpigmentation Hypopigmentation Fissures/cracks Retraction Bulging
NIPPLE	Central to areola	Central to areola	Central to areola	Central to areola, circular shape, flush, protruding, or everted from areola Retraction of nipple, which can be everted	Central to areola, circular shape, flush, protruding, or everted from areola Retraction of nipple, which can be everted	Retraction Shape other than circular Cracked Fissured Laceration
LYMPH NODES	Nonpalpable	Nonpalpable	Nonpalpable	Nonpalpable	Nonpalpable	Palpable lymph nodes with fixed, hard, undefined borders

TABLE XI
Clinical Assessment Guide for Various Age Groups: The Abdomen

ABDOMEN	NEWBORN/INFANCY	TODDLER/PRESCHOOL	SCHOOL AGE/PREPUBESCENCE	ADOLESCENCE/ADULTHOOD	ELDERLY	DEVIATIONS FROM NORMAL
SKIN	Translucent in premature Pink in newborn Harlequin sign in newborn Pink to dark brown with even coloration Mottling with stress	Pink to dark brown, even coloration	Pink to dark brown, even coloration Striae associated with obesity or rapid growth spurts	Pink to dark brown, even coloration Linea nigra may be present Striae associated with pregnancy, obesity, or rapid growth spurts; may be reddish to silver in color	Pink to dark brown, may have faded Yellowish coloration Linea nigra Striae associated with pregnancy, obesity, or rapid growth spurts; may be reddish to silver in color	Lack of pigmentation Loss of pigmentation Hyperpigmentation Jaundice Bronze Persistent mottling Patchy pigmentation or depigmented skin Erythema Rashes Cyanosis
	Fine light hair may be present	Fine light hair may be present	Fine light hair may be present	In the mature male, dark coarse terminal hairs in varying amounts may be present. In the mature female, a minimal amount of dark coarse terminal hairs may be present	Abdominal hair thins, softens and grays in color	Folliculitis Loss of hair in adult Presentation of dark, coarse terminal hair prior to 10 years of age
	Smooth	Smooth	Smooth	Smooth	Smooth	Exanthems Excoriations Scars
	Abdominal veins may be visible	Abdominal veins may be visible	Visible abdominal veins begin to lose prominence	Abdominal veins not visible unless pregnant	Abdominal veins may be minimally visible	Prominent distention of vessels Tortuosity of veins
LYMPH NODES	Nonpalpable	Nonpalpable	Nonpalpable	May present shotty inguinal lymph nodes	May present shotty inguinal lymph nodes	Enlarged Tender Matted
ABDOMINAL WALL	Cylindrical, slightly protruding, or rounded	Toddler retains cylindrical shape Preschooler begins to develop a flat contour unless obese Protuberance in standing position	Contour ranges from scaphoid, flat, to rounded protuberance in standing position	Contour ranges from scaphoid, flat, to round	Contour ranges from scaphoid, flat, to round	Extreme scaphoid Extreme rounding Distention Indrawn Bulging Asymmetrical contour Ventral hernia

TABLE XI CONTINUED

398

ABDOMEN	NEWBORN/INFANCY	TODDLER/PRESCHOOL	SCHOOL AGE/PREPUBESCENCE	ADOLESCENCE/ADULTHOOD	ELDERLY	DEVIATIONS FROM NORMAL
ABDOMINAL WALL (cont.)	Abdominal movement with respiration	Abdominal movement with respiration	May have abdominal movement with respiration	Frequently, abdominal movement with respiration in male. May have abdominal movement with respiration in female	Frequently, abdominal movement with respiration in male. May have abdominal movement with respiration in female	Exaggerated abdominal movement with respiration; Splinting of abdomen with inspiration
	Epigastric impulse visible	May have visible an epigastric impulse	May have visible an epigastric impulse	In thin, epigastric impulse may be visible	In thin, epigastric impulse may be visible	Exaggerated epigastric impulse
	Infrequent, low-intensity peristaltic waves	May have infrequent, low-intensity peristaltic waves	Infrequent, low-intensity peristaltic waves generally not seen unless scaphoid contour and weak abdominal musculature	Infrequent, low-intensity peristaltic waves normally not seen unless scaphoid contour and weak abdominal musculature	Infrequent, low-intensity peristaltic waves normally not seen unless scaphoid contour and weak abdominal musculature	Frequent, high-intensity peristaltic waves; Left upper quadrant peristaltic waves proceeding from left to right
	Muscle tone less developed than older child. Abdomen soft to semifirm	Muscle tone developing, semifirm	Muscle tone firm, abdomen soft	Muscle tone firm, abdomen soft	Muscle tone may be decreased, abdomen soft	Atonic; Hypertonic; Absent abdominal musculature
ABDOMINAL ORGANS	Bowel sounds every 10 to 30 seconds. Greater frequency shortly after ingestion of nutrients or when meal long overdue	Bowel sounds every 10 to 30 seconds. Greater frequency shortly after ingestion of nutrients or when meal long overdue	Bowel sounds 5 to 6 per minute. High-pitched gurgling. Greater frequency shortly after meal consumption or when meal long overdue	Bowel sounds 5 to 6 per minute. High-pitched gurgling. Greater frequency shortly after meal consumption or when meal long overdue	Bowel sounds 5 to 6 per minute. High-pitched gurgling. Greater frequency shortly after meal consumption or when meal long overdue	30 or more sounds per minute; Absence of bowel sounds following 5 minutes of auscultation; High-pitched, rushing sounds that increase in intensity
	Absence of sounds other than bowel to auscultation	Absence of sounds other than bowel to auscultation	Absence of sounds other than bowel to auscultation	Absence of sounds other than bowel to auscultation. Pregnancy: fetal heart sounds, souffles, fetal movement	Absence of sounds other than bowel to auscultation	Peritoneal friction rub; Bruits; Venous hum

LIVER	Generally, percussion yields tympany to semidull sound Liver edge at or 1 to 2 cm below right costal margin Superior liver border at sixth intercostal space anteriorly Liver edge smooth, sharp, soft Liver width not assessed	Generally, percussion yields tympany to semidull sound Liver edge may be at or 1 to 2 cm below costal margin Superior liver border at sixth intercostal space anteriorly Liver edge smooth, sharp, soft Variable with size of child	Generally, percussion yields tympany to semidull sound Liver edge at or 1 to 2 cm below costal margin Superior liver border at sixth intercostal space anteriorly Liver edge smooth, sharp, soft Variable with size of child	Generally, percussion yields tympany to semidull sound Liver edge at or 1 cm below costal margin Superior liver border at sixth intercostal space anteriorly Liver edge smooth, sharp, soft Liver width midclavicular line 8 to 10 cm	Generally, percussion yields tympany to semidull sound Liver edge at costal margin Superior liver border at sixth intercostal space anteriorly Liver edge smooth, sharp, soft Liver width of 8 to 10 cm	Flat Marked dullness Infant liver edge exceeding 2 cm below costal margin In adult, liver edge 2 cm below costal margin Liver border markedly above or below sixth intercostal space Rounded edge Firm Nodular Width greater than 10 cm or less than 7 cm
KIDNEY	Kidney is palpable bilaterally Smooth, firm, and lobular in the newborn	Kidney is palpable bilaterally Smooth and firm	Kidney may be palpable bilaterally More frequently right kidney is palpable	Kidney nonpalpable unless thin with moderate muscle tone, then only lower pole, especially right	Kidney nonpalpable unless thin with moderate muscle tone, then only lower pole, especially right	Cystic Nodular Irregular Asymmetrical enlargement
SPLEEN	Soft, smooth, spleen may be palpable in newborn. In infancy spleen generally not palpable	Spleen nonpalpable	Spleen nonpalpable	Spleen nonpalpable	Spleen nonpalpable	Readily palpable spleen after newborn period of life Hard Nodular Enlarged
ABDOMINAL AORTA	Aortic pulsation palpable if thin or mildly obese	Aortic pulsation palpable if thin or mildly obese	Aortic pulsation palpable if thin or mildly obese	Aortic pulsation palpable if thin or mildly obese	Aortic pulsation palpable if thin or mildly obese	Nonpalpable aortic pulsations in thin or mildly obese Markedly palpable aortic pulsations

TABLE XI CONTINUED

ABDOMEN	NEWBORN/INFANCY	TODDLER/PRESCHOOL	SCHOOL AGE/PREPUBESCENCE	ADOLESCENCE/ADULTHOOD	ELDERLY	DEVIATIONS FROM NORMAL
ABDOMINAL AORTA (cont.)	Full pulsation intensity Regular rhythm	Full pulsation intensity Regular rhythm	Full pulsation intensity Regular rhythm	Full pulsation intensity Regular rhythm	Full pulsation intensity Regular rhythm	Decreased pulsatile sensations Bounding pulsations Marked localized distention during pulsation Irregular rhythm Discrepant pulse rate between aorta and carotid artery or apical pulse rate
BLADDER	Bladder may be to level of umbilicus	With growth the height of the superior margin lowers	With growth the height of the superior margin lowers	Superior margin approximately at the upper level of the symphasis pubis Displacement during pregnancy	Superior margin approximately at the upper level of the symphasis pubis	Marked and prolonged distention yielding a high and tense superior bladder margin
BOWEL	Loop of colon rounded over pelvic brim may be palpable	Segments of colon may be palpable in lateral margins of abdomen as round, tubular segments	Segments of colon may be palpable in lateral margins of abdomen as round, tubular segments	Segments of colon may be palpable in lateral margins of abdomen as round, tubular segments	Segments of colon may be palpable in lateral margins of abdomen as round, tubular segments	Localized distention, tenderness Localized, hard masses
UMBILICUS	Umbilical cord possesses three vessels Newborn (day 3 to 14)-cord stump dry and hard Inverted, even, or slightly protruding (0.5 cm)	Toddler: may have slight protrusion (0.5–1 cm) Even with abdomen or inverted	Even with abdomen or inverted	Even with abdomen or inverted During pregnancy may protrude	Even with abdomen or inverted	Newborn: contains other than three vessels Exudate of cord Herniation Denudation Erosion Patent Urachus

400

TABLE XII

Clinical Assessment Guide for Various Age Groups: The Male Genitalia

MALE GENITALIA	NEWBORN/INFANCY	TODDLER/PRESCHOOL	SCHOOL AGE/PREPUBESCENCE	ADOLESCENCE/ADULTHOOD	ELDERLY	DEVIATIONS FROM NORMAL
PUBIC HAIR	Normally absent	Normally absent	Normally absent	Pubic hair beginning between 12 to 16 years of age	Hair present	Failure to develop secondary sexual characteristics of pubic hair
				At completion of puberty, hair pattern is diamond shaped with point toward umbilicus	Retains diamond-shaped pattern	Development of pubic hair prior to 10 years of age
				Covers pubis, scrotum, perineum, and lower abdomen	Covers pubis, scrotum, perineum, and lower abdomen	Loss of pubic hair
				Dense	Generally thins	Abnormal hair pattern
				Coarse Curly Generally darkly pigmented	Becomes fine May straighten Decrease in pigmentation, graying in color	Folliculitis Parasitic infestation
PENIS SHAFT	Infantile in appearance	Infantile in appearance	Infantile in appearance	At puberty increases in length and diameter to adult size	May atrophy, decreasing in size	Edematous Micro or macro in size Misplacement Incomplete formation
	Soft in texture	Soft in texture	Soft in texture	Firm in texture	May become flabby after the age of 50	Flabby prior to age 50, hard nodular or soft areas
	Possesses pigmentation of the surrounding tissue	Possesses pigmentation of the surrounding tissue	Possesses pigmentation of the surrounding tissue	Skin reddens during pubertal growth changes Increased pigmentation compared to skin of thigh and abdomen at the completion of puberty	May have a decrease in pigmentation	Increase or loss of pigmentation Erythema Petechiae Extravasation of blood
	Smooth consistency	Smooth consistency	Smooth consistency	Smooth consistency	Smooth consistency	Hard Nodular Irregular indurations Warts Vesicles Ulcerations Papules or other lesions

401

TABLE XII CONTINUED

MALE GENITALIA	NEWBORN/INFANCY	TODDLER/PRESCHOOL	SCHOOL AGE/PREPUBESCENCE	ADOLESCENCE/ADULTHOOD	ELDERLY	DEVIATIONS FROM NORMAL
PENIS SHAFT (cont.)	Superficial vessels generally not visible	Superficial vessels generally not visible	Superficial vessels generally not visible	Superficial vessels may be visible	Superficial vessels may be visible	Vessels tortuously dilated Rupture of vessels Abnormal curvature of shaft
	Nontender	Nontender	Nontender	Nontender	Nontender	Tender or painful to palpation
GLANS	Infantile in appearance	Infantile in appearance	Infantile in appearance	Glans broadens during puberty	May have atrophy with decrease in diameter	Conical shaped Swelling Edema
	Pinkish-red in color Reddened following circumcision	Pinkish-red in color	Pinkish-red in color	Pink to pinkish-blue in color	Pale pink	Erythema Cyanosis Petechiae
	Exposed if circumcised	Exposed if circumcised	Exposed if circumcised	Exposed if circumcised	Exposed if circumcised	
	Covered by prepuce if not circumcised	Covered by prepuce if not circumcised	Covered by prepuce if not circumcised	With growth of penis and glans prepuce may or may not cover glans	Prepuce may or may not cover glans	
	Prepuce may be adherent to glans up to 6 months of age	Prepuce is retractable	Prepuce is retractable	Prepuce is retractable	Prepuce is retractable	Adhesion of prepuce to glans; nonretractable after 6 months to 1 year: phimosis Constriction of prepuce behind glans: paraphimosis Deposits of smegma
	Smooth	Smooth	Smooth	Smooth	Smooth	Indurations Ulcerations Vesicles Warts Erosions
MEATUS	Meatus midline on tip of glans	Meatus midline on tip of glans	Meatus midline on tip of glans	Meatus midline on tip of glans	Meatus midline on tip of glans	Meatus anterior to tip of glans: epispadias Meatus posterior to tip of glans: hypospadias
	Patent: determined by first voiding	Patent	Patent	Patent	Patent	Stenotic Atresia

					Abnormal Findings
Lips approximate in smooth contour No secretions	Lips approximate in smooth contour No secretions	Lips approximate in smooth contour No secretions	Lips approximate in smooth contour Generally no secretions, although may have crystal-clear droplet	Lips approximate in smooth contour Generally no secretions, from urethral meatus; may have crystal-clear droplet	Pouting medial lips Ulcers Vesicles Exudate that is opaque, whitish, or greenish
SCROTUM					
Smooth, small, and nonrugated if premature	Pendulous Smooth and rugated	Pendulous Smooth and rugated	Pendulous Increases in size and length during puberty	Pendulous Smooth and rugated	Edema Abnormal enlargement unilateral or bilateral
Rugated and pendulous if full term	Smooth and rugated	Smooth and rugated	Smooth and rugated	Smooth and rugated	Pendulous and weighted in appearance Warts Sebaceous cyst Hematoma Ulcerations Vesicles
Hairless	Hairless	Hairless	Development of hair over scrotum between ages 12 and 16 Generally, hair darkly pigmented	Decrease in the amount of hair over scrotum with aging Graying of scrotal hair	Infestation of hairy regions by parasites Loss of hair after puberty up to aged
Superficial vasculature not readily noted	Superficial vasculature structures or may not be readily noted	Superficial vascular structures or may not be readily noted	Superficial vascular structures easily recognized in relaxed, pendulous state	Superficial vascular structures easily recognized in relaxed, pendulous state	Tortuous and dilated veins Rupture of veins
Pigmentation similar to surrounding skin	Pigmentation similar to surrounding skin	Pigmentation similar to surrounding skin	Reddened during pubertal changes Pigmentation darker than skin of thighs or abdomen at completion of puberty	Pigmentation may decrease	Loss of pigmentation Increased pigmentation Erythema Shiny Bluish discoloration
Raphe appears almost as suture line	Raphe appears almost as suture line	Raphe appears almost as suture line	Raphe may not be as prominent	Raphe may not be as prominent	Right side lower than left Bulging of scrotum
Left side slightly lower than right	Left side slightly lower than right	Left side slightly lower than right	Left side slightly lower than right	Left side slightly lower than right	

TABLE XII CONTINUED

TESTIS	In premature infant, located in inguinal ring / In full-term infant, descended into scrotum	Bilaterally descended into scrotum	Bilaterally descended into scrotum	Bilaterally descended into scrotum	Unilaterally or bilaterally absent / Failure to descend into scrotum
	Slightly firm in consistency	Firm in consistency	Firm in consistency	Firm to rubbery in consistency	Softening prior to age 50 / Hard / Loss of resilience / Fluid or cystic feeling surrounding testis
	Smooth	Smooth	Smooth	Smooth	Nodular / Irregular surface
	Tender to pressure	Tender to pressure	Tender to pressure	Tender to pressure	Absence of tenderness when pressure applied
	Symmetrical size and shape (minimal variance)	Symmetrical size and shape	Symmetrical size and shape	Symmetrical size and shape	Asymmetrical in size and shape
	Mobile in its cleft	Mobile in its cleft	Mobile in its cleft	Mobile in its cleft	Restriction or loss of mobility
EPIDIDYMUS	Epididymus not assessed	Epididymus not assessed	Smooth / Soft, tubular, distinct from testis	Smooth / Soft, tubular, distinct from testis	Nodular / Cystic / Swollen / Pain on palpation
SPERMATIC CORD	Spermatic cord not assessed	Soft, cordlike, and smooth	Soft, cordlike, and smooth	Soft, cordlike, and smooth	Cordlike and smooth / Left longer than right	Nodular / Cystic / Numerous cordlike structures; simulates feeling of dried noodles or bag of worms
INGUINAL RING	Inguinal ring usually not assessed	Rarely assessed due to small diameter of inguinal ring	Assessed with little finger taught; bounce against finger	Tight to admission of one finger	Tight to admission of one finger tip	Envelopment of finger with mass or sliding sensation
				Sharp bounce against fingertip	Sharp bounce against fingertip	Sharp bounce against fingertip

PROSTATE					
Prostate not assessed	Prostate not assessed	Prostate not assessed	Firm to rubbery consistency Smooth	Firm to rubbery consistency Smooth	Hard Soft Boggy Nodular
			Minimal projection into rectum	Projection of 1 to 2 centimeters into rectum	Generalized enlargement Asymmetrical enlargement Nodular
			Uncomfortable sensation to palpation	Uncomfortable sensation to palpation	Pain upon palpation
ANUS					
Patent Smooth with puckered borders	Patent Smooth with puckered borders	Patent Smooth with puckered borders	Patent Smooth with puckered borders	Patent Smooth with puckered borders	Dilated tortuous veins Stenosis Obstruction Skin tag Excoriation Sinuses Ulceration Fistulas Bulges
Increased pigmentation compared to surrounding tissue	Increased pigmentation compared to surrounding tissue	Increased pigmentation compared to surrounding tissue	Increased pigmentation compared to surrounding tissue	Increased pigmentation compared to surrounding tissue	Erythema Petechiae
Sphincter tone taut to firm	Sphincter tone taut to firm	Sphincter tone taut to firm	Sphincter tone taut to firm	Sphincter tone taut to firm	Sphincter tone relaxed Weak Spastic Tight
RECTUM					
Rectal walls smooth Resilient walls	Rectal walls smooth Resilient walls	Rectal walls smooth Resilient walls	Rectal walls smooth Resilient walls	Rectal walls smooth Resilient walls	Ridged walls Wall without tonus Inability to palpate rectal walls Protrusion of rectal mucosa through sphincter Protrusion of internal hemorrhoids with increased intra-abdominal pressure Stricture Polyps Fecal impactions Tubular

TABLE XIII
Clinical Assessment Guide for Various Age Groups: The Female Genitalia

FEMALE GENITALIA	NEWBORN/INFANCY	TODDLER/ PRESCHOOL	SCHOOL AGE/ PREPUBESCENCE	ADOLESCENCE/ ADULTHOOD	ELDERLY	DEVIATIONS FROM NORMAL
PUBIC HAIR	Absent	Absent	Absent	Puberty: fine, dark hairs begin developing At completion of puberty, hair pattern is of an inverted triangle Hair is dense, coarse, and curly	Hair present, thinning, fine, soft texture, graying in color	Development of pubic hair prior to age 10 Failure to develop secondary sexual characteristic of pubic hair by age 16 Total or patchy loss of pubic hair Folliculitis Nits on hair shaft
LABIA MAJORA	Premature: small, edges not approximated, may appear underdeveloped Full-term infant: small, edges of labia approximated, may appear edematous	Small with symmetrical, approximating lips	Small with symmetrical, approximating lips	At puberty, symmetrical enlargement Adulthood, large and prominent Lips are approximated until after vaginal delivery	Atrophy less prominent Retiring in appearance Labia symmetrical in size and shape	Hypertrophy Unilateral enlargement Failure to develop in prominence during puberty Atrophy during adulthood Asymmetrical size and shape
	Skin is smooth	Skin is smooth	Skin is smooth	Skin is smooth	Skin appears wrinkled after menopause	Atrophy of skin and subcutaneous tissue prior to menopause Warts Ulcers Erosions Papules Nodules
	External labial color resembles surrounding tissue	External labial color resembles surrounding tissue	External labial color resembles surrounding tissue	External labial color increases in pigmentation during puberty At completion of puberty, pigmentation is darker than surrounding tissue	External labial pigmentation decreases, becoming more like surrounding tissue	Erythema Cyanosis Complete or patchy loss of pigmentation Hyperpigmentation Bluish swelling

	Newborn/Infant	Child	Adolescent	Adult	Older Adult	Abnormal Findings
	External surface free of hair Internal surface pink, smooth, and free of hair	External surface free of hair Internal surface pink, smooth, and free of hair	External surface free of hair Internal surface pink, smooth, and free of hair	External surface covered with thick, coarse, curly hair Internal surface pink, smooth, and free of hair	External surface covered with less dense, fine, graying hairs Internal surface pink, smooth, and free of hair	...dense hair prior to age 10 Patchy or complete loss of hair Erythema Cyanosis Pallid Irregular, rough surface Warts Cysts Lesions
LABIA MINORA	Premature: protrusion of labia minora between lips of labia majora Full-term infant: labia minora hidden by labia majora Pink in color Wrinkled Labia minora surfaces closely approximated	Hidden by labia majora Pink in color Wrinkled Labia minora surfaces closely approximated	Hidden by labia majora Pink in color Wrinkled Labia minora surfaces closely approximated	Hidden by labia majora Increased pigmentation following puberty Wrinkled Labia minora surfaces closely approximated	Generally covered by labia majora, although minimal exposure may occur with atrophy of labia majora Decreased pigmentation Wrinkled Atrophy with aging; labia minora may appear retracted from each other	Protrusion of labia minora beyond the labia majora Erythematous Pallid Hypo- or hyperpigmentation in symmetrical or asymmetrical locations Smooth Swollen Tense appearing Separation or atrophy of labia minora prior to aging
CLITORIS	Premature: protrudes through labia majora Full-term infant: some hypertrophy, may protrude through labia minora	Small, retired	Small, retired	Following biological maturity, approximately 2 cm in length and 1 cm in diameter Generally remains nonprominent	Involution of size Nonprominent	Hypertrophy Atrophy Hyperplasia

TABLE XIII CONTINUED

FEMALE GENITALIA	NEWBORN/INFANCY	TODDLER/PRESCHOOL	SCHOOL AGE/PREPUBESCENCE	ADOLESCENCE/ADULTHOOD	ELDERLY	DEVIATIONS FROM NORMAL
CLITORIS (cont.)	Involutes after neonatal period to nonprominent status					
URETHRA	Located midline between clitoris and vaginal orifice	Located midline between clitoris and vaginal orifice	Located midline between clitoris and vaginal orifice	Located midline between clitoris and vaginal orifice	Located midline between clitoris and vaginal orifice	Congenital misplacements Absence
	Patent	Patent	Patent	Patent	Patent	Stenotic Obstruction
	Circular or slitlike with meatal lips smooth, pink, and approximated	Circular or slitlike with meatal lips smooth, pink, and approximated	Circular or slitlike with meatal lips smooth, pink, and approximated	Circular or slitlike with meatal lips smooth, pink, and approximated	Circular or slitlike with meatal lips smooth, pink, and approximated	Erythematous Cyanosis Pallid Pouting of lips Gaping of meatal lips Vesicles Ulcerations Presence of discharge Protrusion of urethral mucosa through meatal lips
PARAURETHRAL	Nonvisible Nonpalpable	Nonvisible Nonpalpable	Nonvisible Nonpalpable	Nonvisible Nonpalpable	Nonvisible Nonpalpable	Visible duct opening Palpable Nodular Tender Erythematous
HYMEN	Hymenal tag may be present, involutes by 4 weeks of age Hymen perforated	Perforated hymen or hymen may be torn, leaving hymenal tags	Perforated hymen or hymen may be torn, leaving hymenal tags	Perforate Tears with sexual activity, vaginal delivery of fetus, or trauma, leaving hymenal tags Increased fragmentation with each vaginal delivery	May be intact or perforate if no tearing has occurred Hymenal tags involute	Imperforate (rare) Cribriform Absence

						Obstructed Stenotic
VAGINAL ORIFICE	Walls of vaginal orifice approximated	Walls of vaginal orifice approximated	Walls of vaginal orifice approximated	Walls of vaginal orifice approximated until onset of sexual activity Open, especially after vaginal delivery of fetus	Walls of vaginal orifice approximated if not sexually active or vaginal deliveries Open	Visible Palpable Swollen Erythematous Fluctuant mass Small palpable cyst
BARTHOLIN'S GLANDS	Not visible Not palpable Not assessed	Not visible Not palpable Not assessed	Not visible Not palpable Not assessed	Not visible Not palpable	Not visible Not palpable	Visible Palpable Swollen Erythematous Fluctuant mass Small palpable cyst
VAGINA	Pink in color Not assessed	Pink in color Not assessed	Pink in color Not assessed	Pink in color May be red in color if breast feeding Bluish in color with pregnancy	Pale pink in color	Cyanotic in non-pregnant state Erythematous Pallid
	Smooth walled Not assessed	Smooth walled Not assessed	Smooth walled Not assessed	Vaginal walls rugated Decreasing numbers of rugations with each vaginal delivery	Vaginal wall rugations decrease; walls may appear smooth	Adhesion of vaginal walls White, curdy, irregular patches Ulcerations
	Muscle tone not assessed	Muscle tone not assessed	Muscle tone not assessed	Firm musculature may present some minor relaxation following vaginal delivery	Muscle tone decreases	Related muscle tone Cystocele Rectocele Vaginal prolapse
UTERUS	Uterine size not assessed	Uterine size not assessed	Uterine size not assessed	At completion of biological maturity, 5.5 to 8 cm in length and 3.5 to 4 cm in width Increases in size during pregnancy	Atrophies in size, becoming notably smaller	Generalized enlargement in non-pregnant state Failure to develop during biological maturation
	Uterine consistency not assessed	Uterine consistency not assessed	Uterine consistency not assessed	Smooth, firm Softening at the junction of the cervix and uterus body during first trimester of pregnancy	Smooth, firm	Nodular Irregular Hard Boggy Soft Fibrotic
	Uterine position not assessed	Uterine position not assessed	Uterine position not assessed	Anteverted Retroverted Mid-position Antiflexed Retroflexed	Anteverted Retroverted Mid-position Antiflexed Retroflexed	Lateral displacement

TABLE XIII CONTINUED

FEMALE GENITALIA	NEWBORN/INFANCY	TODDLER/PRESCHOOL	SCHOOL AGE/PREPUBESCENCE	ADOLESCENCE/ADULTHOOD	ELDERLY	DEVIATIONS FROM NORMAL
CERVIX	Not assessed	Not assessed	Not assessed	Smooth	Smooth	Ulceration Polyp Nodular Irregular surface Erosions Lacerations Fissures Notches Nabothian follicles
				Pink Bluish color in pregnancy	Pink	Cyanotic in non-pregnant state Erythematous Pallid
				Glistening	Glistening	Dull Lusterless Serous
				Round and symmetrical in shape	Round and symmetrical in shape	Assymmetrical shape Cylindrical shape Effaced in nonpregnant state
				Firm	Firm Softens in pregnancy	Soft in nonpregnant state Boggy
				Protrusion into vaginal vault 1 to 2 cm nongravid, 2 to 3 cm gravid	Becomes even with vaginal wall	Protrusion into vaginal vault more than 3 cm
				2.5 to 3.5 cm in diameter	Atrophy results in diameter of 2.5 cm or less	Diameter greater than 4 cm or smaller than 2 cm
				Mobile in anterior, posterior, and lateral directions	Mobile in anterior, posterior, and lateral directions	Immobility
CERVICAL OS	Not assessed	Not assessed	Not assessed	Centrally located Closed, round, and symmetrical in nulliparous	Centrally located Closed, round, and symmetrical in nulliparous	Open Asymmetrical

410

Structure				Adult	Older Adult	Abnormal Findings
SQUAMOCOLUMNAR JUNCTION	Not assessed	Not assessed	Not assessed	Slitlike or stellate, partially everted lower lip with minimal asymmetry in parus uterus	Slitlike or stellate, partially everted lower lip with minimal asymmetry in parus uterus	Open / Marked asymmetry
(Cervix — shape/surface)	Not assessed	Not assessed	Not assessed	Endocervical / Ectocervical / Round / Symmetrical / Smooth	Endocervical / Ectocervical / Round / Symmetrical / Smooth	Noncircular shape / Irregular borders / Nodular / Ulcerated / Eroded
(Cervix — color)			Pinkish red	Pinkish red	Pinkish red	Bright red / Pallid
OVARY	Not assessed	Not assessed	Not assessed	3 to 4 cm in size / Up to 6 cm in size prior to ovulation	Atrophic	Ovarian size greater than 6 cm or continuous size of 6 cm
(Ovary — palpation)				Almond shaped / Firm / Smooth / Frequently nonpalpable	Generally, nonpalpable	Fluctuant, cystic mass
FALLOPIAN TUBE	Not assessed	Not assessed	Not assessed	Frequently nonpalpable / Smooth / Firm	Nonpalpable	Irregular surface / Asymmetrical enlargement / Bilateral enlargement
(Fallopian — tenderness)				Nonpainful with cervical or uterine movement	Nonpainful with cervical or uterine movement	Pain with cervical or uterine movement
ANUS — patency	Patent	Patent	Patent	Patent	Patent	Stenotic / Obstruction
ANUS — surface	Smooth, with puckered border	Smooth, with puckered border	Smooth	Smooth	Smooth	Skin tags (hemorrhoids) / Excoriation / Ulceration / Dilated, tortuous veins / Sinuses / Fistulas / Bulges
ANUS — pigmentation	Increased pigmentation compared to surrounding tissue	Increased pigmentation compared to surrounding tissue	Increased pigmentation compared to surrounding tissue	Increased pigmentation compared to surrounding tissue	Increased pigmentation compared to surrounding tissue	Erythema / Petechiae

TABLE XIII CONTINUED

	FEMALE GENITALIA					
ANUS (cont.)	Sphincter tone taut to firm	Sphincter tone taut to firm	Sphincter tone taut to firm	Sphincter tone taut to firm	Sphincter tone taut to firm	Sphincter tone weak Relaxed Spastic Tight
RECTUM	Rectal walls smooth and resilient Not assessed	Rectal walls smooth and resilient Not assessed	Rectal walls smooth and resilient Not assessed	Rectal walls smooth and resilient	Rectal walls smooth and resilient	Protrusion of rectal mucosa through sphincter Ridged walls Lack of tone Inability to palpate rectal walls Protrusion of internal hemorrhoids with increased intra-abdominal pressure Stricture polyps Fecal impaction Tubular

TABLE XIV

Clinical Assessment Guide for Various Age Groups: The Musculoskeletal System

MUSCULOSKELETAL	NEWBORN/INFANCY	TODDLER/ PRESCHOOL	SCHOOL AGE/ PREPUBESCENCE	ADOLESCENCE/ ADULTHOOD	ELDERLY	DEVIATIONS FROM NORMAL
LONGITUDINAL HEIGHT	Newborn/term: 45 to 52.5 cm in length 1 year: increases from birth length 50 to 75%	2 years: height increase of 12 to 13 cm 3 to 5 years: height increase of 5 to 6 cm per year	Increase of 5 to 6 cm per year Occasionally, a mid-growth spurt occurs between 6 and 7 years of age	Height increases markedly. May be up to 20 cm. Growth ceases at age 18 for females and age 20 for males. Height maintained throughout adulthood	Height decreases with aging	Marked height increase other than during adolescence. Failure to grow
MUSCLE STRENGTH	Assessed using the Denver Developmental Screening Test	Assessed using the Denver Developmental Screening Test	Able to move against gravity and overcome a subjective amount of resistance added by examiner	Able to move against gravity and overcome a subjective amount of resistance added by examiner	Able to move against gravity and overcome a subjective amount of resistance added by examiner	Delayed development of muscular strength. Inability to overcome added resistance. Inability to move against gravity. No muscle contraction. Hypertonic muscle contraction
NECK	Bilateral symmetry of angles and general contour with numerous fat folds; may appear asymmetrical	Bilateral symmetry of angles and general contour. With numerous fat folds may appear asymmetrical	Bilateral symmetry of angles and general contour. With numerous fat folds may appear asymmetrical	Bilateral symmetry of angles and general contour. With numerous fat folds may appear asymmetrical	Bilateral symmetry of angles and general contour. With numerous fat folds may appear asymmetrical	Asymmetrical Enlargement Unilateral mass Atrophy Torticollis
	Neck structure short, almost nonexistent	1 to 2 years: neck structure short, almost nonexistent 2 years: neck becomes more visible	Neck structure is prominent, length variable	Neck structure is prominent, length variable	Neck structure is prominent, length variable	Brevicollis
	Muscles firm to palpation	Muscles firm to palpation	Muscles firm to palpation	Muscles firm to palpation	Muscles firm to palpation	Rigid Soft Flabby Atonic Hypertonic

413

TABLE XIV CONTINUED

NECK (cont.)	Full range of motion without tenderness	Full range of motion without tenderness	Full range of motion without tenderness	Full range of motion without tenderness	Full range of motion without tenderness	Limited range of motion Torticollis Splinting with range of motion Asymmetrical movement Tenderness with movement
UPPER EXTREMITIES	Bilateral symmetry of size, shape, and posture of arms and hands	Bilateral symmetry of size, shape, and posture of arms and hands	Bilateral symmetry of size, shape, and posture of arms and hands	Bilateral symmetry of size, shape, and posture of arms and hands	Bilateral symmetry of size, shape, and posture of arms and hands	Asymmetrical size, shape, posture, or length Unilateral hypertrophy Lateral or medial displacement Accentuated or abnormal curvature
ARM LENGTH	Appears short relative to total body height	Appears appropriate for body length, extending to upper- or mid-thigh	Appears appropriate for body length, extending to upper- or mid-thigh	Appears appropriate for body length, extending to upper- or mid-thigh	May appear long relative to total body height	Extreme length or shortness Total or partial absence Asymmetrical arm length
POSTURE	Arms flexed, held close to body	Arms held in extension, closely approximated to body	Arms held in extension, closely approximated to body	Arms held in extension, closely approximated to body	Arms held in extension, closely approximated to body	Abduction or adduction of arms to body Splinting Contracture Ankylosis of joint
SHOULDERS	Full, rounded, and smooth	Full, rounded, and smooth	Full, rounded, and smooth	Full, rounded, and smooth	Full, rounded, and smooth	Drooping contracture, atrophy, hypertrophy, protruding mass, hollows, swollen, irregular surface
	Full range of motion without tenderness	Full range of motion without tenderness	Full range of motion without tenderness	Full range of motion without tenderness	Full range of motion without tenderness	Limited movement Splinting of movement Asymmetrical movement Tenderness with

Region						Abnormal Findings
	Firm to palpation	Firm to palpation	Firm to palpation	Firm to palpation	Firm to palpation	alized softness, flabbiness, hardness, rigidity, hollows, cystic, tense, hypotonic, hypertonic
BICEPS AND TRICEPS	Possess a slight longitudinal rounding	Possess a slight longitudinal rounding	Possess a slight to prominent longitudinal rounding	Possess a moderate to prominent longitudinal rounding	Possess a moderate to prominent longitudinal rounding	Localized bulging mass in mid-anterior arm Swelling, protrusions Cleft
	Firm to palpation	Firm to palpation	Firm to palpation	Firm to palpation	Firm to palpation	Localized or generalized softness, flabbiness, hardness, rigidity, cystic, tense, hypotonic, hypertonic
	Bilaterally, muscle strength equal	Bilaterally, muscle strength equal	Bilaterally, muscle strength equal	Bilaterally, muscle strength equal	Bilaterally, muscle strength equal	Bilaterally, unequal muscle strength Spasticity Flaccidity
ROTATOR CUFF	Not assessed	Routinely not assessed; firm and nontender	Routinely not assessed; firm and nontender	Firm and nontender	Firm and nontender	Soft Rigid Tense Tender
SCAPULA	Bilaterally symmetrical in position, closely approximated to chest wall and triangular in shape	Bilaterally symmetrical in position, closely approximated to chest wall and triangular in shape	Bilaterally symmetrical in position, closely approximated to chest wall and triangular in shape	Bilaterally symmetrical in position, closely approximated to chest wall and triangular in shape	Bilaterally symmetrical in position, closely approximated to chest wall and triangular in shape	Scapula displaced upward, downward, or laterally. Winging or protrusion from chest wall. Scapular shape other than triangular in shape
	Bilaterally, scapulae are of equal distance from mid-spinal column	Bilaterally, scapulae are of equal distance from mid-spinal column	Bilaterally, scapulae are of equal distance from mid-spinal column	Bilaterally, scapulae are of equal distance from mid-spinal column	Bilaterally, scapulae are of equal distance from mid-spinal column	Unequal distance from mid-spinal column
	Smooth, bony surface to palpation	Smooth, bony surface to palpation	Smooth, bony surface to palpation	Smooth, bony surface to palpation	Smooth, bony surface to palpation	Nodular Irregular surface Crepitation
ELBOW	Carrying angle usually not assessed	Carrying angle approximately 5°	Carrying angle approximately 5° or slightly more	Carrying angle ranges between 5 to 15°	Carrying angle ranges between 5 to 15°	Carrying angle less than 5° or greater than 15°

TABLE XIV CONTINUED

MUSCULOSKELETAL	NEWBORN/INFANCY	TODDLER/PRESCHOOL	SCHOOL AGE/PREPUBESCENCE	ADOLESCENCE/ADULTHOOD	ELDERLY	DEVIATIONS FROM NORMAL
ELBOW (cont.)	Rounded posterior cubital surface	Rounded posterior cubital surface	Rounded posterior cubital surface	Rounded posterior cubital surface	Rounded posterior cubital surface	Irregular surfaces Nodular, irregular Dislocation Protrusions Swelling Marked grooves Pitting
	Elbow joint is firm and smooth to palpation	Elbow joint is firm and smooth to palpation	Elbow joint is firm and smooth to palpation	Elbow joint is firm and smooth to palpation	Elbow joint is firm and smooth to palpation	Localized or generalized tenseness, hardness, doughiness Fluctuant Cystic
	Full range of motion without tenderness	Full range of motion without tenderness	Full range of motion without tenderness	Full range of motion without tenderness	Full range of motion without tenderness	Limited movement Splinting movement Asymmetrical movement Tenderness with movement
WRIST	Radial and ulnar processes symmetrical in contour, shape, and position	Radial and ulnar processes symmetrical in contour, shape, and position	Radial and ulnar processes symmetrical in contour, shape, and position	Radial and ulnar processes symmetrical in contour, shape, and position	Radial and ulnar processes symmetrical in contour, shape, and position	Absence Swelling Pitting edema Generalized enlargement Cystic Fibrotic Irregular surfaces
	Full range of motion without tenderness	Full range of motion without tenderness	Full range of motion without tenderness	Full range of motion without tenderness	Full range of motion without tenderness	Limited movement Splinting movement Asymmetrical movement Tenderness with movement
HANDS	Symmetrical in size, shape, and position	Symmetrical in size, shape, and position	Symmetrical in shape and position; may possess slight asymmetry in size with dominant hand slightly larger	Symmetrical in shape and position; may possess slight asymmetry in size with dominant hand slightly larger	Symmetrical in shape and position; may possess slight asymmetry in size with dominant hand slightly larger	Hypertrophy Atrophy Proportional enlargement Short, thick, fat, slender, and elongated
	Dorsal surface smooth	Dorsal surface smooth	Dorsal surface smooth with beginning prominence of vascular and tendinous structures	Dorsal surface smooth with prominence of vascular and tendinous structures	Dorsal surface smooth with prominence of vascular and tendinous structures	Hollows between tendons Localized or generalized swelling Bulges Edema Ulceration Erosions Hypertrophy

416

				Normal	Deviations from Normal
FINGERS	...geal joints round and slightly raised	geal joints round and slightly raised	geal joints round and slightly raised	geal joints round and slightly raised	Joint enlargement Tenseness Irregular surface Bulges Protrusions
	Metacarpophalangeal joints smooth, firm, and nontender to palpation	Metacarpophalangeal joints smooth, firm, and nontender to palpation	Metacarpophalangeal joints smooth, firm, and nontender to palpation	Metacarpophalangeal joints smooth, firm, and nontender to palpation	Hard Fluctuant Boggy Doughy Tender Fibrotic
	Intermetacarpophalangeal joint depressions are shallow	Intermetacarpophalangeal joint depressions become prominent	Intermetacarpophalangeal joint depressions are prominent	Intermetacarpophalangeal joint depressions are prominent	Decreased depth Absence of depression
	Thenar and hypothenar eminences prominent, forming a central palmar depression	Thenar and hypothenar eminences prominent, forming a central palmar depression	Thenar and hypothenar eminences prominent, forming a central palmar depression	Thenar and hypothenar eminences prominent, forming a central palmar depression	Atrophy of thenar and/or hypothenar eminences Absence or decreased depth of central palmar depression
	Bilateral symmetry of shape, position, and number	Bilateral symmetry of shape, position, and number	Bilateral symmetry of shape, position, and number	Bilateral symmetry of shape, position, and number	Nodules Supernumerary digits Absence and/or partial absence of digit(s)
	Fingers held in close approximation	Fingers held in close approximation	Fingers held in close approximation	Fingers held in close approximation	Fingers in opposition or adduction
	Fingers straight with minimal interphalangeal joint enlargement	Fingers straight with minimal interphalangeal joint enlargement	Fingers straight with minimal interphalangeal joint enlargement	Fingers straight with minimal interphalangeal joint enlargement	Deviation toward ulnar side of hand Hyperextension or flexion of joints Joint enlargement Tense Irregular surface Bulges Protrusions
	Variable finger length with third digit being longest	Variable finger length with third digit being longest	Variable finger length with third digit being longest	Variable finger length with third digit being longest	Slender, elongated fingers Proportionally enlarged fingers Short, thick, fat fingers Absence and/or partial absence of digit Extension of interdigital webbing

417

TABLE XIV CONTINUED

MUSCULOSKELETAL	NEWBORN/INFANCY	TODDLER/PRESCHOOL	SCHOOL AGE/PREPUBESCENCE	ADOLESCENCE/ADULTHOOD	ELDERLY	DEVIATIONS FROM NORMAL
FINGERS (cont.)	Full range of motion without tenderness	Full range of motion without tenderness	Full range of motion without tenderness	Full range of motion without tenderness	Full range of motion without tenderness	Limited movement Splinted movement Asymmetrical movement Tenderness with movement
ARTERIAL PULSATIONS	Bilateral symmetry of rate, rhythm, and quality Impulse attains maximal intensity quickly with a slower decrescendo	Bilateral symmetry of rate, rhythm, and quality Impulse attains maximal intensity quickly with a slower decrescendo	Bilateral symmetry of rate, rhythm, and quality Impulse attains maximal intensity quickly with a slower decrescendo	Bilateral symmetry of rate, rhythm, and quality Impulse attains maximal intensity quickly with a slower decrescendo	Bilateral symmetry of rate, rhythm, and quality Impulse attains maximal intensity quickly with a slower decrescendo	Bilateral inequality of rate, rhythm, and quality Forceful, rapid attainment of maximal impulse Minimal pulsation Waxing and waning of impulse Alternating strong and weak impulses
	Rate: Newborn, 120 to 140 Infancy, 80 to 140	Rate: Toddler, 80 to 130 Preschool, 70 to 115	Rate: 60 to 110	Rate: 60 to 110	Rate: 60 to 110	Pulsations above or below those indicated as normal or: Newborn ↑180 or ↓90 Infancy ↑160 or ↓80 Toddler ↑140 or ↓80 Preschool ↑125 or ↓70 School Age ↑120 or ↓60 Adolescent ↑110 or ↓60 Adult and elderly ↑110 or ↓60

BACK

| SPINAL COLUMN | Term newborn: C-shaped contour. Cervical curvature forms with ability to hold head midline. Lumbar curvature originates with sitting up, accentuates when learning to walk | Concave cervical curve, convex thoracic curve, concave lumbar curve, convex pelvic curve; possesses an accentuated lumbar curve until approximately 4 years of age | Concave cervical curve, convex thoracic curve, concave lumbar curve, convex pelvic curve | Concave cervical curve, convex thoracic curve, concave lumbar curve, convex pelvic curve | Concave cervical curve, convex thoracic curve, may be exaggerated, concave lumbar curve, convex pelvic curve | Scoliosis
Kyphosis
Poker spine |

418

					Abnormal Findings
PARASPINUS MUSCLES	Firm, smooth, and nontender to palpation	Firm, smooth, and nontender to palpation	Firm, smooth, and nontender to palpation	Firm, smooth, and nontender to palpation	nontender to palpation	Flabby / Tense / Bulging / Rigid / Atrophic / Hypertrophic / Tender / Marked grooving or arching
	Full range of motion without tenderness	Full range of motion without tenderness	Full range of motion without tenderness	Full range of motion without tenderness	Full range of motion without tenderness	Limited / Splinted motion / Asymmetrical movement / Tenderness with movement
LOWER EXTREMITIES	Bilateral symmetry of size, shape, and posture	Bilateral symmetry of size, shape, and posture	Bilateral symmetry of size, shape, and posture	Bilateral symmetry of size, shape, and posture	Bilateral symmetry of size, shape, and posture	Discrepant leg length / Atrophy / Hypertrophy / Dislocation
	Gait not assessed	Toddler: gait consists of wide stance and marked shifting of weight from side to side, "cautious waddling" Preschool: stance with legs close together, gait is smooth, coordinated, and deliberate	Stance with legs close together, gait smooth, coordinated, and deliberate	Stance with legs close together, gait smooth, coordinated, and deliberate	Stance with legs close together, gait smooth, coordinated, and deliberate	Wide stance following toddlerhood / Gait awkward, uncoordinated, non-deliberate
PELVIS	Lies on a horizontal plane	Lies on a horizontal plane	Lies on a horizontal plane	Lies on a horizontal plane	Lies on a horizontal plane	Tilting of sacral triangle / Tilting of pelvic crest plane
HIP JOINT	Hip joint stable. Does not dislocate	Hip joint stable	Hip joint stable	Hip joint stable	Hip joint stable	Ortolani's sign
	Full range of motion without tenderness	Full range of motion without tenderness	Full range of motion without tenderness	Full range of motion without tenderness	Full range of motion without tenderness	Limited movement / Splinted movement / Asymmetrical movement / Tenderness with movement

419

TABLE XIV CONTINUED

MUSCULOSKELETAL	NEWBORN/INFANCY	TODDLER/PREPUBESCENCE	SCHOOL AGE/PREPUBESCENCE	ADOLESCENCE/ADULTHOOD	ELDERLY	DEVIATIONS FROM NORMAL
BUTTOCKS	Rounded with symmetry of size, shape, position, and gluteal folds	Rounded with symmetry of size, shape, position, and gluteal folds	Rounded with symmetry of size, shape, position, and gluteal folds	Rounded with symmetry of size, shape, position, and gluteal folds	Rounded with symmetry of size, shape, position, and gluteal folds	Localized or generalized atrophy and hypertrophy Protrusions Bulging Indurated Deviated curvature Asymmetry of gluteal folds
	Smooth and firm to palpation	Smooth and firm to palpation	Smooth and firm to palpation	Smooth and firm to palpation	Smooth and firm to palpation	Nodular Soft Flabby Rigid Cystic
THIGH	Bilateral symmetry of size and shape with tapering of muscle mass from hip to knee	Bilateral symmetry of size and shape with tapering of muscle mass from hip to knee	Bilateral symmetry of size and shape with tapering of muscle mass from hip to knee	Bilateral symmetry of size and shape with tapering of muscle mass from hip to knee	Bilateral symmetry of size and shape with tapering of muscle mass from hip to knee	Asymmetrical size greater than 0.5 cm Anasarca Bulges Indurated Protrusion Irregular surface Scar
	Firm, smooth, and contiguous to palpation	Firm, smooth, and contiguous to palpation	Firm, smooth, and contiguous to palpation	Firm, smooth, and contiguous to palpation	Firm, smooth, and contiguous to palpation	Nodular Flabby Soft Rigid Gaping between/-within muscle mass Atrophic Hypertrophic Irregular Fibrotic Fluctuant Cystic Pitting edema Crepitation
KNEE	Bilaterally patellae are at same level with slight valgus of the tibia	Bilaterally patellae are at same level with slight valgus of the tibia	Bilaterally patellae are at same level with slight valgus of the tibia	Bilaterally patellae are at same level with slight valgus of the tibia	Bilaterally patellae are at same level with slight valgus of the tibia	Genu valgum Genu varum Genu recurvatum

Region							Abnormal
	Patella blends into rounding contour of knee	Patella prominent, encircled by hollows	Patella prominent encircled by hollows	Patella prominent encircled by hollows	Patella prominent encircled by hollows	Patella prominent encircled by hollows	Marked patellar protrusion; Subluxation of patella; Localized or generalized loss of hollows or bulging of hollows
	Smooth, firm and nontender to palpation	Smooth, firm and nontender to palpation	Smooth, firm and nontender to palpation	Smooth, firm and nontender to palpation	Smooth, firm and nontender to palpation	Smooth, firm and nontender to palpation	Boggy; Cystic; Pitting edema; Doughy; Hard; Tense; Crepitant
	Knee joint stability not assessed	Knee joint stable	Knee joint stable	Knee joint stable	Knee joint stable	Knee joint stable	Opposing forces produce palpable gap; Marked forward gliding of knee
	Full range of motion without tenderness	Full range of motion without tenderness	Full range of motion without tenderness	Full range of motion without tenderness	Full range of motion without tenderness	Full range of motion without tenderness	Limited movement; Splinted movement; Asymmetrical movement; Tenderness with movement
ANKLE	Malleolar prominences smooth, rounded, and firm	Malleolar prominences smooth, rounded, and firm	Malleolar prominences smooth, rounded, and firm	Malleolar prominences smooth, rounded, and firm	Malleolar prominences smooth, rounded, and firm	Malleolar prominences smooth, rounded, and firm	Absence of malleolar prominence; Edema; Pitting; Generalized or localized swelling; Enlargement; Cystic; Fibrotic
	Ankle stability not assessed	Ankle stable	Ankle stable	Ankle stable	Ankle stable	Ankle stable	Notable gapping with eversion
	Full range of motion without tenderness	Full range of motion without tenderness	Full range of motion without tenderness	Full range of motion without tenderness	Full range of motion without tenderness	Full range of motion without tenderness	Limited; Splinted movement; Asymmetrical movement; Tenderness with movement
FOOT	Dorsal surface smooth and rounded. Bony, vascular, and tendinous structures not readily visible	Dorsal surface smooth, slightly rounded with bony, vascular, and tendinous structures not readily visible. Increase in prominence with growth toward preschool years	Dorsal surface smooth with prominent vascular, tendinous, and bony structures	Dorsal surface smooth with prominent vascular, tendinous, and bony structures	Dorsal surface smooth with prominent vascular, tendinous, and bony structures	Dorsal surface smooth with prominent vascular, tendinous, and bony structures	Marked atrophy in spaces between tendons; Edematous; Pitting edema; Inflammation; Tense; Bulges; Indurated; Ulcerations; Erosions

TABLE XIV CONTINUED

MUSCULOSKELETAL	NEWBORN/INFANCY	TODDLER/PRESCHOOL	SCHOOL AGE/PREPUBESCENCE	ADOLESCENCE/ADULTHOOD	ELDERLY	DEVIATIONS FROM NORMAL
FOOT (cont.)	Plantar surface smooth and rounded with fat pads. Heel prominent, ball of foot visible	Plantar surface smooth and rounded with fat pads during early toddlerhood. Late toddlerhood and preschool age, plantar surface smooth, longitudinal arch present, prominent ball and heel	Plantar surface smooth, possesses a longitudinal arch, prominent ball and heel	Plantar surface smooth, possesses a longitudinal arch, prominent ball and heel	Plantar surface smooth, possesses a longitudinal arch, prominent ball and heel	Plantar warts Bunions Heel spurs Pes cavus Pes planus Irregular surface Inflammation Scars Ulceration
	Preterm (28 weeks gestation to term): creases become visible from ball to heel. Multiple creases in full term	Multiple creases on plantar surface	Multiple creases on plantar surface	Multiple creases on plantar surface	Multiple creases on plantar surface	Absence of creases
	Foot in straight alignment	Foot in straight alignment	Foot in straight alignment	Foot in straight alignment	Foot in straight alignment	Pes varus Pes valgus
	Full range of motion without tenderness	Full range of motion without tenderness	Full range of motion without tenderness	Full range of motion without tenderness	Full range of motion without tenderness	Limited movement Splinted movement Asymmetrical movement Tenderness with movement
TOES	Bilateral symmetry of size, shape, contour	Bilateral symmetry of size, shape, contour	Bilateral symmetry of size, shape, contour	Bilateral symmetry of size, shape, contour	Bilateral symmetry of size, shape, contour	Hallux valgus Claw toe Hammer toe Absence and/or partial absence of digits Supernumerary digit
	Interphalangeal joints smooth, firm, and nontender to palpation	Interphalangeal joints smooth, firm, and nontender to palpation	Interphalangeal joints smooth, firm, and nontender to palpation	Interphalangeal joints smooth, firm, and nontender to palpation	Interphalangeal joints smooth, firm, and nontender to palpation	Nodular Hard Fluctuant Boggy Tense Irregular surface Bulges

					Deviations from Normal
Full range of motion without tenderness	Full range of motion without tenderness	Full range of motion without tenderness	Full range of motion without tenderness	Full range of motion without tenderness	Limited movement Splinted movement Asymmetrical movement Tenderness with movement
Bilateral symmetry of rate, rhythm, and quality Impulse attains maximal intensity quickly with a slower decrescendo	Bilateral symmetry of rate, rhythm, and quality Impulse attains maximal intensity quickly with a slower decrescendo	Bilateral symmetry of rate, rhythm, and quality Impulse attains maximal intensity quickly with a slower decrescendo	Bilateral symmetry of rate, rhythm, and quality Impulse attains maximal intensity quickly with a slower decrescendo	Bilateral symmetry of rate, rhythm, and quality Impulse attains maximal intensity quickly with a slower decrescendo	Bilateral inequality in rate, rhythm, and quality Forceful rapid attainment of maximal impulse Minimal pulsation Waxing and waning of impulse Thready impulse Alternately strong and weak impulses
Rate: Newborn, 120 to 140 Infancy, 80 to 140	Rate: Toddler, 80 to 130 Preschool, 70 to 115	Rate: 60 to 110	Rate: 60 to 110	Rate: 60 to 110	Rates above or below those indicated as normal
Superficial veins not readily apparent. When visualized are smooth, full, and possess an even course of travel	Superficial veins not readily apparent. When visualized are smooth, full, and possess an even course of travel	Superficial veins are smooth, full, and possess an even course of travel	Superficial veins are smooth, full, and possess an even course of travel	Superficial veins are smooth, full, and possess an even course of travel	Dilated Distended Tortuous Varicose
Saphenous and communicating vein valves competent, although generally not assessed	Saphenous and communicating vein valves competent, although generally not assessed	Saphenous and communicating vein valves competent, although generally not assessed	Saphenous and communicating vein valves competent	Saphenous and communicating vein valves competent	Incompetent venous valves. Hollowing of veins with legs elevated. Veins fill in downward direction with removal of tourniquet. Emptied veins fill from below while client stands with tourniquet on upper thigh

ARTERIAL PULSATION

VENOUS STRUCTURES

TABLE XV

Clinical Assessment Guide for Various Age Groups: The Neurological System

NEUROLOGICAL	NEWBORN/INFANCY	TODDLER/PRESCHOOL	SCHOOL AGE/PRE-PUBESCENCE	ADOLESCENCE/ADULTHOOD	ELDERLY	DEVIATIONS FROM NORMAL
GENERAL APPEARANCE	Dependent upon care giver	Dependent upon care giver	General appearance is one of being clean and in accordance with peer group, background, and sex	General appearance is one of being clean and in accordance with peer group, background, and sex	General appearance is one of being clean and in accordance with peer group, background, and sex	General appearance is markedly incongruent with expected
	Absence of gross abnormalities or body disproportion	Absence of gross abnormalities or body disproportion				
LEVEL OF CONSCIOUSNESS	Newborn/young infant: alert prior to feeding. Immediately after feeding, alertness decreases	Alert, responsive. Facial expression reflects mood. Irritable and less cooperative when tired or hungry	Facial expression reflects situation, content, and direction of conversation. Responds to environmental stimuli	Facial expression reflects situation, content, and direction of conversation. Responds to environmental stimuli	Facial expression reflects situation, content, and direction of conversation. Responds to environmental stimuli	Lethargy Stupor Light coma Deep coma
POSTURAL POSITIONING	While prone, neonate turns head to the side and draws knees up under the abdomen. In supine position, arms flexed, held close to chest, knees drawn up to abdomen	Toddler: While standing, arms rest at sides, stands with wide base. Overall posture is relaxed, although frequent motions are carried out Preschool: While standing, arms rest at sides, stands with a narrow base. Overall posture is relaxed	While standing, arms rest at sides, stands with narrow base. Overall posture is relaxed	While standing, arms rest at sides, stands with narrow base. Overall posture is relaxed	While standing, arms rest at sides, stands with narrow to medium base. Overall posture is relaxed. May present kyphosis of the thoracic spine	Marked extension of an extremity or all extremities. Continuously turning head to one side. Retraction of head. Stiff neck
SPEECH	Birth to 4 weeks Cries; throaty noises 4 to 16 weeks Begins to coo, gurgle, and grunt	Approximately 15 months Uses at least 3 to 5 words meaningfully	Able to use language and speech to articulate thoughts, ideas, and experiences	Able to use language and speech to articulate thoughts, ideas, and experiences	Able to use language and speech to articulate thoughts, ideas, and experiences	Noise production that ceases. Speech delayed beyond 2 1/2 and 3 years of age.

16 to 28 weeks Continues cooing and gurgling. Laughs

28 to 40 weeks M sounds. Different vowel sounds. By 36 weeks uses words such as mama and dada and understands name

40 weeks to 1 year Repetitive sounds. Responds to name

Approximately 18 months Uses 10 words plus own name. Comprehends and follows simple instructions

Approximately 24 months Speaks with 3 word sentences. Beginning to express verbally wants, desires, and basic emotions

Approximately 36 months Speech includes plurals. Describes events in a picture. Expresses ideas, thoughts, and emotions using a small repertoire of words. Speaks in 4 word phrases. Comprehends and uses concepts of on, under, in front of, in back of, and beside.

Approximately 48 months Expresses ideas, thoughts, and emotions. Requests clarification and meaning of words. Talks in sentences

1 Year May use some words understandably

18 months Understandable words

2 years Speech understandable 50%

Early school age Expression of thoughts, feelings are generally clear, may be disorganized with minimal logic, although are essentially followed through until complete. As growth occurs organization and logic increases

Expression of thoughts, feelings, and beliefs are clear, minimally disorganized, logical, sequential, and followed through until complete

Speech is easy and free flowing

Speech is easy and free flowing

Speech is easy and free flowing

Speech, articulation not assessed

speech. Vague use of speech. Uncertain in choice of words. Marked deliberation in use of speech. Inability to find a certain word. Inability to verbalize words

Disorganized expression. Partial or total lack of clarity. Illogical. Nonsequential. Incomplete expressions. Flight of ideas

Markedly slow speech. Poorly articulated speech. Deletion of words in sentences. Verbalization of sounds that have no meaning. Parroting. Inability to formulate words

TABLE XV CONTINUED

NEUROLOGIC AREA	NEWBORN/INFANCY	TODDLER/PRESCHOOL	SCHOOL-AGE/PREADOLESCENCE	ADOLESCENCE/ADULTHOOD	DEVIATIONS FROM NORMAL
SPEECH (cont.)		3 years Four-word phrases understandable 75% 4 years Understandable sentences 5 years Few articulation errors in speech			
AFFECT	3 months Smiles Laughs Progresses to next stage with additional emotional responses	Affect is congruent with verbal or nonverbal communications (congruence of the expected and observed)	Affect is congruent with verbalizations and content of discussion (congruence of expected and observed)	Affect is congruent with verbalizations and content of discussion (congruence of expected and observed)	Blunt Bland Indifferent Rapid swings of behavior (e.g., laughing to crying). Inappropriate behaviors (e.g., cries when told a joke, laughs when told of significant other's death)
ORIENTATION	Not assessed as such. Developmental milestones achieved are identified specifically in the areas of self-help and personal-social	At 2 years, may give first name 2 1/2 to 3 1/2 years Able to state first and last name. Discriminates self from others	Knows day, month, and year Identifies present setting, city or rural area, and state in which residence is located and home address Identifies self and significant others. Discriminates self from others. Recognizes who people in the immediate setting are (e.g., the nurse)	Knows and states day, month, and year Identifies present setting, city or rural area, and state in which residence is located and home address Identifies self and significant others. Discriminates self from others. Recognizes who people in the immediate setting are (e.g., the nurse)	Unable to state day, month, and year. Guesses wrong by the day, month and year Unaware of present setting. Inability to name city, rural area, or state in which residence is located and home address Unable to state name. Does not respond when name called. Unable to recognize significant others. Unable to discriminate between

another name.

Category	Developmental level	Normal findings	Abnormal findings
MEMORY	Not assessed **6 months** Knows familiar persons from strangers **9 months** Performs learned activities, (e.g., pat-a-cake) Preschooler recognizes who people in the immediate setting are (e.g., the nurse) **1 to 2 years** imitates **2 to 4 years** Immediate recall, appropriate for development	Recalls distant events that are of significance to the client Recalls recent events and experiences	Inability to recall remote or distant events that would be significant to the client Unable to recall recent events (e.g., contents of breakfast). Unable to recall a series of 5 digits presented 5 minutes earlier
KNOWLEDGE FUND	Not assessed **3 to 4 years** Comprehends cold, tired, hungry, in back of, in front of, and on top of **3 1/2 to 4 1/2 years** Identifies city of residence. Recognizes some colors **3 1/2 to 5 years** Comprehends opposite analogies. Able to define words **5 years** May be able to judge similarities and differences between objects **Toddler** Not assessed **Preschool** Although it varies with individuals, able to count or recite numbers in correct sequence	Names current president of the United States. Identifies and describes recent critical community, national, or peer-group events Identifies major cities in the United States Describes abstractly a commonly known metaphor Judges similarities and differences between objects Following elementary education of abstract math concepts, correctly calculates simple mathematical problems of addition and subtraction Correctly calculates simple mathematical problems of addition and subtraction	Inability to identify, name or list general known facts, places, and events Concrete interpretation of metaphor Able to identify similarities but not differences. Able to identify differences but not similarities. Unable to identify similarities and differences In school age through the elderly, incorrect calculation of simple mathematical problems of addition and subtraction

427

TABLE XV CONTINUED

CRANIAL NERVES

NEUROLOGICAL	NEWBORN/INFANCY	TODDLER/PRESCHOOL	SCHOOL AGE/PRE-PUBESCENCE	ADOLESCENCE/ADULTHOOD	ELDERLY	DEVIATIONS FROM NORMAL
I, olfactory	Not assessed	Seldom assessed	Discriminates between and identifies familiar aromatic substances or places them into a category such as a seasoning, perfume, etc. Females discriminate and identify more accurately than males	Discriminates between and identifies familiar aromatic substances or places them into a category such as a seasoning. Females discriminate and identify more accurately than males	Discriminates between and identifies familiar aromatic substances or places them into a category such as a seasoning. Females discriminate and identify more accurately than males. Olfaction may be decreased with aging	Inability to determine the presence of an odor unilaterally or bilaterally. Unable to discriminate between odors. Inability to place a familiar odor into a category. Inability to smell secondary to atrophic rhinitis or polyps
II, optic	3 to 7 months 20/200 10 to 12 months 20/100 Second month Stares at bright objects. Able to fixate gaze Third month Follows objects if removed from sight suddenly, acts as if object is gone Fourth month Recognizes significant other(s) Visual fields not assessed Optic nerve is round or oval in shape, creamy pink or grayish in color with a	18 months to 2 years 20/40 2 to 3 years 20/30 (Snellen symbol chart) Visual fields of: 60° nasalward 50° upward 90° temporally 70° downward Optic nerve is round or oval in shape, creamy pink in color with	20/20 (Snellen letter chart) with corrective lenses if worn Visual fields of: 60° nasalward 50° upward 90° temporally 70° downward Optic nerve is round or oval in shape, creamy pink in color with	20/20 (Snellen letter chart) with corrective lenses if worn Visual fields of: 60° nasalward 50° upward 90° temporally 70° downward Optic nerve is round or oval in shape, creamy pink in color with	20/20 (Snellen letter chart) with corrective lenses if worn Visual fields of: 60° nasalward 50° upward 90° temporally 70° downward Optic nerve is round or oval in shape, creamy pink in color	20/40 in one or both eyes from the developmental stages of preschool to the elderly No response to bright objects by 3 months Disconjugate eye movements during attempts to fixate gaze By fourth month of age, does not follow bright objects Scotomatous Homonomous Hemianopsia Heteronomous Distortion of or shapes other than round or oval. Blurred or inter-

				Abnormal Findings
clearly defined temporal margin. Centrally located or slightly temporal within the disc is the physiologic cup, which may or may not be seen.*	defined temporal margin. Centrally located or slightly temporal within the disc is the physiologic cup, which may or may not be seen.*	temporal margin. Centrally located or slightly temporal within the disc is the physiologic cup, which may or may not be seen.*	ral margin. Centrally located or slightly temporal within the disc is the physiologic cup, which may or may not be seen.*	of disc margins. Diffuse or localized pallor of disc color. Erythema. Grayish coloration of disc
Retinal color is uniform and varies with racial characteristics, ranging from light reddish-orange to a deep brownish color as growth occurs.	Retinal color is uniform and varies with racial characteristics, ranging from light reddish-orange to a deep brownish color.	Retinal color is uniform and varies with racial characteristics, ranging from light reddish-orange to a deep brownish color.	Retinal color is uniform and varies with racial characteristics, ranging from light reddish-orange to a deep brownish color.	Varied shapes and diameters of coloration. Bilaterally symmetrical, round, gray or yellow spots. Fading of color
Macula is avascular, reddish in color, and contains a yellow depression, the fovea centralis	Macula is avascular, reddish in color, and contains a yellow depression, the fovea centralis	Macula is avascular, reddish in color, and contains a yellow depression, the fovea centralis	Macula is avascular, reddish in color, and may contain a visible yellow depression, the fovea centralis	Neovascularizations Pigmentation Irregularities Red spots Yellow waxy patches
Vascular structures are smooth with veins being dark red or bluish in color and one-third wider than the arteries	Vascular structures are smooth with veins being dark red or bluish in color and one-third wider than the arteries	Vascular structures are smooth with veins being dark red or bluish in color and one-third wider than the arteries	Vascular structures are smooth with veins being dark red or bluish in color and one-third wider than the arteries	Inability to visualize vascular structures Engorgement Distention Tortuosity Diminished numbers of vessels
Lids cover eyes up to the limbus	Lids cover eyes up to the limbus	Lids cover eyes up to the limbus	Lids cover eyes up to the limbus	Ptosis Retraction
Third month Eyes converge on an object as it approaches nose Pupils accommodate and react to light	Pupils accommodate and react to light	Pupils accommodate and react to light	Pupils accommodate and react to light	Asymmetrical reaction to light Absence of reaction to light
				Failure to accommodate
Conjugate movement with slow moving objects at approximately six weeks of age	Smooth and conjugate movements in six cardinal positions of gaze	Smooth and conjugate movements in six cardinal positions of gaze	Smooth and conjugate movements in six cardinal positions of gaze	Nystagmus. Limited or disconjugate movement in one or more of the six cardinal positions of gaze. Diplopia. Failure of globe to move in any of the six cardinal positions
III, oculomotor IV, trochlear VI, abducens				

TABLE XV CONTINUED

NEUROLOGICAL	NEWBORN/INFANCY	TODDLER/PRESCHOOL	SCHOOL AGE/PRE-PUBESCENCE	ADOLESCENCE/ADULTHOOD	ELDERLY	DEVIATIONS FROM NORMAL
V, trigeminal	Not assessed	Bilateral symmetry of masseter and temporal muscle strength. If cooperative, able to clench teeth and with jaws approximated tightly, the masseter muscle bulges and client is able to resist examiner's attempts to separate jaws.	Bilateral symmetry of masseter and temporal muscle strength. Able to clench teeth with jaws approximated tightly; the masseter muscle bulges and client is able to resist examiner's attempts to separate jaws	Bilateral symmetry of masseter and temporal muscle strength. Able to clench teeth with jaws approximated tightly; the masseter muscle bulges and client is able to resist examiner's attempts to separate jaws	Bilateral symmetry of masseter and temporal muscle strength. Able to clench teeth with jaws approximated tightly; the masseter muscle bulges and client is able to resist examiner's attempts to separate jaws	Unilateral or bilateral muscle weakness. Hollowing over the masseter and or temporal muscles. Inability to move the jaws sideways
	Not assessed	If cooperative, between the ages of 3 and 4 years begins to discriminate between sharp and blunt objects touching facial skin of forehead, cheeks, and chin. Results questionable	Discriminates between sharp and blunt objects touching facial skin of forehead, cheeks, and chin	Discriminates between sharp and blunt objects touching facial skin of forehead, cheeks, and chin	Discriminates between sharp and blunt objects touching facial skin of forehead, cheeks, and chin	Unilateral or bilateral loss of sharp and blunt sensations. Asymmetrical loss of sensation
	Not assessed	Between ages of 3 and 4, if cooperative, able to discriminate between hot and cold sensations on forehead, cheeks, and chin. Results questionable	Discriminates between hot and cold sensations on forehead, cheeks, and chin	Discriminates between hot and cold sensations on forehead, cheeks, and chin	Discriminates between hot and cold sensations on forehead, cheeks, and chin	Unilateral or bilateral loss of hot and cold sensations. Asymmetrical loss of sensation
	Prompt blinking when cornea is touched with fine wisp of cotton	Prompt blinking when cornea is touched with fine wisp of cotton	Prompt blinking when cornea is touched with fine wisp of cotton	Prompt blinking when cornea is touched with fine wisp of cotton	Prompt blinking when cornea is touched with fine wisp of cotton	Absence of blink reflex
VII, facial	Newborn: smiles responsively 2 to 3 months: smiles spontaneously. Symmetry of wrinkles, nasolabial folds, and facial contours	Uses face for purposes of expression. Symmetry of wrinkles, nasolabial folds, and facial contours	Uses face for purposes of expression. Symmetry of wrinkles, nasolabial folds, and facial contours	Uses face for purposes of expression. Symmetry of wrinkles, nasolabial folds, and facial contours	Uses face for purposes of expression. Symmetry of wrinkles, nasolabial folds, and facial contours	Asymmetrical facial movement Tics Grimaces Tremors Facial masking

Cranial nerve	Infant					Abnormal findings
	Purses lips for sucking	Purses lips, puffs out cheeks, and shows teeth	Purses lips, puffs out cheeks, and shows teeth	Purses lips, puffs out cheeks, and shows teeth	out cheeks, and shows teeth	...ing of lips. Retraction at corner of mouth. Inability to show teeth. Inability to retain puffed cheeks against pressure
	If able to cooperate, retains eyelids in closed position against examiner's attempts to open them	Retains eyelids in closed position against examiner's attempts to open them	Retains eyelids in closed position against examiner's attempts to open them	Retains eyelids in closed position against examiner's attempts to open them	Retains eyelids in closed position against examiner's attempts to open them	Lid fails to descend when attempting to close them. Absent or weak resistance to examiner's attempts to open eyelid
	Generally not assessed	Not assessed	Identifies the tastes of sweet, sour, bitter, and salt when anterior two-thirds of tongue is stimulated	Identifies the tastes of sweet, sour, bitter, and salt when anterior two-thirds of tongue is stimulated	Identifies the tastes of sweet, sour, bitter, and salt when anterior two-thirds of tongue is stimulated	Absence of taste
VIII, acoustic	Newborn: responds to noise with body or facial movement; 3 months: turns head or eyes toward source of sound; 6 months: turns entire head toward source of sound; 9 to 12 months: determines specific source of sound; above, below, behind the ear	Hearing is equal in both ears; Sound originating from tuning fork placed midline on head is heard equally in both ears	Hearing is equal in both ears; Sound originating from tuning fork placed midline on head is heard equally in both ears	Hearing is equal in both ears; Sound originating from tuning fork placed midline on head is heard equally in both ears	Hearing is equal in both ears; Sound originating from tuning fork placed midline on head is heard equally in both ears	Asymmetrical hearing; Lateralization of sound
	Air versus bone conduction of sound not assessed	If able to cooperate, sound conducted via air is heard twice as long as bone-conducted sound	Sound conducted by air is heard twice as long as bone-conducted sound	Sound conducted by air is heard twice as long as bone-conducted sound	Sound conducted by air is heard twice as long as bone-conducted sound	Inability to hear sound via air following sound reception via bone. Air conduction time less than twice that of bone conduction
IX, glossopharyngeal, and X, vagus	Swallowing is smooth and coordinated.	Swallowing is smooth and coordinated.	Swallowing is smooth and coordinated.	Swallowing is smooth and coordinated.	Swallowing is smooth and coordinated.	Dysphagia; Choking

TABLE XV CONTINUED

NEUROLOGICAL	NEWBORN/INFANCY	TODDLER/PRESCHOOL	SCHOOL AGE/PRE-PUBESCENCE	ADOLESCENCE/ADULTHOOD	ELDERLY	DEVIATIONS FROM NORMAL
IX, glossopharyngeal, and X, vagus (cont.)	Soft palate and uvula rise midline upon phonation (crying)	Soft palate and uvula rise midline upon phonation	Soft palate and uvula rise midline upon phonation	Soft palate and uvula rise midline upon phonation	Soft palate and uvula rise midline upon phonation	Palate pulls to one side, the affected side. Uvula deviates to one side, the unaffected side, or does not move with phonation
	Gags with stimulation of the lateral pharyngeal wall	Gags with stimulation of the lateral pharyngeal wall	Gags with stimulation of the lateral pharyngeal wall	Gags with stimulation of the lateral pharyngeal wall	May or may not gag with stimulation of the lateral pharyngeal wall	Absence of gag reflex when lateral pharyngeal wall stimulated, with the exception of the elderly
XI, spinal accessory	Not assessed	If able to cooperate, lifts shoulders against added resistance	Lifts shoulders against added resistance	Lifts shoulders against added resistance	Lifts shoulders against added resistance	Unable to lift shoulders against resistance or without resistance. Minimal elevation.
		If able to cooperate, turns head to side against added resistance	Turns head to side against added resistance	Turns head to side against added resistance	Turns head to side against added resistance	Unable to turn head to the side against resistance or without resistance
XII, hypoglossal	Newborn and Young Infant: with nares obstructed, mouth opens and tip of tongue rises	Little or no activity with tongue at rest on floor of mouth	Little or no activity with tongue at rest on floor of mouth	Little or no activity with tongue at rest on floor of mouth	Little or no activity with tongue at rest on floor of mouth	Fasciculations. Deviation of tongue to one side
	Tongue protrusion difficult to assess and therefore generally not done	Tongue protrudes from mouth in midline or with minimal deviations. May present minor tremors	Tongue protrudes from mouth in midline or with minimal deviations. May present minor tremors	Tongue protrudes from mouth in midline or with minimal deviations. May present minor tremors	Tongue protrudes from mouth in midline or with minimal deviations. May present minor tremors	Deviation of tongue to one side, the affected side. Inability to protrude tongue from mouth
	Strength of tongue not assessed	Preschooler is able to push tongue strongly against cheek	Tongue pushes strongly against added resistance of hand on cheek	Tongue pushes strongly against added resistance of hand on cheek	Tongue pushes strongly against added resistance o hand on cheek	Weak or inability to push tongue against added resistance of hand on cheek. Asymmetrical tongue

432

MOTOR COORDINATION					
Birth to 1 month: uses extremities alternately, making crawling motions. By end of first month, attempts are made at holding head erect	If able to cooperate, protrusion of tongue in and out of mouth and movement from side to side is rapid and coordinated	Protrusion of tongue in and out of mouth, movement from side to side is rapid and coordinated	Protrusion of tongue in and out of mouth, movement from side to side is rapid and coordinated	Protrusion of tongue in and out of mouth, movement from side to side is rapid and coordinated	Slow alternating motions. Movement only toward one side and the midline
Third month: holds head erect and in midline. Lifts head and chest when prone					Asymmetrical movement of extremities
3 to 6 months: Rolls over completely. Raises chest off a flat surface. Able to sit for a variable period of time, holding head erect in midline					Head lag
Unable to right head
6 to 7 months: sits without support. Able to pull self up to a sitting position. May scoot in a backward direction					Generalized or localized hypotonia or hypertonia. Spasticity
7 to 9 months: creeps, crawls, pulls self up to standing position. Side stepping or cruising					Significant developmental delay for age
9 to 12 months: begins to walk with wide base, waddling movements					
13 to 14 months: walks with broad-based station, maintain balance. Stoops and recovers objects. May walk backward	Stance with legs close together, gait smooth, coordinated, and deliberate	Stance with legs close together, gait smooth, coordinated, and deliberate	Stance with legs close together, gait smooth, coordinated, and deliberate	Stance with legs close together, gait smooth, coordinated, and deliberate	Wide stance following toddlerhood. Gait awkward, uncoordinated, and nondeliberate
Jerky, dancing movements
Shuffling short steps
Staggering
Excessive high elevation of hip and knee
Waddling
15 to 19 months: walks up steps, walks backward. Able to kick a ball					

TABLE XV CONTINUED

NEUROLOGICAL	NEWBORN/INFANCY	TODDLER/PRESCHOOL	SCHOOL AGE/PRE-PUBESCENCE	ADOLESCENCE/ADULTHOOD	ELDERLY	DEVIATIONS FROM NORMAL
MOTOR COORDINATION (cont.)		20 to 24 months: may jump in place. Balance on one foot for 1 second				Dragging ball of foot. Leg stiff and extended in swing phase
		25 to 30 months: balance on one foot for 1 second. Jumps in place. Broad jumps				
		3 to 4 years: balance on 1 foot for 5 seconds. May be able to walk heel to toe				
	Walking heel to toe not assessed	3 1/2 to 5 years of age, able to maintain balance and performs smoothly walking heel to toe with practice	Maintains balance and performs smoothly when walking heel to toe on a straight line	Maintains balance and performs smoothly when walking heel to toe on a straight line	Elderly may find this maneuver somewhat difficult. Maintains balance and in general performs smoothly when walking heel to toe on a straight line	Side stepping loss of balance
	Standing with feet close together with eyes closed not assessed	Stands with feet close together, eyes closed, with minimal or no swaying	Stands with feet close together, eyes closed, with minimal or no swaying	Stands with feet close together, eyes closed, with minimal or no swaying	Stands with feet close together, eyes closed, with minimal or no swaying	Marked swaying Falling
	Hopping on one foot not assessed	Between ages of 3 to 4 1/2, able to hop on one foot staying in place and maintaining balance	Hops on one foot, staying in place and maintaining balance	Hops on one foot, staying in place and maintaining balance	Hops on one foot, staying in place and maintaining balance; however this may normally be difficult.	Hits heel hard when landing. Loss of balance. Inability to get off the floor. Lands more than several inches from take off spot. Inability to drop foot after take off. Awkward performance
	Shallow knee bend not assessed	Performance of shallow knee bend generally not assessed	Performs shallow knee bend on one foot with ease and balance	Performs shallow knee bend on one foot with ease and balance	Shallow knee bend may be difficult to perform	Asymmetrical performance of shallow knee bend

Infant	Young Child (Toddler/Preschooler)				Abnormal Findings
				If able, performs shallow knee bend on one foot with ease and able to step up on a footstool with ease and balance	Loss of balance. Difficulty rising from squatting position. Difficulty or inability to raise self onto footstool
Walking on heels and on toes not assessed	Walking on heels and toes generally not assessed	Walks on heels and on toes in a smooth and balanced manner	Walks on heels and on toes in a smooth and balanced manner	Walks on heels and on toes in a smooth and balanced manner with some difficulty	Heel drop while walking on toes. Ball of foot drops while walking on heel
3 to 4 months: grasp rattle; 6 to 7 months: passes object from hand to hand; 7 to 10 months: thumb finger grasp	Symmetrical hand grip strength. Toddler: pincer grasp well developed. Preschooler: able to resist examiner's attempts to remove fingers from grasp	Symmetrical hand grip strength and able to resist examiner's attempts to remove fingers from grasp	Symmetrical hand grip strength and able to resist examiner's attempts to remove fingers from grasp	Symmetrical hand grip strength and able to resist examiner's attempts to remove fingers from grasp	Asymmetrical hand grip strength. Weak hand grip. Inability to retain examiner's grasp of fingers
Voluntary motor control of raising arms and supination/pronation of hands not assessed	If able to cooperate, raises both arms horizontal to the shoulder with palms pronated and supinated for several seconds	Raises both arms horizontal to the shoulder with palms pronated and supinated and holds each position for 20 to 30 seconds	Raises both arms horizontal to the shoulder with palms pronated and supinated and holds each position for 20 to 30 seconds	Raises both arms horizontal to the shoulder with palms pronated and supinated and holds each position for 20 to 30 seconds	Drooping of one or both arms. Arm or hand flexes and internally rotates. Extremity drifts down and outward. Postural changes
Voluntary motor control of raising arms above head not assessed	Playing "so big" with toddler, raises arms above head. Preschooler able to raise arms above head and holds for several seconds	Raises arms above head, holds for 20 to 30 seconds and lowers arms into extension	Raises arms above head, holds for 20 to 30 seconds and lowers arms into extension	Raises arms above head, holds for 20 to 30 seconds and lowers arms into extension	Tremors of the fingers with fingers abducted and palms facing downward
Proprioception not assessed	Toddler: alternating finger-nose touching not assessed. Preschool: accurate, smooth alternating finger-nose touching with the forefinger (proprioception)	Accurate, smooth alternating finger-nose touching with the forefinger (proprioception)	Accurate, smooth alternating finger-nose touching with the forefinger (proprioception)	Accurate, smooth alternating finger-nose touching with the forefinger (proprioception)	Jerky, incoordinated movements. Tremors of the hand when slowing movement as nose is approached. Persistent inaccuracy. Persistent missing

TABLE XV CONTINUED

NEUROLOGICAL	NEWBORN/INFANCY	TODDLER/PRESCHOOL	SCHOOL AGE/PRE-PUBESCENCE	ADOLESCENCE/ADULTHOOD	ELDERLY	DEVIATIONS FROM NORMAL
MOTOR COORDINATION (cont.)	Alternating hand movements not assessed	Toddler: alternating hand movements not assessed. Preschool: rapidly and smoothly supinates and pronates hands or smoothly taps leg with hand. Nondominant hand is generally slower	Rapidly and smoothly supinates and pronates hands or rapidly and smoothly taps leg with hand. Nondominant hand is generally slower	Rapidly and smoothly supinates and pronates hands or rapidly and smoothly taps leg with hand. Nondominant hand is generally slower	Rate may be slower than during adulthood, performs supination and pronation of hands smoothly or at a variable rate, smoothly taps leg with hand. The nondominant hand is generally slower	Awkwardness. Slow rate of motion. Unable to stabilize proximal portion of extremity while engaged in the alternating movement
DEEP REFLEXES	Newborn and Early Infancy: stimulation of tendon produces variable responses, ranging from exaggerated to absent. Ankle jerk may be accompanied by quick alternating plantar and dorsiflexion of the foot. Clonus is unsustained. Triceps reflex is present at approximately 6 months	Pectoralis, biceps, triceps, brachioradials, finger flexor, patellar, and Achilles reflexes present a quick, nonsustained contracture of muscles when stimulated	Pectoralis, biceps, triceps, brachioradials, finger flexor, patellar, and Achilles reflexes present a quick, nonsustained contracture of muscles when stimulated	Pectoralis, biceps, triceps, brachioradials, finger flexor, patellar, and Achilles reflexes present a quick, nonsustained contracture of muscles when stimulated	Pectoralis, biceps, triceps, brachioradials, finger flexor, patellar, and Achilles reflexes present a quick, nonsustained contracture of muscles when stimulated	Asymmetrical response to stimuli. A change in response from previous testing. Absence of response. Diminished response. Slightly hyperactive. Brisk with intermittent clonus. Very brisk with sustained clonus
SUPERFICIAL REFLEXES	Gagging occurs with stimulation of lateral pharyngeal wall	Gagging occurs with stimulation of lateral pharyngeal wall	Gagging occurs with stimulation of lateral pharyngeal wall	Gagging occurs with stimulation of lateral pharyngeal wall	Gagging may or may not occur with stimulation of the lateral pharyngeal wall	Absence of gag reflex when lateral pharyngeal wall stimulated, with the exception of the elderly

PATHOLOGIC REFLEXES						Absence / Abnormal
Prompt blinking when cornea touched with fine wisp of cotton	Prompt blinking when cornea touched with fine wisp of cotton	Prompt blinking when cornea touched with fine wisp of cotton	Prompt blinking when cornea touched with fine wisp of cotton	Prompt blinking when cornea touched with fine wisp of cotton		Absence of blink reflex
By the sixth month, the umbilicus deviates toward the stimulated quadrant unless abdominal wall tautly stretched	Umbilicus deviates toward the stimulated quadrant unless abdominal wall tautly stretched or a large amount of subcutaneous fat exists	Umbilicus deviates toward the stimulated quadrant unless abdominal wall tautly stretched or a large amount of subcutaneous fat exists	Umbilicus deviates toward the stimulated quadrant unless abdominal wall tautly stretched or a large amount of subcutaneous fat exists	Umbilicus deviates toward the stimulated quadrant unless abdominal wall tautly stretched or a large amount of subcutaneous fat exists		Absence. Absence of lower right and left quadrant reflexes with the presence of the upper right and left quadrant reflexes. Unilaterally diminished or absent
Plantar flexion of toes when lateral edge of sole scratched from heel to toe	Plantar flexion of toes when lateral edge of sole scratched from heel to toe	Plantar flexion of toes when lateral edge of sole scratched from heel to toe	Plantar flexion of toes when lateral edge of sole scratched from heel to toe	Plantar flexion of toes when lateral edge of sole scratched from heel to toe		Absence of plantar flexion of toes. Dorsiflexion of toes.
At some point within the first 6 months, there is elevation of the ipsilateral testis when the thigh is stimulated	Elevation of the ipsilateral testis when the thigh is stimulated	Elevation of the ipsilateral testis when the thigh is stimulated	Elevation of the ipsilateral testis when the thigh is stimulated	Elevation of the ipsilateral testis when the thigh is stimulated		Absence of testicular elevation
Contraction of anal sphincter with scratching of perianal area	Contraction of anal sphincter with scratching of perianal area	Contraction of anal sphincter with scratching of perianal area	Contraction of anal sphincter with scratching of perianal area	Contraction of anal sphincter with scratching of perianal area		Absence of anal sphincter contraction
Birth to 12 months, symmetrical rhythmic oscillations of no more than 12 beats may be normal	Oscillations of foot are not elicited with sudden and maintained dorsiflexion of foot	Oscillations of foot are not elicited with sudden and maintained dorsiflexion of foot	Oscillations of foot are not elicited with sudden and maintained dorsiflexion of foot	Oscillations of foot are not elicited with sudden and maintained dorsiflexion of foot		Oscillations with sudden and sustained dorsiflexion of foot. Unilateral oscillations. Spontaneous clonus
Stroking lateral sole of foot from heel to toe and across ball of foot produces fanning of toes and dorsiflexion of great toe (equivocal Babinski)	Up to 2 years of age, stroking lateral sole of foot from heel to toe and across ball of foot may produce fanning of toes and dorsiflexion of great toe. After 2 years of age, stroking lateral sole of foot from heel to toe and across ball of foot produces plantar flexion of toes	Stroking lateral sole of foot from heel to toe and across ball of foot produces plantar flexion of toes	Stroking lateral sole of foot from heel to toe and across ball of foot produces plantar flexion of toes	Stroking lateral sole of foot from heel to toe and across ball of foot produces plantar flexion of toes		After the age of 2 years, fanning of the toes and dorsiflexion of the great toe

TABLE XV CONTINUED

NEUROLOGICAL	NEWBORN/INFANCY	TODDLER/ PRESCHOOL	SCHOOL AGE/ PRE-PUBESCENCE	ADOLESCENCE/ ADULTHOOD	ELDERLY	DEVIATIONS FROM NORMAL
PATHOLOGIC REFLEXES (cont.)	Hoffmann's sign not assessed	Forced flexion of distal phalanx of the middle finger produces no response	Forced flexion of distal phalanx of the middle finger produces no response	Forced flexion of distal phalanx of the middle finger produces no response	Forced flexion of distal phalanx of the middle finger produces no response	Flexion–adduction of the fingers with opposing flexion–adduction. Movement of the thumb
PRIMITIVE REFLEXES	Blink reflex: blinks when bright light flashed into eye	Blink reflex: blinks when bright light flashed into eye	Blink reflex: blinks when bright light flashed into eye	Blink reflex: blinks when bright light flashed into eye	Blink reflex: blinks when bright light flashed into eye	Absence of blink reflex to sudden light; unilateral blinking
	Pupillary reflex: pupil constricts when bright light is placed on eye	Pupillary reflex: pupil constricts when bright light is placed on eye	Pupillary reflex: pupil constricts when bright light is placed on eye	Pupillary reflex: pupil constricts when bright light is placed on eye	Pupillary reflex: pupil constricts when bright light is placed on eye	Absence. Asymmetry of response
	Cochleopalpebral reflex: blinks and may startle with loud noise from birth to 6 to 9 months of age	Cochleopalpebral reflex not present	Cochleopalpebral reflex not present	Cochleopalpebral reflex not present	Cochleopalpebral reflex not present	Absence
	Sucking reflex: automatic sucking when object placed in mouth	Sucking reflex not present	Sucking reflex not present	Sucking reflex not present	Sucking reflex not present	Failure to suck when object placed in mouth
	Rooting reflex: with stroking of the corner of the mouth, or middle upper lip, or middle lower lip, the head and mouth move toward the stimulus until 3 to 4 months of age	Rooting reflex not present	Rooting reflex not present	Rooting reflex not present	Rooting reflex not present	Failure to respond to stimulus. Persistence beyond 3 to 4 months of age
	Absent after 3 or 4 months of age					
	Palmar grasp reflex: reflexively grasp finger forcefully when pressed in palm	Palmar grasp reflex not present	Palmar grasp reflex not present	Palmar grasp reflex not present	Palmar grasp reflex not present	Persistence of reflex beyond 5 or 6 months of age. Weak grasping. Absence of reflex grasp
	Plantar grasp reflex: plantar flexion of toes in response to pressure on ball of foot	Plantar grasp reflex not present	Plantar grasp reflex not present	Plantar grasp reflex not present	Plantar grasp reflex not present	Absent Asymmetry

Crossed extension reflex: while supine, one leg is held in extension and the soles pricked. The opposite leg extends and adducts until infant 1 or 2 months old. Not present after 2 months of life	Crossed extension reflex not present	Crossed extension reflex not present	Crossed extension reflex not present	Crossed extension reflex not present	...to stimuli. Persistence of response beyond the second month of life
Tonic neck reflex: while supine, turning the head to left side results in extension of limbs, and to the right side, vice versa. Not present after 7 months of age	Tonic neck reflex not present	Tonic neck reflex not present	Tonic neck reflex not present	Tonic neck reflex not present	Persistence of reflex beyond 7 months of age
Moro reflex: sudden disalignment of head from spine results in abduction, extension and supination of arms, extension of third and fourth fingers, flexion of thumb and index finger bilaterally. Extension of legs and cry may also occur. Not present after 6 months of age	Moro reflex not present	Moro reflex not present	Moro reflex not present	Moro reflex not present	Absence. Asymmetrical body response. Persistence beyond 6 months of age
Stepping reflex: until 4 months of age, walking movements are made when held erect, with feet on a surface and tilted forward and laterally	Stepping reflex not present	Stepping reflex not present	Stepping reflex not present	Stepping reflex not present	Persistence beyond 4 months of age. Recurrence once reflex has ceased to exist
Placing reflex: from birth to approximately 1 year of age, when held erect and dorsal surface of foot is touched there is flexion of the ipsilateral knee and hip	Placing reflex not present	Placing reflex not present	Placing reflex not present	Placing reflex not present	Absence of flexion of the ipsilateral knee and hip

439

TABLE XV CONTINUED

NEUROLOGICAL	NEWBORN/INFANCY	TODDLER/PRESCHOOL	SCHOOL AGE/PRE-PUBESCENCE	ADOLESCENCE/ADULTHOOD	ELDERLY	DEVIATIONS FROM NORMAL
PRIMITIVE REFLEXES (cont.)	Landau reflex: 1 to 2 months not present. 3 to 12 months, flexion of legs occurs when infant is held prone over one hand and chin is tucked to chest	Landau reflex: up to 2 years of age, flexion of the legs may occur when prone and chin tucked to chest. Not present after 2 years of age	Landau reflex not present	Landau reflex not present	Landau reflex not present	Absence of leg flexion
	Parachute reflex: while prone above a surface, a sudden downward thrust results in extension of arms, fingers, and legs toward surface	Parachute reflex: while prone above a surface, a sudden downward thrust results in extension of arms, fingers, and legs toward surface. Not assessed	Parachute reflex: while prone above a surface, a sudden downward thrust results in extension of arms, fingers, and legs toward surface. Not assessed	Parachute reflex: while prone above a surface, a sudden downward thrust results in extension of arms, fingers, and legs toward surface. Not assessed	Parachute reflex: while prone above a surface, a sudden downward thrust results in extension of arms, fingers, and legs toward surface. Not assessed	Absence or asymmetry of arm, finger, and leg extension toward surface
SUPERFICIAL SENSATION	Discrimination between the sensations of sharp and blunt not assessed	If cooperative, between the ages of 3 and 4 years, begins to discriminate between sharp and blunt sensations. Results may be questionable	Discriminates between the sensations of sharp and blunt over the entire body	Discriminates between the sensations of sharp and blunt over the entire body	Discriminates between the sensations of sharp and blunt over the entire body	Decreased pain sensation (hypoalgesia). Loss of pain sensation (analgesia). Unpleasant cutaneous sensations (paresthesia). Overresponse to pain (hyperalgesia)
	Discrimination between the sensations of hot and cold not assessed	If cooperative, between the ages of 3 and 4, able to discriminate between hot and cold sensations. Results may be questionable	Discriminates between the sensations of hot and cold over the entire body	Discriminates between the sensations of hot and cold over the entire body	Discriminctes between the sensations of hot and cold over the entire body	Inability to identify sensations of hot or cold. Persistent inaccurate identification of sensation. Unilateral loss of sensation
	Newborn to 28 weeks: gentle stroking on body may produce withdrawal from the stimuli, gross motor movement, or change in facial expression. By the fifth month, response to gentle stroking is more localized	Toddler: light touch generally not assessed. May look to the areas being lightly touched

Preschool: identifies when being touched lightly on body | Identifies when being touched lightly anywhere on body | Identifies when being touched lightly anywhere on body | Identifies when being touched lightly anywhere on body | Inability to identify light stroking |

440

DEEP SENSATION					
Vibratory sense not assessed	Vibratory sense difficult to assess and therefore not generally done	Able to detect vibrations over the bony prominences of the trunk, upper and lower extremities	Able to detect vibrations over the bony prominences of the trunk, upper and lower extremities	Able to detect vibrations over the bony prominences of the trunk, upper and lower extremities. Vibratory sense may be diminished in lower extremities	Absence of vibratory sensation
Position sense not assessed	Position sense not assessed	Identifies position in which great toe has been placed while eyes are closed	Identifies position in which great toe has been placed while eyes are closed	Identifies position in which great toe has been placed while eyes are closed	Inability to identify spatial relationship of body parts
Crys with vigorous pin sticking	Responds to pain with vocalization and withdrawal with light pinching of Achilles tendon or firm squeezing of calf	Identifies pain with light pinching of Achilles tendon or firm squeezing of calf	Identifies pain with light pinching of Achilles tendon or firm squeezing of calf	Identifies pain with light pinching of Achilles tendon or firm squeezing of calf	Failure to detect pain. Increased amounts of pressure needed to elicit pain. Absence of withdrawal from painful stimuli. Crying or vocalization of pain without withdrawal from stimuli. Withdrawal from painful stimuli without change of facial expression or vocalization

CORTICAL SENSORY					
Stereognosis not assessed	Stereognosis not assessed	With eyes closed, uses fingers and palms of hand to identify and name familiar objects (stereognosis)	With eyes closed, uses fingers and palms of hand to identify and name familiar objects (stereognosis)	With eyes closed, uses fingers and palms of hand to identify and name familiar objects (stereognosis)	Inability to identify familiar objects placed in hand
Graphesthesia not assessed	Graphesthesia not assessed	While eyes are closed, identifies numerals drawn on the palm of the hand (graphesthesia)	While eyes are closed, identifies numerals drawn on the palm of the hand (graphesthesia)	While eyes are closed, identifies numerals drawn on the palm of the hand (graphesthesia)	Failure to identify 7 out of 9 numerals
Perception of testicular pain not assessed	Experiences testicular pain with gentle squeezing of the testis	Experiences testicular pain with gentle squeezing of the testis	Experiences testicular pain with gentle squeezing of the testis	Experiences testicular pain with gentle squeezing of the testis	Absence of testicular pain upon gentle squeezing

* For a more complete description of the ophthalmoscopic exam, refer to Table IV.

Index

W

X

Y

Z